W9-BTJ-447

CLINICAL CHALLENGES IN HEART FAILURE

CLINICAL CHALLENGES IN HEART FAILURE

Edited by

Mandeep R. Mehra
Herbert Berger Professor of Medicine and Head of Cardiology
University of Maryland School of Medicine
Baltimore, Maryland, USA

CLINICAL PUBLISHING

OXFORD

Clinical Publishing
an imprint of Atlas Medical Publishing Ltd

Oxford Centre for Innovation
Mill Street, Oxford OX2 0JX, UK
Tel: +44 1865 811116
Fax: +44 1865 251550
Email: info@clinicalpublishing.co.uk
Web: www.clinicalpublishing.co.uk

Distributed in USA and Canada by:
Clinical Publishing
30 Amberwood Parkway
Ashland OH 44805, USA
Tel: 800-247-6553 (toll free within US and Canada)
Fax: 419-281-6883
Email: order@bookmasters.com

Distributed in UK and Rest of World by:
Marston Book Services Ltd
PO Box 269
Abingdon
Oxon OX14 4YN, UK
Tel: +44 1235 465500
Fax: +44 1235 465555
Email: trade.orders@marston.co.uk

A catalogue record for this book is available from the British Library

ISBN 13   978 1 84692 044 8
ISBN e-book   978 1 84692 608 2

Project manager: Gavin Smith, GPS Publishing Solutions, Hertfordshire, UK
Typeset by Mizpah Publishing Services Private Limited, Chennai, India
Printed by BookMasters, Inc., Ashland, Ohio, USA

Contents

Editor

MANDEEP R. MEHRA, MBBS, FACC, FACP, Herbert Berger Professor of Medicine and Head of Cardiology, University of Maryland School of Medicine, Baltimore, MD, USA

Contributors

KIRKWOOD F. ADAMS, JR, MD, Associate Professor of Medicine and Radiology, Division of Cardiology, Department of Medicine, University of North Carolina School of Medicine, Chapel Hill, NC, USA

ANDREW AMBROSY, BS, Center for Cardiovascular Innovation, Northwestern University, Feinberg School of Medicine, Chicago, IL, USA

The late KENNETH L. BAUGHMAN, MD, Formerly Professor of Medicine, Harvard Medical School, Director, Advanced Heart Disease Section, Brigham & Women's Hospital, Boston, MA, USA

FILIPPO BRANDIMARTE, MD, Cardiologist, Department of Cardiovascular Diseases, San Giovanni - Addolorata Community Hospital, Rome, Italy

LEONARDO DE LUCA, MD, PhD, FACC, Department of Cardiovascular Sciences, Laboratory of Interventional Cardiology, European Hospital, Rome, Italy

CHRISTOPHER DE FILIPPI, MD, FACC, Associate Professor of Medicine, Division of Cardiology, University of Maryland School of Medicine, Baltimore, MD, USA

TIMM M. DICKFELD, MD, PhD, FACC, Associate Professor of Medicine, Division of Cardiology, University of Maryland School of Medicine, Baltimore, MD, USA

KENNETH DICKSTEIN, MD, PhD, University of Bergen, Stavanger University Hospital, Stavanger, Rogaland, Norway

GERASIMOS S. FILIPPATOS, MD, FACC, FCCP, FESC, Head, Heart Failure Unit, Department of Cardiology, Athens University Hospital Attikon, Athens, Greece

MIHAI GHEORGHIADE, MD, FACC, Professor of Medicine and Surgery, Director of Experimental Therapeutics, Center of Cardiovascular Innovation, Northwestern University Feinberg School of Medicine, Co-Director, Cardiovascular Center for Drug Development, Duke University, Chicago, IL, USA

JOSHUA M. HARE, MD, FACC, FAHA, Louis Lemberg Professor of Medicine, Director, Interdisciplinary Stem Cell Institute, University of Miami Miller School of Medicine, Miami, FL, USA

KONSTANTINOS E. HATZISTERGOS, PhD, Post-Doctoral Fellow, University of Miami, Miller School of Medicine, Interdisciplinary Stem Cell Institute, Miami, FL, USA

LIVIU KLEIN, MD, MS, The Bluhm Cardiovascular Institute, The Feinberg School of Medicine, Northwestern Memorial Hospital, Chicago, IL, USA

CARL J. LAVIE, MD, FACC, FACP, FCCP, Medical Director, Cardiac Rehabilitation and Prevention, Director, Stress Testing Laboratory, John Ochsner Heart and Vascular Institute, Ochsner Health System, New Orleans, LA, USA

DENNIS M. MCNAMARA, MD, Professor of Medicine, Director, Heart Failure/Transplantation Program, Cardiovascular Institute, University of Pittsburgh Medical Center, Pittsburgh, PA, USA

MANDEEP R. MEHRA, MBBS, FACC, FACP, Dr Herbert Berger Professor of Medicine and Head of Cardiology, Assistant Dean for Clinical Services, Division of Cardiology, University of Maryland School of Medicine, Baltimore, MD, USA

RICHARD V. MILANI, MD, FACC, FAHA, Vice-Chairman, Department of Cardiology, John Ochsner Heart and Vascular Institute, Ochsner Health System, New Orleans, LA, USA

THOMAS J. MULHEARN IV, MD, Fellow in Cardiovascular Medicine, Division of Cardiology, Duke University Medical Center, Durham, NC, USA

JOHN B. O'CONNELL, MD, Executive Director, Heart Failure Program, St Joseph's Hospital, Atlanta, GA, USA

MYUNG H. PARK, MD, FACC, Associate Professor of Medicine, Director, Pulmonary Vascular Disease Program, Division of Cardiology, University of Maryland School of Medicine, Baltimore, MD, USA

JAMES G. PREMPEH, MD, Clinical Research Fellow, Section of Cardiology, San Francisco Veterans Affairs Medical Center, School of Medicine, University of California, San Francisco, CA, USA

GAUTAM V. RAMANI, MD, Assistant Professor of Medicine, Division of Cardiology, University of Maryland School of Medicine, Baltimore, MD, USA

MADHAVI T. REDDY, MD, Fellow in Cardiology, University of Illinois, Chicago, IL, USA

JOSEPH G. ROGERS, MD, Associate Professor of Medicine, Division of Cardiology, Duke University School of Medicine and the Duke Clinical Research Institute, Durham, NC, USA

STUART D. RUSSELL, MD, FACC, Associate Professor of Medicine, Chief, Heart Failure and Transplantation, Division of Cardiology, Johns Hopkins School of Medicine, Baltimore, MD, USA

KEYUR B. SHAH, MD, FACC, Assistant Professor of Medicine, Division of Cardiology, Virginia Commonwealth University, Richmond, VA, USA

JOHN R. TEERLINK, MD, FACC, FAHA, FESC, Professor of Medicine (UCSF), Director, Heart Failure (SFVAMC), Director, Clinical Echocardiography (SFVAMC), Section of Cardiology, San Francisco Veterans Affairs Medical Center, School of Medicine, University of California, San Francisco, CA, USA

KONSTANTINOS TZIOMALOS, MD, PhD, Cardiovascular Division and Interdisciplinary Stem Cell Institute, University of Miami Miller School of Medicine, Miami, FL, USA

PATRICIA A. UBER, BS, PharmD, Assistant Professor of Medicine, Division of Cardiology, University of Maryland School of Medicine, Baltimore, MD USA

HECTOR O. VENTURA, MD, FACC, FACP, FASH, Section Head, Cardiomyopathy and Heart Transplantation, John Ochsner Heart and Vascular Institute, Ochsner Health System, New Orleans, LA, USA

1

Digoxin in heart failure: an ancient potion?

K. F. Adams, Jr

INTRODUCTION

Controversy over clinical effectiveness surrounds many treatments and consensus at the level of guidelines and quality of care measures is difficult to reach for most therapies. But few therapies have induced such a historically rich and long lived dispute as digoxin concerning their basic medical value and best indications for use. Our deep and rationale commitment to evidence from randomized clinical trials is understandable, but centuries of positive observational data with various digitalis preparations remain difficult to fully dismiss. Following a long period dominated by non-randomized results and a poor understanding of the physiological actions of the drug, a number of potentially beneficial properties have been identified and randomized clinical trials of digoxin have been performed that provide additional support for efficacy of this agent. However, even as stronger evidence accumulates, controversy continues to surround this agent, engendering ongoing analyses of critical randomized trial data. Digoxin is still attractive to many, given that heart failure (HF) remains a therapeutic challenge and substantial public health problem in spite of recent advances in therapy. This chapter will attempt to make sense of the current evidence in a way that, in total, supports a continued therapeutic role for this agent, while simultaneously presenting a number of caveats concerning drug use. Be forewarned that absolute conclusions are not possible, but the thoughtful reader should be able to take a position on the role of this drug in their practice after consideration of the material presented.

HISTORICAL PERSPECTIVE

No account of the use of digoxin in HF could be considered complete without some historical considerations. The concept of taking external substances as remedies for human maladies must predate written history. The Egyptians are known to have used many herbal preparations for medicinal purposes and one, called squill, contained rather weak cardiac glycosides and does appear to have been given to patients with dropsy. The name digitalis was used in 1542 by the German scholar Fuchsius as a term for the plant known as the Foxglove which has blossoms that resembled the fingers of a glove. The drug was used from the late Middle Ages by Welsh physicians under the name menygellydon [1]. The 'modern' history of the drug begins in 1785 with the publication of the famous memoir by Sir William Withering *'An Account of the Foxglove and Some of its Medical Uses: With Practical Remarks on*

Kirkwood F. Adams, Jr, MD, Associate Professor of Medicine and Radiology, Division of Cardiology, Department of Medicine, University of North Carolina School of Medicine, Chapel Hill, NC, USA.

Table 1.1 Effects of digoxin (with permission from [58])

Hemodynamic effects in HF
  Increased cardiac output
  Decreased PCWP
  Increased LVEF
Neurohormonal effects
  Vagomimetic action
  Improved baroreceptor sensitivity
  Decreased norepinephrine serum concentration
  Decreased activation of renin-angiotensin system
  Direct sympathoinhibitory effect
  Increased sympathetic CNS outflow at high-doses
  Decreased cytokine concentrations
  Increased release of ANP and BNP
Electrophysiological effects
  S-A node: slowing of the sinus rate
  Atrium: no effect or decreased refractory period
  AV node: slowed conduction
  Ventricle and Purkinje fibers: practically no electrophysiological effects at
  low therapeutic doses

ANP = atrial natriuretic peptide; AV = atrioventricular; BNP = B-type natriuretic peptide; CNS = central nervous system; LVEF = left ventricular ejection fraction; PCWP = pulmonary capillary wedge pressure.

Dropsy and Other Diseases', justifiably recognized as a medical classic. Withering advocated for the utility of digoxin, in a pioneering way, presenting carefully recorded observations on the clinical effects of the drug which he prescribed to patients with edematous states, irregular heartbeats and chronic HF [2]. According to Withering, digitalis was believed to slow heart rate in patients with irregular pulse and result in diuresis. Only in the twentieth century were digitalis preparations considered useful in patients with HF and sinus rhythm. Digoxin, only one of many cardiac glycosides that could be considered for therapeutic use, was popularized during the 1930s by Burroughs Wellcome, presumably due to the advantages of lower protein binding and faster clearance. Digoxin was not approved by the U.S. Food and Drug Administration (FDA) under its new regulations until the 1990s with an indication for the treatment of mild to moderate HF and for control of ventricular response rate in atrial fibrillation.

MECHANISM OF ACTION

POSITIVE INOTROPIC EFFECTS

Controversy continues concerning the primary mechanism of action that accounts for the clinical improvement associated with digoxin therapy in HF (Table 1.1). Traditional explanations have focused on the positive inotropic effect of the drug. This favorable action on contractility originates from inhibition of membrane-bound alpha subunits of sodium-potassium ATPase that are primarily, but not exclusively, located in human myocardium. As a result of this inhibition, sodium-calcium exchange is augmented and there is a corresponding rise in intracellular calcium concentration that enhances activation of the contractile apparatus and produces an increase in the force of myocardial contraction [3, 4]. There is reasonable evidence to indicate that even 'low' serum digoxin concentrations (< 1.0 ng/ml) are associated with a measurable inotropic effect. Although sodium-potassium ATPase receptor density is reduced in HF, sodium-calcium exchanger protein levels remain the same [5]. There is no evidence for up-regulation of the sodium-potassium ATPase pump in human myocardium during chronic digoxin therapy [6].

NEUROHORMONAL MODULATION

Recognition that abnormal neurohormonal regulation plays a critical role in the pathophysiology of HF represented a major conceptual advance and helped to promote development of life saving drugs that counteract these systems. In addition to its inotropic properties, digoxin is well known to modulate many neurohormonal abnormalities noted in HF, especially those involving the autonomic nervous system. These additional mechanisms of action make it more plausible that digoxin could be beneficial in patients with HF [7]. In low-output HF models, there is attenuation of carotid sinus baroreceptor discharge sensitivity that may occur due to augmentation of sodium-potassium ATPase pump activity. Administration of digoxin in these models produces improvement in baroreceptor function that may result in decreased activation of the sympathetic nervous system [8]. Digoxin, at therapeutic doses, increases vagal tone and decreases sinoatrial and atrioventricular conduction [9]. Digoxin has a direct sympathoinhibitory effect that does not appear to be related to any increase in cardiac output produced by the drug. Both dobutamine and digoxin cause a similar acute increase in cardiac output in patients with HF, but only digoxin decreases sympathetic nerve discharge. Therapeutic doses of digoxin also decrease serum norepinephrine concentration [10, 11]. A low dose of digoxin, that has no effect on cardiac contractility or hemodynamics, decreases cardiac norepinephrine spillover in patients with severe HF [12]. Interestingly, higher doses of digoxin may result in stimulation of sympathetic nerve activity. Other studies have shown that increasing the dose of digoxin, when serum concentration is within therapeutic range, improves hemodynamics but produces no further improvement in neurohormonal profile [13].

Although the clinical significance of these effects is not known, digoxin also lessens activation of neurohormones related to the renin-angiotensin system and appears to increase circulating natriuretic peptides. Both acute and chronic administration of digoxin has been shown to reduce plasma renin, angiotensin II, and aldosterone levels [11, 14]. Aldosterone stimulation of the sodium-potassium pump may lead to perivascular fibrosis which can be prevented in experimental models by digoxin administration [15]. Digitalis was found to produce a modest increase (approximately 10%) in atrial natriuretic peptide and B-type natriuretic peptide during acute treatment of severe HF, even as filling pressures decline, which suggests a direct effect of the drug on the myocardial release of these peptides [14].

CARDIOVASCULAR ACTIONS OF DIGOXIN

HEMODYNAMIC EFFECTS

Digitalis administration does not alter cardiac output in normal control subjects even though the drug causes a significant increase in cardiac contractility. In normals, this lack of effect on cardiac output is likely due to increased systemic vascular resistance which also occurs with drug administration. In patients in HF, normal sinus rhythm, and reduced systolic function, digoxin administration improves left ventricular ejection fraction, reduces pulmonary capillary wedge pressure, and increases cardiac output both at rest and during exercise [16]. These favorable acute effects are particularly evident in patients who continue to have elevated pulmonary capillary wedge pressure or decreased cardiac output in the face of other treatments. If hemodynamics improve substantially with diuretics and vasodilators,

Table 1.2 Effect of Digoxin in Patients in Sinus Rhythm With Stable Heart Failure and Reduced Systolic Function Receiving Diuretics (PROVED Study) or Diuretics and ACE Inhibitors (RADIANCE Study) (with permission from [52])

	On diuretics	On ACE inhibitors and diuretics
Treadmill time	Improved	Improved
Six-minute walk	No change	Improved
Incidence of treatment failure	Decreased	Decreased
Time to treatment failure	Decreased	Decreased
Change in signs and symptoms of HF	No change	Improved
Quality of life (Minnesota Living With Heart Failure Questionnaire)	No change	Improved
CHF score	No change	Improved
Global evaluation of progress	No change	Improved
LVEF	Improved	Improved
HR and BP	Decreased	Decreased
Body weight	Decreased	Decreased

BP = blood pressure; CHF = congestive heart failure; HR = heart rate; LVEF = left ventricular ejection fraction.

acute administration of digoxin produces no further benefit [17]. Improvement in hemodynamics is sustained during chronic therapy, likely partly related to lack of up-regulation of sodium-potassium ATPase site during digoxin treatment [18].

ELECTROPHYSIOLOGICAL EFFECTS

Digoxin has a predominant parasympathomimetic action on the atrial myocardium and it slows conduction and prolongs the AV node refractory period. Digoxin has practically no electrophysiological effect in the Purkinje system of ventricular muscle. Digoxin toxicity is well known to produce a variety of arrhythmias some of which may be lethal. Maintaining serum concentrations < 1 ng/ml is the best way to prevent therapeutic doses of digoxin from increasing the risk of arrhythmias. Ischemia seems to promote arrhythmia risk with digoxin [19].

EVIDENCE CONCERNING CLINICAL UTILITY IN HF

Digoxin has been extensively studied in small trials, but the most important data concerning efficacy in HF come from two moderate-sized studies that have a common design: the Prospective Randomized study Of Ventricular failure and Efficacy of Digoxin (PROVED) study and the Randomized Assessment of Digoxin on Inhibitors of Angiotensin-Converting Enzyme (RADIANCE) study and one large scale outcomes trial, the Digitalis Investigation Group study (DIG study) [20–22]. As much as these trial data were needed, their results have not been easy to interpret and, in the spirit of earlier observational results, have been fiercely debated by proponents and opponents of this medication. The PROVED and RADIANCE trials do not provide meaningful data on major outcomes, but they do provide considerable supportive data concerning clinically relevant endpoints like exercise tolerance and left ventricular function (Table 1.2). In addition, they allow some insight into the effect of the drug on short-term outcomes. Data was collected on worsening HF during follow-up using a common definition: a decline in clinical status sufficient to require one of the following therapeutic interventions: change in background therapy, visit to an emergency room for increasing HF or hospital admission for HF. Furthermore, any suspected events were independently adjudicated by a committee unaware of treatment assignment in both studies.

PROVED

The PROVED study was designed to investigate whether digoxin was effective in patients with chronic, stable, mild to moderate HF due to systolic dysfunction, who were treated with diuretic [20]. In this multicenter study, digoxin was withdrawn ($n = 46$) or continued ($n = 42$) in a prospective, randomized, double-blind, and placebo-controlled design. All patients enrolled were in normal sinus rhythm and had received long-term treatment with diuretics and digoxin. Several detrimental effects of digoxin withdrawal were noted in this study. Maximal exercise capacity declined in the withdrawal group, but was maintained in patients who continued on digoxin (median decrease −96 seconds vs. +4.5 seconds, $P = 0.003$). Patients withdrawn from digoxin were significantly more likely to experience treatment failure (39%, digoxin withdrawal group vs. 19%, digoxin maintenance group, $P = 0.039$). In addition, patients who continued on digoxin had lower body weight ($P = 0.044$), reduced heart rate ($P = 0.003$), and higher left ventricular ejection fraction ($P = 0.016$).

RADIANCE

The RADIANCE study addressed the therapeutic role of digoxin in the angiotensin-converting-enzyme (ACE) inhibitor era [21]. This trial investigated 178 patients with New York Heart Association (NYHA) class II or III HF and left ventricular ejection fractions $\leq 35\%$. Study patients were in normal sinus rhythm and clinically stable while receiving digoxin, diuretics, and an ACE inhibitor (captopril or enalapril). Patients were randomly assigned, after a stabilization period of approximately 2 months, to either continue digoxin (85 patients) or withdraw from this therapy (93 patients). The design was double-blind with a follow-up period of 12 weeks after randomization. Worsening HF occurred in 23 patients in the digoxin withdrawal group, but in only four patients who continued digoxin (hazard ratio [HR] 5.9; 95% confidence interval [CI] 2.1–17.2; $P < 0.001$). In addition, functional capacity deteriorated, in a similar manner to the PROVED study, when patients discontinued digoxin ($P = 0.033$ for maximal exercise tolerance, $P = 0.01$ for submaximal exercise endurance, and $P = 0.019$ for NYHA class). Other measures of clinical response differed as well, with patients who discontinued digoxin having lower quality of life scores ($P = 0.04$), decreased ejection fractions ($P = 0.001$), and increases in heart rate ($P = 0.001$) and body weight ($P < 0.001$).

The common design of PROVED and RADIANCE allowed a combined analysis of the worsening HF endpoint which provides clear evidence of the short-term effectiveness of digoxin and the utility of 'triple' therapy in these study populations (Figure 1.1).

DIG

The modest sized withdrawal studies provided convincing evidence to many of the short-term efficacy of digoxin, but they lacked definitive results concerning the long-term effects of this drug on morbidity and mortality. This issue was addressed in the DIG trial, which was designed to test the effect of digoxin on the risk of major adverse outcomes in HF in a randomized, double-blind design [22]. This HF trial had two arms: 6800 patients with left ventricular systolic dysfunction (left ventricular ejection fraction $\leq 45\%$) and 988 patients with preserved left ventricular ejection fraction ($> 45\%$) [23]. In the systolic dysfunction arm, patients were randomly assigned to digoxin or placebo in addition to diuretics and ACE inhibitors, as tolerated. Of note, the median dose of digoxin used in the trial was 0.25 mg per day. There were

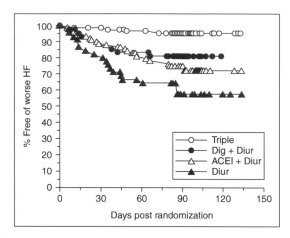

Figure 1.1 Likelihood of deterioration in HF status in the four treatment groups: triple therapy with ACE inhibitor, digoxin and diuretic, digoxin and diuretic, ACE inhibitor and diuretic, and diuretic alone. Patients receiving triple therapy were significantly less likely to experience treatment failure compared to any of the other three groups (all $P<0.01$).

1181 deaths (34.8%) in the digoxin group and 1194 deaths (35.1%) in the placebo group (HR 0.99; 95% CI 0.91–1.07; $P=0.80$). Although overall these findings clearly indicated no effect of digoxin on survival, interestingly there was a trend toward a decrease in the risk of death attributed to worsening HF in patients randomized to digoxin (HR 0.88; 95% CI 0.77–1.01; $P=0.06$). In terms of morbidity, the picture was also mixed. Overall there was a modest reduction in all-cause hospitalization (6% fewer hospitalizations overall in the digoxin group compared to the placebo group), but hospitalization for worsening HF was substantially reduced in digoxin treated patients (26.8% vs. 34.7%, HR 0.72; 95% CI 0.66–0.79; $P<0.001$).

Of particular importance, there was no difference in drug effect between patients who had digoxin withdrawn or prospectively added (randomized to digoxin but not receiving the drug at baseline). Results showed that the absolute risk of death or hospitalization for HF in those previously taking digoxin was −8.6% (HR 0.74; 95% CI 0.66–0.83) compared to −6.2% (HR 0.77; 95% CI 0.68–0.86) in those with the drug added. This important finding reinforced the validity of the PROVED and RADIANCE withdrawal trial findings to many observers.

INTERPRETATION OF KEY CLINICAL TRIAL RESULTS

For many clinicians, the outcome of the DIG study signaled a major reinterpretation of the role of digoxin in the treatment of HF [24]. By the time these results were announced, improving morbidity and mortality had become the major focus of clinical HF research. Landmark trials of ACE inhibitor therapy were proving that better outcomes were possible with medical therapy, not only in patients with mild to moderate clinical HF, but even in patients with NYHA functional class IV symptoms and severe left ventricular dysfunction; a population many considered beyond the reach of medical therapeutics. The lack of even a trend toward improvement in all-cause mortality in the DIG trial stood in marked contrast to published results with ACE inhibitors and data emerging concerning a substantial beneficial effect of beta blockade on these outcomes. Others maintain that reduction in HF morbidity in the DIG trial, improvement in exercise tolerance and quality of life in short-term studies, and low cost and convenience, continue to make digoxin attractive [25].

Our research group, composed of several investigators with a longstanding clinical interest in digoxin who were involved in the PROVED and RADIANCE studies, took yet another approach. The idea was to re-examine results of the three key efficacy trials to better understand the factors that influence benefit from this medication. This analysis, presented in detail below, suggested that the serum concentration necessary for clinical benefit needed revision and that there was a relationship between severity of HF present and clinical efficacy of the drug. In addition, the role of digoxin in women and patients with HF and preserved ejection fraction was clarified.

As further support for re-interpretation of the DIG study, the careful reader is invited to reconsider the major outcome results in this trial (Figure 1.2A,B). The simultaneous findings that digoxin failed to reduce overall mortality, but reduced the risk of death due to worsening HF does not fit with the usual consistent effect a therapy should have on these two endpoints. In addition, the marked reduction in hospitalization for worsening HF is difficult to reconcile with a modest effect on all-cause hospitalization.

At a more fundamental philosophical level, the debate about the efficacy of digoxin highlights the two major prevailing approaches to the interpretation of the cardiovascular clinical trials by opinion leaders. One side takes the position that cardiovascular diseases are, for practical purposes, homogeneous, that drug response in these conditions is essentially uniform across demographic and clinical subgroups, and that dose response is overrated. This perspective generally promotes a simple interpretation of clinical trial data based on overall results, essentially eschewing subgroup analysis and concerns about factors like drug dose. There certainly do appear to be a number of cardiovascular diseases and therapies that can be evaluated successfully in this straightforward way, but many advocates of digoxin take the opposite perspective. This view recognizes significant heterogeneity in cardiovascular disease states, allows for some difference in effectiveness among demographic and clinical subgroups, and acknowledges the need to pay attention to dose-response relationships.

Of course, there are pitfalls and limitations inherent to both perspectives and which perspective is correct cannot be resolved here. The purpose of the review of the randomized trial data on digoxin that follows is not to reach a definitive conclusion about the effectiveness of this agent, especially its ability to improve clinical outcomes. Although when properly performed and interpreted, retrospective cohort analyses should not be lightly discarded, but they cannot achieve this level of certainty. Rather, the goal is to present a thorough and rigorous analysis of the existing randomized trial data so that the thoughtful clinician can make the most informed decision about utilization of digoxin. HF remains expensive to treat due to poor outcomes despite recent advances in therapy. Inexpensive and convenient therapies that show at least some evidence for effectiveness are not easily discounted.

SERUM CONCENTRATION AND EFFICACY AND SAFETY OF DIGOXIN

BACKGROUND

Although digitalis glycosides have been used for 200 years in the treatment of HF, the serum digoxin concentration required for optimal clinical efficacy and acceptable toxicity remains controversial [25, 26]. Previous work has established that higher serum concentrations exert greater positive effects on left ventricular function [27–30]. However, there is no evidence that increasing dose to improve left ventricular function will result in greater clinical benefit. In addition, digitalis appears to exert a favorable effect on abnormalities of autonomic tone present in HF, which calls into question a pure inotropic mechanism of action for the drug [9, 11]. Recent work suggests these favorable neurohormonal effects occur at low doses of digoxin, and that increasing the serum digoxin concentration beyond modest levels (i.e., 0.7 ng/ml), may not produce additional neurohormonal benefits [13, 31].

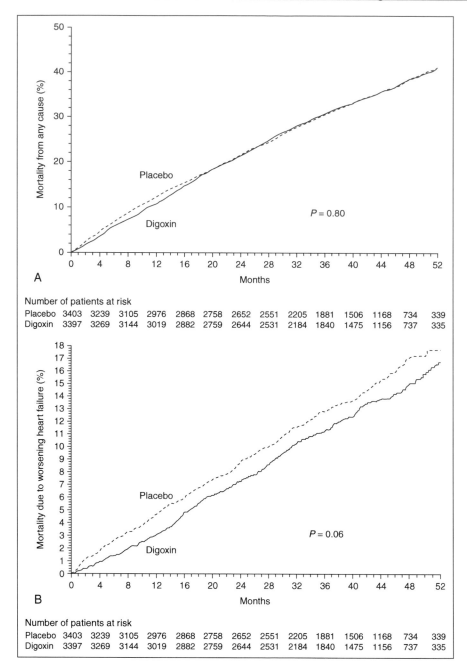

Figure 1.2 (A) Mortality in the digoxin and placebo groups. The number of patients at risk at each 4-month interval is shown below the figure. (B) Mortality due to worsening HF in the digoxin and placebo groups. The number of patients at risk at each 4-month interval is shown below the figure.

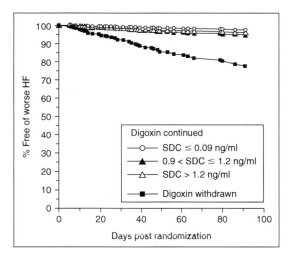

Figure 1.3 Adjusted likelihood of worsening HF in the four patient groups defined by either withdrawal from digoxin or serum digoxin concentration at randomization in those who continued the drug. Patients who continued digoxin in any category of serum concentration were significantly less likely (all *P* < 0.02) to experience treatment failure than patients withdrawn from digoxin.

SERUM CONCENTRATION IN PROVED AND RADIANCE

To determine whether there was a relationship between serum digoxin concentration, including serum digoxin concentrations typically regarded as low, and clinical efficacy of digoxin, combined data from the PROVED and RADIANCE studies were reviewed [32]. Major endpoints were worsening HF, change in left ventricular ejection fraction and treadmill time after randomization. The primary analysis investigated the relationship between serum digoxin concentration at randomization and these endpoints. A secondary categorical analysis compared these endpoints in patients who discontinued digoxin vs. patients who continued digoxin and had low (0.5 to 0.9 ng/ml), moderate (0.9 to 1.2 ng/ml) or high (1.2 ng/ml) serum digoxin concentrations at randomization. Multiple regression analysis failed to find a relationship between randomization serum digoxin concentration, considered as a continuous variable, and any study endpoint (all $P > 0.236$). Multivariable Cox analysis found that the risk of worsening HF was significantly less (all $P < 0.02$) for patients in any category of serum digoxin concentration who continued digoxin, as compared with patients withdrawn from digoxin (Figure 1.3). Specifically, patients in the low serum digoxin concentration category were significantly less likely than placebo patients to experience worsening HF during follow-up ($P = 0.018$). Overall, the beneficial effects of digoxin on common clinical endpoints were similar, regardless of serum digoxin concentration.

SERUM CONCENTRATION IN DIG TRIAL

Thus analysis of the PROVED and RADIANCE studies raised the possibility that low serum concentrations may be effective in improving outcomes as well as short-term clinical endpoints. The DIG trial provided the opportunity to prospectively address this issue in a retrospective, cohort analysis, since blinded serum concentrations were obtained in patients who returned for a 1-month follow-up visit. Several groups have had access to the trial data and have reported various analyses on the relationship of serum concentration to outcomes. Rathore *et al.* [33] published a categorical analysis which only considered the men enrolled in the study. They divided men randomized to digoxin into three groups according to serum concentration obtained at the 1-month time point: 0.5 to 0.8 ng/ml ($n = 572$), 0.9 to 1.1 ng/ml ($n = 322$) and ≥ 1.2 ng/ml ($n = 277$). These groups were compared with all male study patients randomly assigned to receive placebo ($n = 2611$). The primary endpoint in their cohort analysis was all-cause mortality over a mean follow-up of 37 months. Higher serum digoxin concentrations were associated with increased crude all-cause mortality rates (0.5 to 0.8 ng/ml, 29.9%; 0.9 to 1.1 ng/ml, 38.8%; and ≥ 1.2 ng/ml, 48.0%; $P = 0.006$). Serum concentration was still significantly related to mortality after adjustment for many clinical characteristics that could have differed among the study groups. Hazard ratios relative to placebo were as follows: serum concentrations 0.5 to 0.8 ng/ml, 0.80 (95% CI 0.68–0.94), from 0.9 to 1.1 ng/ml, 0.89 (95% CI 0.74–1.08) and concentrations ≥ 1.2 ng/ml, 1.16 (95% CI 0.96–1.39).

We were addressing the issue of serum concentration in the DIG trial data at the same time with a different approach. Our analysis included both men and women and modeled the relationship between serum digoxin concentration and outcome in a continuous fashion to avoid potential bias from arbitrary cut-points. We found a highly significant ($P < 0.001$) linear relationship between serum concentration and the prespecified endpoints from the original DIG trial, death and the combined endpoint of death or hospitalization for worsening HF. Outcomes differed significantly for serum concentrations traditionally considered to be within the therapeutic range of the drug. Relative to placebo, serum digoxin concentrations from 1.5 to 2.0 ng/ml were associated with a higher risk of death (HR 1.30; $P = 0.002$), and even more importantly, there was no effect on the combined endpoint of mortality and hospitalization for HF (HR 0.97; $P = 0.715$). In contrast, serum digoxin concentrations from 0.5 to 0.9 ng/ml were associated with lower risk of death (HR 0.81; $P < 0.001$) and the combined endpoint (HR 0.70; $P < 0.001$).

RATIONALE FOR DOSE-RESPONSE

Accepting the limitations of retrospective analyses, these results concerning serum concentration and efficacy resonated with ongoing concern about the potential risk of inotropic therapy in patients with HF. Adverse effects of chronic inotropic therapy could take several forms. Sudden death, most commonly due to presumed rapid ventricular arrhythmia, remains an important unresolved problem for patients with chronic HF [34]. Despite beneficial hemodynamic effects, inotropic therapy for HF has been associated with an adverse effect on mortality, which appears to be related to an increased risk of sudden death. Data from several clinical trials support the concept that the risk of sudden death is dose-dependent – more likely to occur at higher doses [35–37]. Interestingly, data already suggested that serum digoxin concentration > 1 ng/ml, but still within the therapeutic range, may sometimes be associated with classic digoxin toxicity [38–41]. There is substantial evidence that even short-term therapy with inotropic agents in acute HF may be associated with worse outcomes [42]. Patients with ischemic heart disease may be at particular risk from inotropic agents. Analysis of 60-day outcomes from an acute HF trial demonstrated that patients randomized to milrinone who had an ischemic etiology of their HF were at increased risk of adverse events [43].

Taken together, results from PROVED and RADIANCE trials and the DIG study indicate that serum digoxin concentrations classically considered to be low are, in fact, effective in patients with HF due to systolic dysfunction [44]. Dosing patients to achieve serum digoxin concentrations < 1 ng/ml is suggested as an attractive strategy to achieve beneficial clinical effects and potentially avoid adverse effects due to inotropic or other unknown effects from this drug.

DIGOXIN IN WOMEN

A retrospective analysis of results from all patients with reduced ejection fraction in the DIG trial suggested that digoxin may increase mortality in women [45]. In the multivariable analysis, digoxin was associated with a significantly higher risk of death among women (adjusted HR for the comparison with placebo 1.23, with 95% CI 1.02–1.47), but it had no significant effect among men (adjusted HR 0.93, with 95% CI 0.85–1.02; $P = 0.014$ for the interaction).

A major concern about this conclusion was that serum digoxin concentration was not taken into account in this analysis [46]. Women had higher serum digoxin concentrations compared to men in the DIG trial, making it even more important to account for this factor. To address this issue, Adams *et al.* [47] performed a retrospective analysis with data from the DIG trial. The principal study analysis reviewed 4944 patients with HF due to systolic dysfunction who survived for at least 4 weeks (all 3366 patients randomized to placebo and the 1578 of 3372 patients randomized to digoxin who had serum concentration measured from 6 to 30 h after the last dose of study drug at 4 weeks). Continuous multivariable analysis demonstrated a significant, linear relationship between serum digoxin concentration and mortality in women ($P = 0.008$) and men ($P = 0.002$, $P = 0.766$ for gender interaction). Averaging HRs across serum concentrations from 0.5 to 0.9 ng/ml in women produced a HR for death of 0.8 (95% CI 0.62–1.13; $P = 0.245$) and for death or hospital stay for worsening HF of 0.73 (95% CI 0.58–0.93; $P = 0.011$). In contrast, serum digoxin concentrations from 1.2 to 2.0 ng/ml were associated with a HR for death for women of 1.33 (95% CI 1.001–1.76; $P = 0.049$). This retrospective analysis of data from the DIG trial indicates a beneficial effect of digoxin on morbidity and no excess mortality in women at serum concentrations from 0.5 to 0.9 ng/ml, whereas serum concentrations ≥1.2 ng/ml seem harmful (Figure 1.4). For now, it seems prudent to administer digoxin in low doses in women with HF and to obtain a level once a steady state is reached to ensure that serum digoxin concentration is less than 1 ng/ml. In addition, traditional dosing strategies (0.25 mg daily) are associated with higher serum digoxin concentrations in women, likely due to their reduced body mass and the fact that lower serum creatinine can be associated with a greater reduction in renal function in women. Dosing is discussed in detail later but 0.125 mg daily, or often every other day, appears to be the best approach.

SEVERITY OF HF AND RESPONSE TO DIGOXIN

EARLY WORK

An important small trial reported by Lee *et al.* [48] suggested that digoxin may be more effective in severe HF. In this study, patients who responded to digoxin had more severe HF of longer duration, greater left ventricular dilation and ejection-fraction depression, and a third heart sound. Analysis of a much larger cohort of PROVED and RADIANCE patients found that those with more congestive symptoms, worse ventricular function, greater cardiac enlargement, or who were not taking an ACE inhibitor were significantly more likely to worsen early after digoxin discontinuation [49]. An additional retrospective analysis of PROVED and RADIANCE data investigated whether patients with mild HF (defined by an objective prospective HF score) due to left ventricular systolic dysfunction were at risk of worsening during digoxin withdrawal [50]. Potential differences in treatment failure, left ventricular ejection fraction and exercise capacity were evaluated in three groups of patients: those with mild HF (HF score ≤ 2) who were withdrawn from digoxin, those with moderate HF (HF score > 2) who were withdrawn from digoxin, and patients who continued receiving digoxin regardless of HF score. HF score at randomization did not

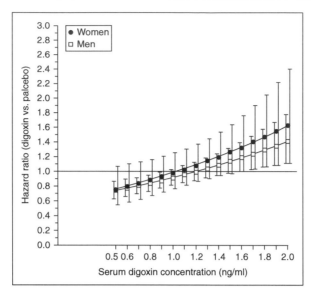

Figure 1.4 Plot of the adjusted point estimates and 95% CI of women and men for the HR for death on digoxin vs. placebo at various serum digoxin concentrations (ng/ml) with concentration modeled as a continuous variable. The 95% CI for the women are offset to allow better depiction of results.

predict outcome during follow-up in patients who continued digoxin. Patients withdrawn from digoxin who had mild HF at baseline were at increased risk of treatment failure and had deterioration of exercise capacity and left ventricular ejection fraction compared with patients who continued digoxin (Figure 1.5, all *P*< 0.01). Patients withdrawn from digoxin who had moderate HF were significantly more likely to experience treatment failure than patients withdrawn from digoxin with mild failure or those who continued digoxin (both *P*<0.05). This analysis suggested that patients with systolic left ventricular dysfunction were at risk of clinical deterioration after digoxin withdrawal despite mild clinical evidence of congestive HF, but that more severe HF at baseline further increased risk during withdrawal.

Results from the DIG study have never been rigorously analyzed, including consideration of serum concentration, in order to address the issue of clinical severity and efficacy of digoxin. A limited analysis based on the combined study endpoint of risk of death or hospitalization due to worsening HF included in the main report of this trial suggested that usual indicators of greater clinical severity (functional class, ejection fraction, cardiothoracic ratio) were modestly predictive of drug efficacy [22]. In contrast, a preliminary report suggests that patients with severe HF (clinical class IV) clearly derived greater benefit in this study [51]. In addition, results of an analysis conducted by the FDA based on the prespecified 2-year time point in the DIG study is of interest [52]. This modeling considered two combined endpoints, death and all-cause hospitalization and death and hospitalization for worsening HF (Table 1.3). Results from this analysis suggested that clinical severity was strongly associated with benefit for the endpoint of death and all-cause hospitalization. Taken as a whole, available results suggest the clinical severity of HF should be a factor when considering the use of digoxin in patients with HF due to systolic dysfunction. Hopefully, additional rigorous and comprehensive analyses of data from the DIG trial, taking into account serum concentration, will provide additional data to help clinicians select patients most likely to respond favorably to digoxin.

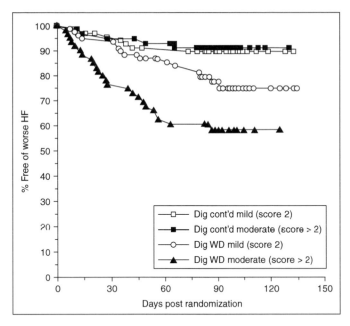

Figure 1.5 Likelihood of deterioration of HF status in patients continuing digoxin therapy who had mild or moderate HF by clinical score vs. patients withdrawn from digoxin who had mild or moderate HF at baseline by the same score criteria. Life-table analysis revealed no difference in the risk of treatment failure by HF score category in patients who continued receiving digoxin ($P=0.944$). The risk of worsening was significantly greater in patients with mild HF who were withdrawn from digoxin than in all patients who continued receiving digoxin ($P=0.011$). Patients withdrawn from digoxin who had moderate HF were significantly more likely to experience treatment failure during follow-up than either patients who continued receiving digoxin ($P<0.001$) or patients in the mild HF group ($P=0.028$).

PRESERVED SYSTOLIC FUNCTION

Ahmed *et al.* [53] reported the effects of digoxin in patients with HF and preserved ejection fraction enrolled in the DIG trial. Their analysis reported in detail on this arm of the DIG trial that included 988 ambulatory, chronic HF patients in normal sinus rhythm with a left ventricular ejection fraction > 45% (median, 53%). During a mean follow-up period of 37 months, 102 patients (21%) in the digoxin group and 119 patients (24%) in the placebo group experienced the primary combined outcome of HF hospitalization or HF mortality (HR 0.82; 95% CI 0.63–1.07; $P=0.136$). Use of digoxin was associated with a trend toward a reduction in hospitalizations resulting from worsening HF (HR 0.79; 95% CI 0.59–1.04; $P=0.094$), but also a trend toward an increase in hospitalizations for unstable angina (HR 1.37, 95% CI 0.99–1.91; $P=0.061$). Despite some favorable trends in the data, this arm of the DIG trial failed to establish clear evidence that digoxin had a favorable effect on natural history endpoints such as mortality and all-cause or cardiovascular hospitalizations in patients with HF and preserved ejection fraction.

Table 1.3 Subgroup analyses of mortality and hospitalization during the first 2 years after randomization in the Digitalis Investigation Trial (with permission from [52])

Variable	No. patients	Risk of all-cause mortality or all-cause hospitalization			Risk of HF-related mortality or HF-related hospitalization*		
		Placebo	Digoxin	RR (95% CI)	Placebo	Digoxin	RR (95% CI)
All patients (EF ≤0.45)	6801	604	593	0.94 (0.88 to 1.00)	294	217	0.69 (0.63 to 0.76)
NYHA FC I/II	4571	548	541	0.96 (0.89 to 1.04)	242	178	0.70 (0.62 to 0.80)
NYHA FC III/IV	2224	719	696	0.88 (0.80 to 0.97)	402	295	0.65 (0.57 to 0.75)
EF ≥0.45†	987	571	585	1.04 (0.88 to 1.23)	179	136	0.72 (0.53 to 0.99)
EF 0.25 to 0.45	4543	568	571	0.99 (0.91 to 1.07)	244	190	0.74 (0.66 to 0.84)
EF <0.25	2258	677	637	0.84 (0.76 to 0.93)	394	270	0.61 (0.53 to 0.71)
Cardiothoracic ratio on chest x-ray ≤0.55	4455	561	569	0.98 (0.91 to 1.06)	239	180	0.71 (0.63 to 0.81)
Cardiothoracic ratio on chest x-ray >0.55	2346	687	650	0.55 (0.77 to 0.94)	398	287	0.65 (0.57 to 0.75)

CI=confidence interval; EF=ejection fraction; NYHA FC=New York Heart Association Functional Class; RR=relative risk. †DIG Ancillary Study.
*No. of patients with an event during the first 2 years per 1000 randomized patients.

OTHER ASPECTS OF DIGOXIN IN HF

DIGOXIN IN THE MULTI-DRUG APPROACH TO HF

By necessity, digoxin is widely used with thiazide and loop diuretics in the management of HF. These diuretics may cause hypokalemia and possibly hypomagnesemia that may increase the tendency for digoxin to cause serious arrhythmia. Thus adequate potassium and magnesium levels should be maintained when these agents are used together. In contrast, the combination of potassium sparing diuretics and digoxin avoids these electrolyte issues. In the Randomized Aldactone Evaluation Study of severe HF, spironolactone was particularly beneficial in patients receiving digoxin [54].

One major gap in the evidence from randomized trials of digoxin relates to concomitant beta blocker therapy. The efficacy of digoxin in patients with HF treated with beta blockade has not been investigated by placebo-controlled trials. Positive mortality trials with beta blockade have consistently included digoxin as a background therapy and there has been no convincing interaction with efficacy. Experimentally, severe arrhythmia secondary to digoxin is less likely when beta-blocker is present [55]. Digoxin may prevent or lessen the initial negative hemodynamic effects observed with beta-blocker therapy. In contrast, since many of non-inotropic effects of digoxin involve attenuation of the sympathetic nervous system, some have questioned if efficacy would persist when the adrenergic system was inhibited by beta blockade. Current guidelines do not make this assumption and digoxin remains a recommended therapy in patients taking beta blockade.

PRECAUTION IN USING DIGOXIN

Digoxin should not be used when sinoatrial or second/third degree AV block is present, unless the patient has a pacemaker. Digoxin should not be used in Wolf-Parkinson-White syndrome, in patients with hypertrophic or restrictive cardiomyopathy or in amyloid heart disease. The drug should be used with caution in patients with thyroid disorders and acute coronary syndromes. If possible, digoxin should be discontinued a few days prior to electrical cardioversion for atrial arrhythmias. If cardioversion is performed in patients receiving digoxin, potassium levels should be corrected and the lowest energy possible should be used.

PHARMACOLOGICAL ASPECTS

PHARMACOKINETICS AND PHARMACODYNAMICS

Because of the importance of serum concentration, knowledge of basic pharmacokinetics and pharmacodynamics of digoxin is important. Absorption occurs rapidly (1 to 3h) and is followed by a 6 to 8h tissue distribution phase. The great majority of digoxin (84%) is excreted unchanged in the urine so that renal function is a major consideration when dosing this drug. To illustrate this, the half-life of digoxin is 36 to 48h when renal function is normal, but increases to 3.5 to 5 days in anuric patients. Patients with normal renal function will reach steady-state blood levels on oral maintenance dosing in approximately 7 days [56].

DOSING FOR IDEAL SERUM CONCENTRATION

The latest available evidence strongly suggests that digoxin should be administered to attain a serum concentration < 1 ng/ml. Many recommend a daily dose of 0.125 mg in patients with normal renal function not taking drugs that may increase digoxin concentration. Data from the DIG trial suggest that a dose of 0.125 mg daily of digoxin will result in a serum concentration of approximately 0.7 ng/ml in such patients. A dose of 0.125 mg every other day will be more appropriate in HF patients who are elderly, female, or have renal impairment. Even lower doses are indicated in patients with multiple characteristics that may produce higher than expected serum concentrations. In these patients, close monitoring of digoxin level is indicated and dosing may begin at 0.0625 mg one to three times a week. When patients are at steady-state, serum digoxin concentration should be measured at least 12 to 24 h after the last dose of the drug (in the post-distribution phase) [57].

DRUG INTERACTIONS

A number of drugs may significantly affect the absorption, clearance, and volume of distribution of digoxin and reduce or potentiate its effects [52, 58]. A number of these agents, including quinidine, verapamil and amiodarone, frequently produce a significant increase in serum concentration, which may occur rapidly or only after a few weeks. The dose of digoxin is typically reduced approximately 50% when used with these medications, but serum levels should be followed closely as substantial individual variation is common. Oral digoxin is partially inactivated by colonic bacteria in some patients, so certain antibiotics may increase digoxin absorption in these individuals.

INDICATIONS FOR DIGOXIN THERAPY

An individual opinion is given here based on a synthesis of key trial results, retrospective cohort analyses that have emerged to clarify these studies, and discussions with expert colleagues [58–60]. Practice guidelines provide consensus insight concerning the use of digoxin in HF [61]. Digoxin is indicated in patients with HF and reduced left ventricular ejection fraction who continue to have symptomatic HF despite background therapy with ACE inhibitors and beta blockers. Digoxin is also indicated in patients with HF and atrial fibrillation and may be useful in patients with this arrhythmia in the absence of HF. Digoxin should be avoided or used with extreme caution in patients with severe conduction abnormalities or acute coronary syndromes. Available data provide invaluable insights concerning choice of HF patient and appropriate serum concentration for best efficacy of the drug. Digoxin is particularly useful in patients with moderate to severe symptoms, low left ventricular ejection fraction, or cardiac enlargement by chest X-ray. A low dose resulting in a serum concentration of < 1 ng/ml should be used when treating either HF or atrial fibrillation. Serum concentration may trend higher in women with usual dosing, so extra care to achieve concentrations < 1 ng/ml is needed. The drug is likely effective at the lowest traditional serum concentration in the therapeutic range, 0.5 ng/ml, which may be an appropriate target when treating patients who are at risk for higher serum concentrations (elderly, renal insufficiency, specific medications) on currently recommended doses. Digoxin remains a low cost, convenient medication for HF, which much evidence suggests can have important benefits on outcome, if dosed correctly.

REFERENCES

1. Withering W. An account of the foxglove and some of its medical uses, with practical remarks on dropsy, and other diseases. In: Aronson JK, ed. *An Account of the Foxglove and Its Medical Uses 1785–1985*. London: Oxford University Press, 1985, pp 1-193.
2. Lehrer S. *Explorers of the Body: Dramatic Breakthroughs in Medicine from Ancient Times to Modern Science*. Bloomington, Indiana: iUniverse, Inc., 2006, pp 12-19.
3. Smith TW, Antman EM, Friedman PL, Blatt CM, Marsh JD. Digitalis glycosides: mechanisms and manifestations of toxicity. Part I. *Prog Cardiovasc Dis* 1984; 26:413-458.
4. Smith TW, Antman EM, Friedman PL, Blatt CM, Marsh JD. Digitalis glycosides: mechanisms and manifestations of toxicity. Part II. *Prog Cardiovasc Dis* 1984; 26:495-540.

5. Schwinger RH, Wang J, Frank K *et al.* Reduced sodium pump alpha1, alpha3, and beta1-isoform protein levels and Na+,K+-ATPase activity but unchanged Na+-Ca2+ exchanger protein levels in human heart failure. *Circulation* 1999; 99:2105-2112.

6. Schmidt TA, Allen PD, Colucci WS, Marsh JD, Kjeldsen K. No adaptation to digitalization as evaluated by digitalis receptor (Na,K-ATPase) quantification in explanted hearts from donors without heart disease and from digitalized recipients with end-stage heart failure. *Am J Cardiol* 1993; 71:110-114.

7. Ferguson DW. Digitalis and neurohormonal abnormalities in heart failure and implications for therapy. *Am J Cardiol* 1992; 69:24G-32G.

8. Wang W, Chen JS, Zucker IH. Carotid sinus baroreceptor sensitivity in experimental heart failure. *Circulation* 1990; 81:1959-1966.

9. Krum H, Bigger JT Jr, Goldsmith RL, Packer M. Effect of long-term digoxin therapy on autonomic function in patients with chronic heart failure. *J Am Coll Cardiol* 1995; 25:289-294.

10. Ferguson DW, Berg WJ, Sanders JS, Roach PJ, Kempf JS, Kienzle MG. Sympathoinhibitory responses to digitalis glycosides in heart failure patients: direct evidence from sympathetic neural recordings. *Circulation* 1989; 80:65-77.

11. van Veldhuisen DJ, Man in 't Veld AJ, Dunselman PH *et al.* Double-blind placebo-controlled study of ibopamine and digoxin in patients with mild to moderate heart failure: results of the Dutch Ibopamine Multicenter trial (DIMT). *J Am Coll Cardiol* 1993; 22:1564-1573.

12. Newton GE, Tong JH, Schofield AM, Baines AD, Floras JS, Parker JD. Digoxin reduces cardiac sympathetic activity in severe congestive heart failure. *J Am Coll Cardiol* 1996; 28:155-161.

13. Gheorghiade M, Hall VB, Jacobsen G, Alam M, Rosman H, Goldstein S. Effects of increasing maintenance dose of digoxin on left ventricular function and neurohormones in patients with chronic heart failure treated with diuretics and angiotensin-converting enzyme inhibitors. *Circulation* 1995; 92:1801-1807.

14. Tsutamoto T, Wada A, Maeda K *et al.* Digitalis increases brain natriuretic peptide in patients with severe congestive heart failure. *Am Heart J* 1997; 134:910-916.

15. Sundaram S, Zampino M, Gheorghiade M. Is there still a place for digoxin in heart failure? In: van Veldhuisen DJ, Pitt B, eds. *Focus on Cardiovascular Diseases: Chronic Heart Failure.* Amsterdam, The Netherlands: Benecke NI, 2002:219-254.

16. Gheorghiade M, St Clair J, St Clair C, Beller GA. Hemodynamic effects of intravenous digoxin in patients with severe heart failure initially treated with diuretics and vasodilators. *J Am Coll Cardiol* 1987; 9:849-857.

17. Gheorghiade M, Hall V, Lakier JB, Goldstein S. Comparative hemodynamic and neurohormonal effects of intravenous captopril and digoxin and their combinations in patients with severe heart failure. *J Am Coll Cardiol* 1989; 13:134-142.

18. Arnold SB, Byrd RC, Meister W *et al.* Long-term digitalis therapy improves left ventricular function in heart failure. *N Engl J Med* 1980; 303:1443-1448.

19. Lown B, Graboys TB, Podrid PJ, Cohen BH, Stockman MB, Gaughan CE. Effect of a digitalis drug on ventricular premature beats. *N Engl J Med* 1977; 296:301-306.

20. Uretsky BF, Young JB, Shahidi FE, Yellen LG, Harrison MC, Jolly MK. Randomized study assessing the effect of digoxin withdrawal in patients with mild to moderate chronic congestive heart failure: results of the PROVED trial. PROVED Investigative Group. *J Am Coll Cardiol* 1993; 22:955-962.

21. Packer M, Gheorghiade M, Young JB *et al.* Withdrawal of digoxin from patients with chronic heart failure treated with angiotensin-converting-enzyme inhibitors. RADIANCE Study. *N Engl J Med* 1993; 329:1-7.

22. The effect of digoxin on mortality and morbidity in patients with heart failure. The Digitalis Investigation Group. *N Engl J Med* 1997; 336:525-533.

23. Rationale, design, implementation, and baseline characteristics of patients in the DIG trial: a large, simple, long-term trial to evaluate the effects of digitalis on mortality in heart failure. The Digitalis Investigation Group. *Control Clin Trials* 1996; 17:77-97.

24. Packer M. End of the oldest controversy in medicine. Are we ready to conclude the debate on digitalis? *N Engl J Med* 1997; 336:575-576.

25. Gheorghiade M, Pitt B. Digitalis Investigation Group (DIG) trial: a stimulus for further research. *Am Heart J* 1997; 134:3-12.

26. Gheorghiade M, Zarowitz BJ. Review of randomized trials of digoxin therapy in patients with chronic heart failure. *Am J Cardiol* 1992; 69:48G-62G.

27. Carliner NH, Gilbert CA, Pruitt AW, Goldberg LI. Effects of maintenance digoxin therapy on systolic time intervals and serum digoxin concentrations. *Circulation* 1974; 50:94-98.

28. Hoeschen RJ, Cuddy TE. Dose-response relation between therapeutic levels of serum digoxin and systolic time intervals. *Am J Cardiol* 1975; 35:469-472.

29. Buch J, Waldorff S. Classical concentration-response relationship between serum digoxin level and contractility indices. *Dan Med Bull* 1980; 27:287-290.

30. Belz GG, Erbel R, Schumann K, Gilfrich HJ. Dose-response relationships and plasma concentrations of digitalis glycosides in man. *Eur J Clin Pharmacol* 1978; 13:103-111.

31. Slatton ML, Irani WN, Hall SA *et al.* Does digoxin provide additional hemodynamic and autonomic benefit at higher doses in patients with mild to moderate heart failure and normal sinus rhythm? *J Am Coll Cardiol* 1997; 29:1206-1213.

32. Adams KF Jr, Gheorghiade M, Uretsky BF, Patterson JH, Schwartz TA, Young JB. Clinical benefits of low serum digoxin concentrations in heart failure. *J Am Coll Cardiol* 2002; 39:946-953.

33. Rathore SS, Curtis JP, Wang Y, Bristow MR, Krumholz HM. Association of serum digoxin concentration and outcomes in patients with heart failure. *JAMA* 2003; 289:871-878.

34. Stevenson WG, Sweeney MO. Arrhythmias and sudden death in heart failure. *Jpn Circ J* 1997; 61:727-740.

35. Xamoterol in severe heart failure. The Xamoterol in Severe Heart Failure Study Group. *Lancet* 1990; 336:1-6.

36. Packer M, Carver JR, Rodeheffer RJ *et al.* Effect of oral milrinone on mortality in severe chronic heart failure. The PROMISE Study Research Group. *N Engl J Med* 1991; 325:1468-1475.

37. Cohn JN, Goldstein SO, Greenberg BH *et al.* A dose-dependent increase in mortality with vesnarinone among patients with severe heart failure. Vesnarinone Trial Investigators. *N Engl J Med* 1998; 339:1810-1816.

38. Kelly RA, Smith TW. Recognition and management of digitalis toxicity. *Am J Cardiol* 1992; 69:108G-118G.

39. Warren JL, McBean AM, Hass SL, Babish JD. Hospitalizations with adverse events caused by digitalis therapy among elderly Medicare beneficiaries. *Arch Intern Med* 1994; 154:1482-1487.

40. Mahdyoon H, Battilana G, Rosman H, Goldstein S, Gheorghiade M. The evolving pattern of digoxin intoxication: observations at a large urban hospital from 1980 to 1988. *Am Heart J* 1990; 120:1189-1194.

41. Smith TW, Haber E. Digoxin intoxication: the relationship of clinical presentation to serum digoxin concentration. *J Clin Invest* 1970; 49:2377-2386.

42. Abraham WT, Adams KF, Fonarow GC *et al.* ADHERE Scientific Advisory Committee and Investigators; ADHERE Study Group. In-hospital mortality in patients with acute decompensated heart failure requiring intravenous vasoactive medications: an analysis from the Acute Decompensated Heart Failure National Registry (ADHERE). *J Am Coll Cardiol* 2005; 46:57-64.

43. Felker GM, Benza RL, Chandler AB *et al.* OPTIME-CHF Investigators. Heart failure etiology and response to milrinone in decompensated heart failure: results from the OPTIME-CHF study. *J Am Coll Cardiol* 2003; 41:997-1003.

44. van Veldhuisen DJ, de Graeff PA, Remme WJ, Lie KI. Value of digoxin in heart failure and sinus rhythm: new features of an old drug? *J Am Coll Cardiol* 1996; 28:813-819.

45. Rathore SS, Wang Y, Krumholz HM. Sex-based differences in the effect of digoxin for the treatment of heart failure. *N Engl J Med* 2002; 347:1403-1411.

46. Eichhorn EJ, Gheorghiade M. Digoxin – new perspective on an old drug. *N Engl J Med* 2002; 347:1394-1395.

47. Adams KF Jr, Patterson JH, Gattis WA *et al.* Relationship of serum digoxin concentration to mortality and morbidity in women in the digitalis investigation group trial: a retrospective analysis. *J Am Coll Cardiol* 2005; 46:497-504.

48. Lee DC, Johnson RA, Bingham JB *et al.* Heart failure in outpatients: a randomized trial of digoxin versus placebo. *N Engl J Med* 1982; 306:699-705.

49. Adams KF Jr, Gheorghiade M, Uretsky BF *et al.* Clinical predictors of worsening heart failure during withdrawal from digoxin therapy. *Am Heart J* 1998; 135:389-897.

50. Adams KF Jr, Gheorghiade M, Uretsky BF *et al.* Patients with mild heart failure worsen during withdrawal from digoxin therapy. *J Am Coll Cardiol* 1997; 30:42-48.

51. Adams KF, Patterson JH, Gattis WA, O'Connor CM, Schwartz TA, Gheorghiade M. Favorable effects of digoxin on mortality and morbidity inpatients with class IV congestive heart failure due to systolic dysfunction: retrospective analysis of the DIG Study. *J Am Coll Cardiol* (abstr) 2003; 41:164A.

52. Eichhorn EJ, Gheorghiade M. Digoxin. *Prog Cardiovasc Dis* 2002; 44:251-266.
53. Ahmed A, Rich MW, Fleg JL *et al*. Effects of digoxin on morbidity and mortality in diastolic heart failure: the ancillary digitalis investigation group trial. *Circulation* 2006; 114:397-403.
54. Pitt B, Zannad F, Remme WJ *et al*. The effect of spironolactone on morbidity and mortality in patients with severe heart failure. Randomized Aldactone Evaluation Study Investigators. *N Engl J Med* 1999; 341:709-717.
55. Lynch JJ, Kitzen JM, Hoff PT, Lucchesi BR. Reduction in digitalis-associated postinfarction mortality with nadolol in conscious dogs. *Am Heart J* 1988; 115:67-76.
56. Bauman JL, DiDomenico RJ, Viana M, Fitch M. A method of determining the dose of digoxin for heart failure in the modern era. *Arch Intern Med* 2006; 166:2539-2545.
57. Valdes R, Jortani S, Gheorghiade M. Standards of laboratory practice: cardiac drug monitoring. National Academy of Clinical Biochemistry. *Clin Chem* 1998; 44:1096-1109.
58. Gheorghiade M, van Veldhuisen DJ, Colucci WS. Contemporary use of digoxin in the management of cardiovascular disorders. *Circulation* 2006; 113:2556-2564.
59. Williamson KM, Patterson JH. Is there an expanded role for digoxin in patients with heart failure and sinus rhythm? A protagonist viewpoint. *Ann Pharmacother* 1997; 31:888-892.
60. Young JB. Whither Withering's Legacy? Digoxin's role in our contemporary pharmacopeia for heart failure. *J Am Coll Cardiol* 2005; 46:505-507.
61. Adams KF, Lindenfeld J, Arnold JMO *et al*. Heart Failure Society of America. Executive Summary: HFSA 2006 Comprehensive Heart Failure Practice Guideline. *J Card Fail* 2006; 12:10-38.

2

Cell therapy for heart failure: ready for prime time?

K. E. Hatzistergos, K. Tziomalos, J. M. Hare

INTRODUCTION

Heart failure (HF), a major cause of morbidity and mortality worldwide [1], is increasing in prevalence; in the US, it is estimated that the lifetime risk of developing HF is 1 in 5 [1]. Despite the significant advances in the management of HF during the last decade, 1-year mortality rates remain approximately 20%, with even higher rates among patients hospitalized for HF [1]. Coronary heart disease is the predominant cause of HF in developed countries [1]. These sobering statistics are among the key motivations in the quest to find therapies that either ameliorate or reverse structural damage to the heart, ischemic or otherwise, that forms the basis for HF. In this context, there is currently enormous enthusiasm for the possibility of preventing or reversing ischemic cardiac damage with cell-based therapies, and early clinical reports support the idea that treatment with stem cells in acute myocardial infarction (AMI) attenuates remodeling, improves myocardial perfusion and preserves contractility [2]. There are substantially fewer data on the effectiveness of stem cells in patients with established ischemic HF; however, this therapeutic strategy will likely benefit HF patients as well. In this chapter we review the state-of-the art of cell-based therapeutics both in terms of mechanistic insights as well as the latest clinical data.

OVERVIEW

In the past decade, several important observations promoted a revision in understanding the pathophysiology of ischemic cardiac damage. These observations include the discovery of adult cardiomyocyte entry into the cell cycle, the presence of cardiac stem cells (CSCs), and the incorporation of precursor cells from remote locations into the heart. In addition to overturning the paradigm that the heart is a terminally differentiated organ, these observations introduced a new opportunity, of using cells as a therapeutic agent. In this regard, a large number of cell-based therapeutic approaches based upon both embryonic and adult stem cells are currently being evaluated at preclinical and early clinical stages, rendering a

Konstantinos E. Hatzistergos, PhD, Post-Doctoral Fellow, University of Miami, Miller School of Medicine, Interdisciplinary Stem Cell Institute, Miami, FL, USA.

Konstantinos Tziomalos, MD, PhD, Cardiovascular Division and Interdisciplinary Stem Cell Institute, University of Miami Miller School of Medicine, Miami, FL, USA.

Joshua M. Hare, MD, FACC, FAHA, Louis Lemberg Professor of Medicine, Director, Interdisciplinary Stem Cell Institute, University of Miami Miller School of Medicine, Miami, FL, USA.

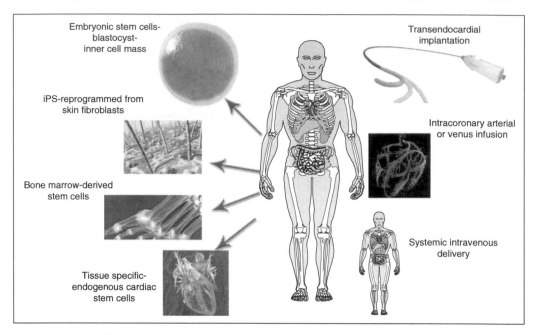

Figure 2.1 Stem cell based therapeutic strategies for cardiac regeneration. The sources for stem cells with cardiac reparative capacities are numerous, including embryonic, BM-derived, and cardiac specific-stem cells. After their expansion into therapeutic quantities, they can be transplanted into the patient using either direct transendocardial implantation, intracoronary infusions, or subcutaneous intravenous delivery.

number of considerations important to achieve a successful cell-based therapeutic. These include issues of stem cell plasticity, as well as practical factors such as dosage, timing and delivery method (Figure 2.1).

> *The goal of cellular cardiomyoplasty is to generate new functional cardiac muscle and vasculature. Can a myocardial scar be completely replaced from functional myocardium?*

CELLULAR CARDIOMYOPLASTY – THE MILESTONES

The idea of a cell-based therapeutic myocardial replacement began in 1993, when Koh and co-workers [3], based upon the premise that cardiomyocytes are terminally differentiated, used murine cardiomyocyte-like tumor cells to create intracardiac grafts. By genetically manipulating murine hearts to overexpress oncogenes such as the simian virus 40 large T antigen (T-Ag), the investigators created a tumorigenic cardiomyocyte cell line that could constantly proliferate *in vitro* and *in vivo*. Implantation of these cells into healthy mouse hearts was accompanied by long-term engraftment in ~50% of the recipients without affecting their heart function, introducing the notion of using cells to replace injured or lost cardiomyocytes. This experiment opened a new field of investigation that has led to the exploration of multiple types and sources of cells as a potential cardiac therapeutic agent. In 1998, Anversa [4] and co-workers reported evidence of mitosis in adult cardiomyocytes, suggesting cellular renewal throughout adult life. This discovery instigated the notion that myocyte renewal may not be attributed only to cardiomyocyte proliferation per se, but also to homing and

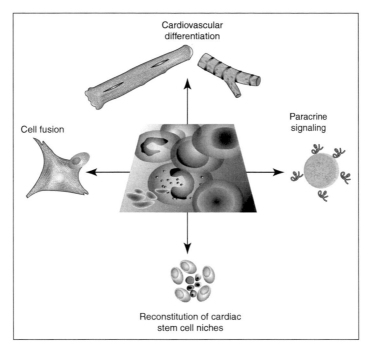

Cardiovascular
differentiation

Cell fusion

Paracrine
signaling

Reconstitution of cardiac
stem cell niches

Figure 2.2 Mechanisms of cardiac repair in cellular cardiomyoplasty. The transplanted grafts have the capacity for trilineage differentiation into cardiac myocytes, endothelial and vascular smooth muscle cells. Fusion with adjoining host cells and paracrine signaling are also critical and stimulate mechanisms for survival and proliferation of the host cells, as well as the mobilization of endogenous stem cells. An intriguing novel hypothesis is that of stem cell niches reconstitution following MSCs transplantation.

differentiation of endogenous stem cells. To address this idea, Orlic [5] and co-workers demonstrated that transplantation of bone marrow (BM) derived lineage-negative (Lin[-]/C-kit[+]) stem cells into the infarcted mouse heart caused differentiation of the BM cells into cardiac myocytes and vessels and substantial recovery of cardiac function.

Cardiac engraftment of cells from distant sites was demonstrated in 2002 by Quaini *et al.* [6] in studies of sex-mismatched heart transplants. In these studies, male cardiomyocytes were demonstrated in female hearts transplanted into male patients. More importantly, the investigators also detected a subpopulation of cardiac precursor cells of donor origin, suggesting for the first time that the heart could contain its own CSC population. These observations opened the field of adult stem cell based therapy and led to a plethora of studies utilizing multiple sources of cells to stimulate post injury cardiac repair. This quest, however, is not without controversy, and other experimental observations have challenged the hypothesis of cell trans-differentiation as a dominant mechanism of action for cell-based cardiac repair [7].

MECHANISMS OF ACTION

Currently there are several contemplated mechanisms of actions, each with varying degrees of experimental support (Figure 2.2). These include differentiation, paracrine signaling, fusion, and cell autonomous niche reconstitution [8]. *Ex vivo* culture of adult and embryonic stem cells (ESC) under specific conditions such as the hanging drop technique, stimulation by biochemical compounds, or co-culture with cardiac myocytes have demonstrated the capacity of stem cells to differentiate into beating cardiomyocytes and vascular lineages [9]. However, many experimental studies suggest that this mechanism is unlikely to account solely for the cardiac repair observed in response to cell-based therapy, since the therapeutic outcomes appear to be in excess of documented levels of cell engraftment and differentiation [10]. Whether the currently employed techniques (i.e. labeling of stem cells with reporter genes, magnetic particles, etc.) are sensitive enough to accurately trace the fate of the implanted cells throughout time is as yet uncertain. Nonetheless, the majority of these studies agree that the exogenously administered stem cells positively regulate the host's cardiac milieu; by fusing with native cells (a very low frequency event) or secreting several cytokines and growth factors, transplanted stem cells can promote angiogenesis and cell survival [11–13]. This concept is further advanced by the discovery of endogenous stem cells, found in cardiac niches. The presence of endogenous stem cells, suggests a broader cell autonomous mechanism of action for successful cell-based therapy [8, 14].

WHERE DO WE STAND NOW?

The field of stem cell research has gained enormous attention during the last decade, and experimental work has employed both embryonic and adult stem cells to treat heart disease. Studies of cardiac development have now discovered that morphogenesis of the mammalian embryonic heart relies strongly on direct differentiation of endogenous cardiac progenitors into cardiovascular elements [15–19]. At the same time, studies from lower vertebrates argue against a similar mechanism producing regeneration of an injured adult heart [20–22]. These studies highlight the common mechanisms between myocardial development and repair, and provide clues for advancing cell therapies in the future. In the clinical setting, while cell-based therapies for heart disease have already advanced substantially, the underlying mechanisms of action remain controversial. In addition to this central issue, other key issues that need to be settled include the role of host factors in cell functionality [23], and the exciting possibility of using allogeneic grafts, possible because of the unique immunoprivileged properties of some cell types.

CARDIOPOIETIC STEM CELLS

Embryonic Stem Cells (ESCs): Murine ESCs were first identified in 1981 by Evans and Kaufman [24] and Martin [25]. These cells arise from the inner cell mass of late mice blastocysts and because of the capacity to differentiate into cell types of all three germ layers including cardiomyocytes, represent a prototypic pluripotent cell. From a practical standpoint, ESCs, because they are pluripotent, have a high probability of causing teratogenicity. However, several groups have employed selective pre-differentiation strategies to enhance cardiopoiesis and reduce the risk of teratoma formation [26–28]. Animal studies suggest that these ESC-derived committed cells have the capacity to improve myocardial function and structure after MI through generation of new cardiomyocytes in the infarcted area. Recently, embryonic cell derived-endothelial cells were described that also improve myocardial contractility in mice following MI through stimulation of angiogenesis. As with cardiogenic cells, teratomas did not form after administration of these cells [29].

Another strategy to obtain pluripotent cells involves adult cell genetic reprogramming, so called induced Pluripotent Stem cells (iPS). In the two pioneering studies conducted by Yu *et al*. [30] and Takahashi *et al*. [31], adult human skin fibroblasts were reprogrammed into pluripotent embryonic-like stem cells, iPS by transfection with stem cell-related genes such as Lin28, c-myc, oct 4, sox 2, klf-4 and Nanog. Importantly, since viral transfection techniques and especially when combined with the induction of the oncogene c-myc into the host genome are accompanied with a high-risk for tumor development, virus-free iPS can be generated by using triplets of the above genes with or without using this specific oncogene [32].

This approach has stimulated enormous enthusiasm given the potential to develop pluripotent cells without using human embryos, offering substantial availability of the cells. Not the least of the advantages of this approach is the prospect of developing host-tailored stem cells that could escape immune rejection, or the development of pluripotent cell lines from hosts with genetic diseases providing an optimal *in vitro* experimental system. Recently, Ieda *et al.* [33] utilized this technology to reprogram murine cardiac fibroblasts into cardiomyocyte-like cells. This approach opens new avenues for regenerative cardiology and provides a valuable tool for further studies of cardiobiology. To date, EPS or iPS cells have not entered the clinic, although a trial for patients with spinal cord injury is reportedly to be initiated shortly [34].

Adult Stem Cells: The field of CSC therapy has been substantially advanced through the discovery that adult stem cells have the capacity to (trans)-differentiate into lineages other than the tissue of origin. This stem cell plasticity allows the use of stem cells isolated from a variety of easily accessible sources such as BM, peripheral blood, fat, umbilical cord or even testis, to be used for cell-based repair of damaged organs. To date, human trials have shown BM-derived mononuclear cells (BMMNCs) and mesenchymal stem cells (MSCs) as the most promising candidates for treating heart disease [35], while tissue-specific CSCs are currently entering trials an offer potential great promise (http://clinicaltrials.gov/ct2/show/NCT00474461).

I. **BM Stem Cells.** Because of its various well-defined stem cell compartments and its ease of access, whole BM and BMMNCs are to date the most widely studied type of cell for cellular cardiomyoplasty. Using different cell-surface markers BMMNCs can be fractionated to hematopoietic (HSCs) or non-hematopoietic stem cells. The latter includes a number of distinct subtypes named as side population (SPs) [36], endothelial progenitors (EPCs) [37], MSCs [38], multipotent adult progenitors (MAPCs) [39], multi-lineage inducible (MIAMI) [40] and Very Small Embryonic Like (VSEL) [41] stem cells.

BMMNCs: Numerous experimental and clinical studies have tested BMMNCs for a range of therapeutic strategies involving their transplantation and/or their mobilization to sites of cardiac injury. The totality of evidence of trials of BM cells and derivatives supports both the safety and provisional efficacy of this approach. Three meta-analyses evaluating data from approximately 18 trials and close to 1000 patients [2, 35, 42] conclude that BM cell-based therapies contribute to modest improvements in cardiac function by reducing infarct size, preserving left ventricular (LV) dimensions and increasing ejection fraction by 2–3% within 6 months after transplantation (Figure 2.3). Long-term follow up data derived from the BOne marrOw transfer to enhance ST-elevation infarct regeneration (BOOST) and TOPCARE-AMI studies have documented that the therapeutic results are sustained up to 5 years post-transplantation [43]. One of the most exciting observations derives from the Data Safety and Monitoring Board (DSMB) data of the Reinfusion of Enriched Progenitor Cells and Infarct Remodelling in Acute Myocardial Infarction (REPAIR-AMI) study [44]. In this study, 204 patients with AMI underwent successful reperfusion of the culprit coronary vessel(s), and 3–7 days later were randomized to receive intracoronary infusion of autologous BMMNCs or placebo. By 4 months patients who had received the cells showed a significantly improved left ventricular ejection fraction (LVEF) compared to the placebo, with the ones having larger infarcts (baseline LVEF < 48.9%) being more responsive to the therapy than the others. Importantly, 1 year follow up data from REPAIR-AMI demonstrates improved event free survival (death, recurrence of MI, revascularization, or re-hospitalization for HF) of the BMMNCs treated patients compared to the placebo (Figure 2.4). In addition to the post-MI setting, several trials have employed BMMNCs for patients with established LV dysfunction and/or HF due to either ischemic or non-ischemic causes; data are sufficiently promising to warrant further study. Based upon the totality of evidence, BMMNCs are poised to enter into pivotal clinical trials [2, 42].

Endothelial Progenitor Cells (EPC): This subset of HSCs can be isolated from BMMNC as well as peripheral blood mononuclear cells, based on the expression of HSC surface markers such as CD34, CD133 and the Vascular Endothelial Growth Factor receptor 2 (VEGF-R2 or kinase

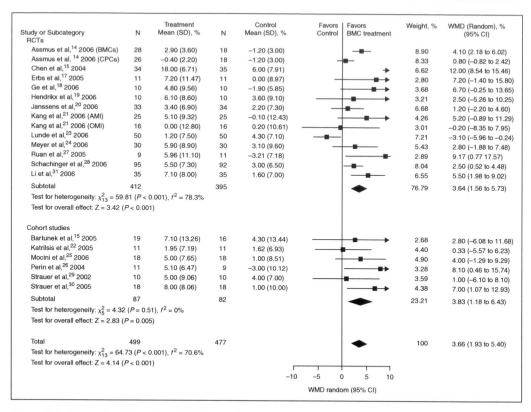

Figure 2.3 Forest plot of unadjusted difference in mean (with 95% confidence intervals [CIs]) improvement in left ventricular ejection fraction (LVEF) in patients treated with bone marrow-derived cells (BMCs) compared with controls (with permission from [2]).

insert domain-containing receptor [KDR]). The main mechanism of action of these cells is the formation of new vessels in the infarcted myocardium, however, little evidence exist for their *in vivo* trans-differentiation into new cardiac myocytes [10]. In rats with AMI, intravenously injected EPC stimulated development of collateral vessels from pre-existing vessels as well as de novo capillary formation [45]. This was associated with decreased apoptosis of myocytes in the borderline zone, reduced fibrosis and scar formation, resulting in prevention of LV remodeling and improvement in myocardial function [45]. It was also reported that infusion of EPC in the infarct-related arteries improves vasomotor function, an effect that could contribute to improved myocardial function [46]. In patients with old MI and chronic coronary total occlusion, intracoronary infusion of EPC after recanalization of the occluded artery improved myocardial perfusion, reduced infarct size and ameliorated myocardial function [47].

> *The decisions for commitment and self renewal of the cardiac stem cells are being taken within the cardiac stem cell niches. But CSC niches are being exhausted and replaced by scar following an MI. Is their reconstitution the missing link in cell-based cardiac repair?*

However, a clinical trial that was comparing the effects of granulocyte-colony stimulating factor (G-CSF) and peripheral blood mononuclear cells (PBMCs) as an alternative approach to

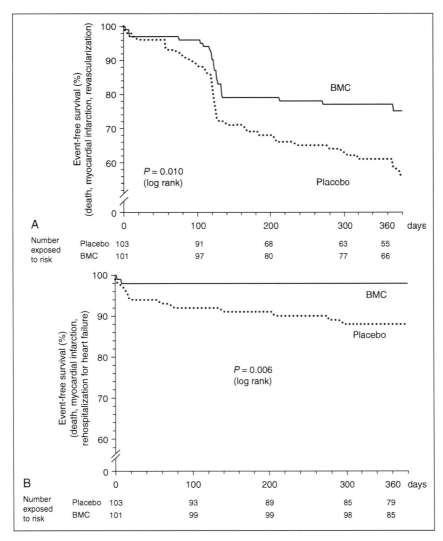

Figure 2.4 Kaplan Meier event free survival analysis of the REPAIR-AMI trial, illustrates that patients who had received BMMNCs had significantly reduced frequences of (A) death, myocardial infarction or revascularization (combined endpoints) and (B) death, myocardial infarction or re-hospitalization (combined endpoints), compared to the patients treated with placebo (with permission from Schachinger, V. *et al. Eur Heart J* 2006; 27:2775-2783; doi:10.1093/eurheartj/ehl388).

recruit EPCs at the sites of myocardial infarction was terminated prematurely due to potential adverse reaction of increased restenosis [48]. Lately, approaches that involve EPC therapies combined with gene therapies or even the genetic manipulation of EPCs before transplantation have been emerged in an attempt to minimize side-effects and improve outcome [49].

Mesenchymal Stem Cells: MSCs, an adult stem cell with self-replication and differentiation capacity, represent a promising adult stem cell for regenerative medicine. MSCs can be isolated from a variety of tissues such as adipose, umbilical cord/umbilical cord blood, and BM, although whether they all share common cardiopoietic and immunomodulatory properties is still not clear. MSCs lack hematopoietic lineage markers such as CD14, CD34 and

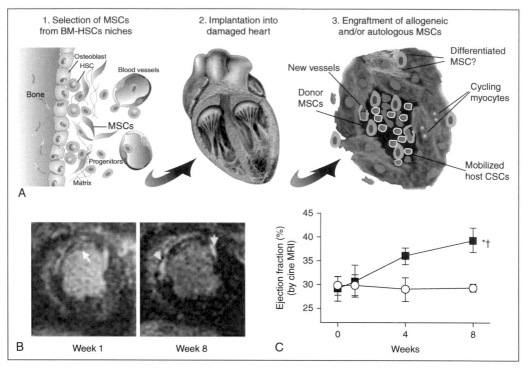

Figure 2.5 (A) MSCs can provide a safe allogeneic source for cell-based therapies. Their mechanisms of action are believed to be multifaceted since activation of innate (stimulation of angiogenesis, cardiomyocytes proliferation, CSCs mobilization) and exogenous (differentiation onto cardiovascular lineages) repair pathways have been reported. (B) Sophisticated multimodality imaging techniques have emerged during the past few years, in order to accurately and non-invasively monitor the effects of cell-based therapies in cardiac repair. Cardiac MRI and multidetector computed tomography (MDCT) document the development of a sub-endocardial rim following MSCs transplantation in the damaged zones of infarcted hearts. The newly formed tissue rendered a ~50% decrease in infarct size and restoration of the heart function (adapted with permission from [48, 49]).

CD45 and express specific stromal cell surface markers such as Stro1, CD105, CD90 and CD71. They adhere to plastic surfaces and grow as cell monolayers without losing their stem cell phenotype. Furthermore, they have reduced expression levels of MHC class-I molecule and absent major histocompatibility complex (MHC) class-II (although Interferon-γ will induce MHC Class II) and co-stimulatory molecules CD80 (B7-1), CD86 (B7-2), and CD40. MSCs are, therefore, the prototypic immunoprivileged cell-based therapy and have entered clinical trials as an allogeneic graft.

The mechanism of action of MSCs as a cardiac regenerative agent remains highly controversial. Lack of definite evidence of their *in vivo* trans-differentiation into cardiovascular elements has led to the conclusion that some of their secreted factors and cytokines evoke the therapeutic response, therefore arguing for the use of MSCs not as a therapeutic agent per se, but rather as a vehicle to deliver such biological molecules at the sites of injury. However, recent data document that MSCs facilitate cardiac regeneration through mechanisms that involve both differentiation and paracrine stimulation of innate repair pathways [8, 50, 51]. Importantly, MSCs also act in a cell-autonomous manner to enhance endogenous cardiac precursor recruitment, differentiation, and regeneration of damaged cardiac muscle [50]. An intriguing hypothesis is that this process employs mechanisms by which MSCs also regulate homeostasis in bone marrow and other niches [52].

In various animal models of AMI, intramyocardial injection of MSC reduced scar formation, attenuated LV remodeling and improved myocardial function (Figure 2.5). However, it should also be mentioned that some studies in mice with AMI failed to show a sustained benefit of MSC therapy despite an early benefit [53, 54]. In patients with AMI, intracoronary MSC infusion improved myocardial perfusion and function and reduced LV end-systolic and end-diastolic volumes [55]. In another small study, combined intracoronary administration of MSC and EPC improved perfusion and contractility of the infarcted area [56]. Even though early uncontrolled animal studies suggested that intracoronary injection of MSC could induce coronary artery occlusion and MI [57], this was not observed in humans [55]. In a rat model of dilated cardiomyopathy, intramyocardial injection of MSC exerted antifibrotic effects and improved myocardial perfusion and function [58]. A number of strategies have been developed in order to enhance the efficacy of MSC. Studies in animals showed that *ex vivo* modification of MSC resulting in over-expression of anti-apoptotic genes augments their regenerative potential [11]. MSC treatment appears to be safe [59–62]. Importantly, allogeneic MSC are not rejected [60, 63] suggesting that MSC may obviate the need for harvesting BM from patients [60]. Furthermore, EPC and BMMNC from patients with established coronary heart disease (CHD) or cardiovascular risk factors show impaired proliferating and migratory capacity [64, 65]. Therefore, treatment of patients with CHD with MSC obtained from healthy patients may be equally safe and more advantageous than using autologous MSC.

The most definitive clinical study of allogeneic MSCs was a 53 patient double-blind placebo-controlled trial of MSCs administered intravenously within 10 days after acute MI. This phase I study confirmed acute and long-term safety of the approach and provided provocative data supporting the conduct of additional phase II studies. Among the possible therapeutic effects of the approach are an increase in LVEF and a reduction in arrhythmic events in treated patients [63].

In conclusion, the mechanism of action of MSCs in cardiac repair remains highly controversial, with some arguing solely for a paracrine effect of these cells. Three proof of concept and one phase I clinical studies using BM-derived MSCs have been completed, illustrating that MSCs can be successfully used either as autologous or allogeneic graft for treating heart disease [55, 56, 63, 66]. While safety has served as the primary endpoint thus far, an overall provisional efficacy of MSCs on reversing heart disease has also been strongly suggested. All four studies recorded significant improvements in cardiac function accompanied by a substantial reduction in scar size whereas, in addition, 42% of the patients that were treated with an allogeneic 'off-the shelf' MSCs preparation showed improvement in their overall condition compared to an 11% of patients that had received the placebo and also improved [63]. Together these promising results have paved the way to a number of phase I/II clinical trials that have already received approvals worldwide and are poised towards efficacy as their primary endpoint (www.clinicaltrials.gov).

II. Myoblasts. Skeletal myoblasts were the first contractile cell type transplanted in the infarcted heart with the goal of restoring cardiac function [67]. These cells can be purified from the skeletal muscle of the patient and, after expansion into therapeutic quantities, can be transplanted into the myocardium. Transplantation of these cells to the heart is accomplished either surgically or by catheter delivery system [68]. There have been two large well-conducted phase I/II clinical studies [69]. The Myoblast Autologous Grafting in Ischemic Cardiomyopathy (MAGIC) trial revealed that there was a dose-dependent attenuation in LV remodeling that, however, was not accompanied by functional improvements in cardiac function (Figure 2.6). In addition, there are ongoing concerns that skeletal myoblast can precipitate arrhythmias [70].

In experimental models of AMI, intramyocardial injection of myoblasts preserves myocardial function and abrogated the remodeling process [71]. Myoblasts can differentiate into slow-twitch myotubes in the infarcted area, which can contribute to myocardial systole [71].

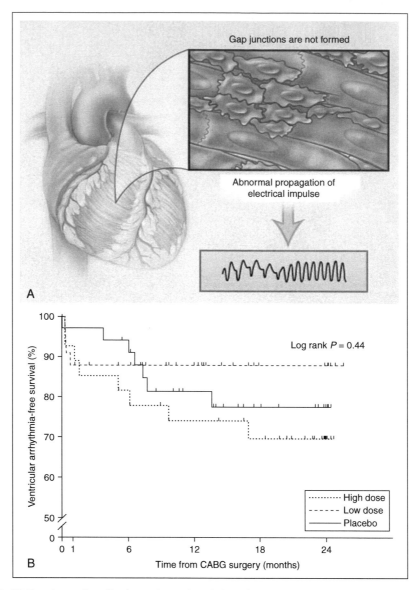

Figure 2.6 (A) Experimental studies have shown that skeletal fibroblasts engraft and survive in the damaged myocardium. However, these contractile cells do not express gap junctional proteins such as Connexin-43 and fail to couple with the host myocytes. As a result, the transplanted cells cannot propagate the conduction signals, giving rise to an arrhythmogenic substrate. (B) In the MAGIC trial, patients with ischemic cardiomyopathy who received skeletal myoblasts were more prone to develop arrhythmias compared to the placebo-treated group ((A) modified with permission from *N Engl J Med* 2008; 358:1397-1398 and (B) adapted with permission from *Circulation* 2008; 117:1189-1200. Epub 2008 Feb 19).

It has been suggested that skeletal muscle-derived stem cells have greater potential for myocyte regeneration than myoblasts and can additionally stimulate innate angiogenesis. This cell population appears to be more effective in improving myocardial perfusion and contractility and attenuating remodeling in animal models of MI [72]. The failure of myoblast

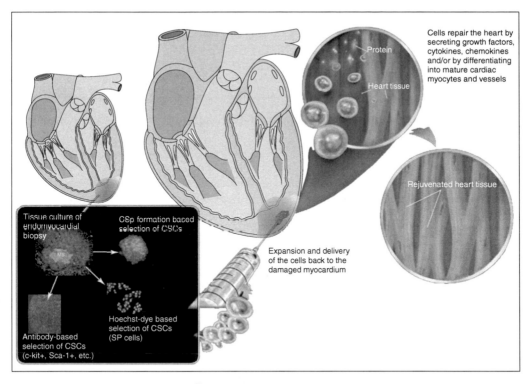

Figure 2.7 Cardiac stem cells represent a heterogenous population of myogenic and vasculogenic progenitor cells. They can be purified from the heart tissue based on the expression of surface molecules (such as c-kit, sca-1, abcg2 and MDR1), their ability to extrude Hoechst-dye or based on a novel identified property to develop cardiospheres. The exact differences and cardiopoietic potentials between these different CSCs populations is not fully understood (modified with permission from: *http://www.mirm.pitt.edu/news/article. asp?qEmpID=110*).

to improve cardiac function in humans has been attributed to their inability to differentiate into cardiac myocytes and the in-situ development of dysfunctional electrical coupling with resident cardiomyocytes (Figure 2.6) [73]. Recent studies are focused towards the identification and characterization of a more cardiogenic skeletal muscle-derived cell population that may improve cardiac repair [74].

III. Cardiac Stem Cells. CSCs are tissue-specific stem cells that reside within the heart itself (Figure 2.7). Cardiac progenitors were first reported in 2002, when Hierlihy *et al.* [75] detected robust SP cells in the post-natal murine heart that expressing the ATP-binding cassette transporter Abcg2 and extruded Hoechst dye. These cells represented ~ 1% of total cardiac cells and differentiated into cardiac myocytes *in vitro*. Following this observation, two different groups in 2003, Beltrami *et al.* [76] and Matsuura *et al.* [77], reported the isolation and characterization of two novel CSCs from the murine heart. These resident stem cells, have been reported to correspond from 0.01% to 2% (or ~1 CSC for every 13 000 cardiomyocytes) of the total cell population of the human heart and are mostly recognized according to the expression of three cell-surface markers: C-kit [the receptor for Stem Cell Factor (SCF)], MDR-1 (Multidrug Resistance protein-1) and/or Sca-1 (Stem cell antigen-1). CSCs are self-renewing, clonogenic, multipotent, and are able to differentiate both *in vitro* and *in vivo* into myogenic, endothelial, and vascular smooth muscle lineages. Two different methods for the isolation of human CSCs have been reported, but whether the purified cells share the same properties is yet unknown. The first method involves the homogenization of relatively large amount of cardiac tissue (~30–60 mg for successful isolation) and subsequent antibody-based selection of CSCs [78]. It is apparent that the applicability of this method is limited only into patients that undergo major cardiac interventions such as coronary artery bypass graft (CABG), left ventricular assist device (LVAD) placement or heart transplantation. The second method has been adapted from the field of neurological sciences and involves the culture of a single biopsy from which CSCs are selected with antibodies as a subpopulation of the outgrowing cells. Alternatively, the CSCs can be selected without the use of antibodies, based on their property to form cardiospheres [79]. The discovery of CSCs represents a major biological discovery furthering understanding of cardiac pathophysiology and facilitating cardiac cell-based therepeutics. Interestingly, in the post-natal senescent human heart CSCs are found to reside in structure with the properties of stem cell niches. These niches are structurally and functionally similar to stem cell niches found in highly regenerating tissues such as the BM, gut, and hair follicles. In cardiac niches, CSCs are regulated by the surrounding cellular and non-cellular constituents so as to maintain homeostasis of both the myocardium and the niche population throughout lifespan. CSCs undergo either symmetric (one CSC gives rise to two CSCs) or asymmetric division (one CSC gives rise to one CSC and one committed cell [i.e. cardiomyocyte precursor]).

Older patients or patients with a developed heart disease may also convey pathological stem cells. Can they all provide the appropriate cellular phenotype in therapeutic quantities or should we aim in the development of a healthy, universal graft?

Following myocardial damage, CSC niches are also damaged and replaced by scarred tissue thereby restricting the capacity of heart to heal itself [8]. Another important concept that arises from the description of CSC niches is that of host related dysfunction of CSCs and or niches due to comorbid diseases or aging [80].

C-kit+ CSCs: c-Kit CSCs represent a highly promising candidate for cardiac-specific stem cell lineages. This cell type is extensively described in multiple species ranging from rodents to large animals to humans, while representing—so far—the only known cell-surface marker with conserved expression between progenitore of pre- and post-natal origin [15, 50, 78]. Endogenous cardiac repair mechanisms involve the mobilization of c-kit+ CSCs to the areas of cardiac injury soon after infarction [81]. In addition, animal studies document how implantation of CSCs in rodent myocardium can reduce infarct size and improve cardiac function through their extensive differentiation into new cardiac muscle and vasculature [76]. Based on these findings c-kit+ CSCs are the first cardiac-specific stem cell population to be approved for human testing in a phase I clinical trial (http://www.clinicaltrials.gov, NCT00474461).

Other CSCs: Sca-1+ CSCs are an alternative adult CSCs. Evaluation of the corresponding human cell is limited by the absence of the Sca-1 antigen in humans [82]. The Islet-1+ CSCs have been isolated only from very young murine cardiac tissues that do not exceed 8 days of age [83], indicating that their presence is possibly ascribed as cell remnants from embryonic development. Therefore, our knowledge in their reparative capacities following cardiac injury is very limited, and more studies are needed in order to assess whether their use can comprise a good therapeutic strategy. Abcg2+ SPs are a well characterized cardiac precursor cell population in rodent hearts [75, 84]. However, although immunohistological studies have documented the existence of MDR1+ and Abcg2+ cells in the post-natal human heart [6, 85] the isolation and expansion of these cells into therapeutic quantities is yet to be reported.

Cardiosphere-forming Cells: There have been several attempts to culture cells from the adult heart. Messina and colleagues reported on 'cardiospheres', structures akin to 'neurospheres'. Cardiospheres are self-aggregating structures arising from cultured cardiac cells, and represent a heterogeneous population, possessing cardiopoietic properties *in vitro* and *in vivo* [86, 87]. Cardiospheres represent a potential advance because of their ability to expand potential cardiac precursor cells from smaller amounts of myocardial tissue, such as a cardiac biopsy. Cardiospheres are incompletely characterized and whether they offer superior regenerative capacities to BM-derived stem cells will require formal testing.

CONCLUSIONS

The prospective of using stem cells to alter the pathophysiology of the heart from a quiescent tissue into an organ with regenerative capacity is a very exciting but highly controversial hypothesis. Whether transplantation of cells with the ability to form new contractile cardiomyocytes and coronary vessels will ultimately lead to a powerful therapeutic strategy to restore a damaged heart's architecture and function is yet unknown. Our current experience has taught us that the use of animal models is an invaluable tool for studying and designing cell-based therapies to cure heart disease. We strongly advocate for rigorous clinical testing using trial designs that establish safety and provisional efficacy. To date, the totality of conducted studies, despite their limitations and variability, document that stem cell therapies are safe and can significantly improve heart function. The strategic design of highly organized multicenter studies is mandatory in order to harness all these confounding factors that could mislead our research in both experimental and clinical settings. In conclusion, stem cell research has significantly advanced our knowledge and understanding of biology. Indeed, the adult organism possesses regenerative pathways that throughout life balance events that destroy or damage organ function, thereby offering a homeostatic mechanism that maintains organ health. This clearly is a new insight with substantial clinical implications for the design of a new wave of therapies for chronic organ dysfunction.

REFERENCES

1. Mosterd A, Hoes AW. Clinical epidemiology of heart failure. *Heart* 2007; 93:1137-1146.
2. Abdel-Latif A, Bolli R, Tleyjeh IM *et al*. Adult bone marrow-derived cells for cardiac repair: a systematic review and meta-analysis. *Arch Intern Med* 2007; 167:989-997.
3. Koh GY, Soonpaa MH, Klug MG, Field LJ. Long-term survival of AT-1 cardiomyocyte grafts in syngeneic myocardium. *Am J Physiol* 1993; 264:H1727-H1733.
4. Anversa P, Kajstura J. Ventricular myocytes are not terminally differentiated in the adult mammalian heart. *Circ Res* 1998; 83:1-14.
5. Orlic D, Kajstura J, Chimenti S *et al*. Bone marrow cells regenerate infarcted myocardium. *Nature* 2001; 410:701-705.
6. Quaini F, Urbanek K, Beltrami AP *et al*. Chimerism of the transplanted heart. *N Engl J Med* 2002; 346:5-15.
7. Guan K, Hasenfuss G. Do stem cells in the heart truly differentiate into cardiomyocytes? *J Mol Cell Cardiol* 2007; 43:377-387.
8. Mazhari R, Hare JM. Mechanisms of action of mesenchymal stem cells in cardiac repair: potential influences on the cardiac stem cell niche. *Nat Clin Pract Cardiovasc Med* 2007; 4(suppl 1):S21-S26.
9. Christoforou N, Gearhart JD. Stem cells and their potential in cell-based cardiac therapies. *Prog Cardiovasc Dis* 2007; 49:396-413.
10. Segers VF, Lee RT. Stem-cell therapy for cardiac disease. *Nature* 2008; 451:937-942.
11. Mangi AA, Noiseux N, Kong D *et al*. Mesenchymal stem cells modified with Akt prevent remodeling and restore performance of infarcted hearts. *Nat Med* 2003; 9:1195-1201.
12. Nygren JM, Jovinge S, Breitbach M *et al*. Bone marrow-derived hematopoietic cells generate cardiomyocytes at a low frequency through cell fusion, but not transdifferentiation. *Nat Med* 2004; 10:494-501.

13. Mirotsou M, Zhang Z, Deb A et al. Secreted frizzled related protein 2 (Sfrp2) is the key Akt-mesenchymal stem cell-released paracrine factor mediating myocardial survival and repair. *Proc Natl Acad Sci USA* 2007; 104:1643-1648.

14. Nakanishi C, Yamagishi M, Yamahara K et al. Activation of cardiac progenitor cells through paracrine effects of mesenchymal stem cells. *Biochem Biophys Res Commun* 2008; 374:11-16.

15. Wu SM, Fujiwara Y, Cibulsky SM et al. Developmental origin of a bipotential myocardial and smooth muscle cell precursor in the mammalian heart. *Cell* 2006; 127:1137-1150.

16. Cai CL, Martin JC, Sun Y et al. A myocardial lineage derives from Tbx18 epicardial cells. *Nature* 2008; 454:104-108.

17. Laugwitz KL, Moretti A, Lam J et al. Postnatal isl1+ cardioblasts enter fully differentiated cardiomyocyte lineages. *Nature* 2005; 433:647-653.

18. Cai CL, Liang X, Shi Y et al. Isl1 identifies a cardiac progenitor population that proliferates prior to differentiation and contributes a majority of cells to the heart. *Dev Cell* 2003; 5:877-889.

19. Zhou B, Ma Q, Rajagopal S et al. Epicardial progenitors contribute to the cardiomyocyte lineage in the developing heart. *Nature* 2008; 454:109-113.

20. Kikuchi K, Holdway JE, Werdich AA et al. Primary contribution to zebrafish heart regeneration by gata4(+) cardiomyocytes. *Nature* 2010; 464:601-605.

21. Jopling C, Sleep E, Raya M, Marti M, Raya A, Belmonte JC. Zebrafish heart regeneration occurs by cardiomyocyte dedifferentiation and proliferation. *Nature* 2010; 464:606-609.

22. Lepilina A, Coon AN, Kikuchi K et al. A dynamic epicardial injury response supports progenitor cell activity during zebrafish heart regeneration. *Cell* 2006; 127:607-619.

23. Kissel CK, Lehmann R, Assmus B et al. Selective functional exhaustion of hematopoietic progenitor cells in the bone marrow of patients with postinfarction heart failure. *J Am Coll Cardiol* 2007; 49:2341-2349.

24. Evans MJ, Kaufman MH. Establishment in culture of pluripotential cells from mouse embryos. *Nature* 1981; 292:154-156.

25. Martin GR. Isolation of a pluripotent cell line from early mouse embryos cultured in medium conditioned by teratocarcinoma stem cells. *Proc Natl Acad Sci USA* 1981; 78:7634-7638.

26. Behfar A, Perez-Terzic C, Faustino RS et al. Cardiopoietic programming of embryonic stem cells for tumor-free heart repair. *J Exp Med* 2007; 204:405-420.

27. Caspi O, Huber I, Kehat I et al. Transplantation of human embryonic stem cell-derived cardiomyocytes improves myocardial performance in infarcted rat hearts. *J Am Coll Cardiol* 2007; 50:1884-1893.

28. Christoforou N, Miller RA, Hill CM, Jie CC, McCallion AS, Gearhart JD. Mouse ES cell-derived cardiac precursor cells are multipotent and facilitate identification of novel cardiac genes. *J Clin Invest* 2008.

29. Li Z, Wu JC, Sheikh AY et al. Differentiation, survival, and function of embryonic stem cell derived endothelial cells for ischemic heart disease. *Circulation* 2007; 116(1 suppl):I46-I54.

30. Yu J, Vodyanik MA, Smuga-Otto K et al. Induced pluripotent stem cell lines derived from human somatic cells. *Science* 2007; 318:1917-1920.

31. Takahashi K, Tanabe K, Ohnuki M et al. Induction of pluripotent stem cells from adult human fibroblasts by defined factors. *Cell* 2007; 131:861-872.

32. Okita K, Nakagawa M, Hyenjong H, Ichisaka T, Yamanaka S. Generation of mouse induced pluripotent stem cells without viral vectors. *Science* 2008; 322:949-953.

33. Ieda M, Fu JD, gado-Olguin P et al. Direct reprogramming of fibroblasts into functional cardiomyocytes by defined factors. *Cell* 2010; 142:375-386.

34. Cyranoski D. Stem cells: 5 things to know before jumping on the iPS bandwagon. *Nature* 2008; 452:406-408.

35. Burt RK, Loh Y, Pearce W et al. Clinical applications of blood-derived and marrow-derived stem cells for nonmalignant diseases. *JAMA* 2008; 299:925-936.

36. Jackson KA, Majka SM, Wang H et al. Regeneration of ischemic cardiac muscle and vascular endothelium by adult stem cells. *J Clin Invest* 2001; 107:1395-1402.

37. Asahara T, Murohara T, Sullivan A et al. Isolation of putative progenitor endothelial cells for angiogenesis. *Science* 1997; 275:964-967.

38. Zimmet JM, Hare JM. Emerging role for bone marrow derived mesenchymal stem cells in myocardial regenerative therapy. *Basic Res Cardiol* 2005; 100:471-481.

39. Jiang Y, Jahagirdar BN, Reinhardt RL et al. Pluripotency of mesenchymal stem cells derived from adult marrow. *Nature* 2002; 418:41-49.

40. D'Ippolito G, Howard GA, Roos BA, Schiller PC. Isolation and characterization of marrow-isolated adult multilineage inducible (MIAMI) cells. *Exp Hematol* 2006; 34:1608-1610.
41. Kucia M, Reca R, Campbell FR *et al*. A population of very small embryonic-like (VSEL) CXCR4(+) SSEA-1(+)Oct-4+ stem cells identified in adult bone marrow. *Leukemia* 2006; 20:857-869.
42. Martin-Rendon E, Brunskill SJ, Hyde CJ, Stanworth SJ, Mathur A, Watt SM. Autologous bone marrow stem cells to treat acute myocardial infarction: a systematic review. *Eur Heart J* 2008; 29:1807-1818. Epub 2008 Jun 3.
43. Dimmeler S, Burchfield J, Zeiher AM. Cell-based therapy of myocardial infarction. *Arterioscler Thromb Vasc Biol* 2008; 28:208-216.
44. Schachinger V, Erbs S, Elsasser A *et al*. Intracoronary bone marrow-derived progenitor cells in acute myocardial infarction. *N Engl J Med* 2006; 355:1210-1221.
45. Kocher AA, Schuster MD, Szabolcs MJ *et al*. Neovascularization of ischemic myocardium by human bone-marrow-derived angioblasts prevents cardiomyocyte apoptosis, reduces remodeling and improves cardiac function. *Nat Med* 2001; 7:430-436.
46. Erbs S, Linke A, Schachinger V *et al*. Restoration of microvascular function in the infarct-related artery by intracoronary transplantation of bone marrow progenitor cells in patients with acute myocardial infarction: the Doppler Substudy of the Reinfusion of Enriched Progenitor Cells and Infarct Remodeling in Acute Myocardial Infarction (REPAIR-AMI) trial. *Circulation* 2007; 116:366-374.
47. Erbs S, Linke A, Adams V *et al*. Transplantation of blood-derived progenitor cells after recanalization of chronic coronary artery occlusion: first randomized and placebo-controlled study. *Circ Res* 2005; 97:756-762.
48. Kang HJ, Kim HS, Zhang SY *et al*. Effects of intracoronary infusion of peripheral blood stem-cells mobilised with granulocyte-colony stimulating factor on left ventricular systolic function and restenosis after coronary stenting in myocardial infarction: the MAGIC cell randomised clinical trial. *Lancet* 2004; 363:751-756.
49. Roncalli J, Tongers J, Renault MA, Losordo DW. Biological approaches to ischemic tissue repair: gene- and cell-based strategies. *Expert Rev Cardiovasc Ther* 2008; 6:653-668.
50. Hatzistergos KE, Quevedo H, Oskouei BN *et al*. Bone Marrow Mesenchymal Stem Cells Stimulate Cardiac Stem Cell Proliferation and Differentiation. *Circ Res* 2010; Jul 29.
51. Quevedo HC, Hatzistergos KE, Oskouei BN *et al*. Allogeneic mesenchymal stem cells restore cardiac function in chronic ischemic cardiomyopathy via trilineage differentiating capacity. *Proc Natl Acad Sci USA* 2009; 106:14022-14027.
52. Mendez-Ferrer S, Michurina TV, Ferraro F *et al*. Mesenchymal and haematopoietic stem cells form a unique bone marrow niche. *Nature* 2010; 466:829-834.
53. Dai W, Hale SL, Martin BJ *et al*. Allogeneic mesenchymal stem cell transplantation in postinfarcted rat myocardium: short- and long-term effects. *Circulation* 2005; 112:214-223.
54. Meyer GP, Wollert KC, Lotz J *et al*. Intracoronary bone marrow cell transfer after myocardial infarction: eighteen months' follow-up data from the randomized, controlled BOOST (BOne marrOw transfer to enhance ST-elevation infarct regeneration) trial. *Circulation* 2006; 113:1287-1294.
55. Chen SL, Fang WW, Ye F *et al*. Effect on left ventricular function of intracoronary transplantation of autologous bone marrow mesenchymal stem cell in patients with acute myocardial infarction. *Am J Cardiol* 2004; 94:92-95.
56. Katritsis DG, Sotiropoulou PA, Karvouni E *et al*. Transcoronary transplantation of autologous mesenchymal stem cells and endothelial progenitors into infarcted human myocardium. *Catheter Cardiovasc Interv* 2005; 65:321-329.
57. Vulliet PR, Greeley M, Halloran SM, MacDonald KA, Kittleson MD. Intra-coronary arterial injection of mesenchymal stromal cells and microinfarction in dogs. *Lancet* 2004; 363:783-784.
58. Nagaya N, Kangawa K, Itoh T *et al*. Transplantation of mesenchymal stem cells improves cardiac function in a rat model of dilated cardiomyopathy. *Circulation* 2005; 112:1128-1135.
59. Lim SY, Kim YS, Ahn Y *et al*. The effects of mesenchymal stem cells transduced with Akt in a porcine myocardial infarction model. *Cardiovasc Res* 2006; 70:530-542.
60. Amado LC, Saliaris AP, Schuleri KH *et al*. Cardiac repair with intramyocardial injection of allogeneic mesenchymal stem cells after myocardial infarction. *Proc Natl Acad Sci USA* 2005; 102:11474-11479.
61. Amado LC, Schuleri KH, Saliaris AP *et al*. Multimodality noninvasive imaging demonstrates in vivo cardiac regeneration after mesenchymal stem cell therapy. *J Am Coll Cardiol* 2006; 48:2116-2124.
62. Hu X, Wang J, Chen J *et al*. Optimal temporal delivery of bone marrow mesenchymal stem cells in rats with myocardial infarction. *Eur J Cardiothorac Surg* 2007; 31:438-443.

63. Hare JM, Traverse JH, Henry TD *et al*. A randomized, double-blind, placebo-controlled, dose-escalation study of intravenous adult human mesenchymal stem cells (prochymal) after acute myocardial infarction. *J Am Coll Cardiol* 2009; 54:2277-2286.

64. Heeschen C, Lehmann R, Honold J *et al*. Profoundly reduced neovascularization capacity of bone marrow mononuclear cells derived from patients with chronic ischemic heart disease. *Circulation* 2004; 109:1615-1622.

65. Vasa M, Fichtlscherer S, Aicher A *et al*. Number and migratory activity of circulating endothelial progenitor cells inversely correlate with risk factors for coronary artery disease. *Circ Res* 2001; 89:E1-E7.

66. Chen S, Liu Z, Tian N *et al*. Intracoronary transplantation of autologous bone marrow mesenchymal stem cells for ischemic cardiomyopathy due to isolated chronic occluded left anterior descending artery. *J Invasive Cardiol* 2006; 18:552-556.

67. Yoon PD, Kao RL, Magovern GJ. Myocardial regeneration. Transplanting satellite cells into damaged myocardium. *Tex Heart Inst J* 1995; 22:119-125.

68. Heldman AW, Hare JM. Cell therapy for myocardial infarction: Special delivery. *J Mol Cell Cardiol* 2008; 44:473-476. Epub 2007 Dec 4.

69. Menasche P. Skeletal myoblasts for cardiac repair: Act II? *J Am Coll Cardiol* 2008; 52:1881-1883.

70. Menasche P, Alfieri O, Janssens S *et al*. The Myoblast Autologous Grafting in Ischemic Cardiomyopathy (MAGIC) trial: first randomized placebo-controlled study of myoblast transplantation. *Circulation* 2008; 117:1189-1200.

71. Ghostine S, Carrion C, Souza LC *et al*. Long-term efficacy of myoblast transplantation on regional structure and function after myocardial infarction. *Circulation* 2002; 106(suppl 1):I131-I136.

72. Oshima H, Payne TR, Urish KL *et al*. Differential myocardial infarct repair with muscle stem cells compared to myoblasts. *Mol Ther* 2005; 12:1130-1141.

73. Reinecke H, Poppa V, Murry CE. Skeletal muscle stem cells do not transdifferentiate into cardiomyocytes after cardiac grafting. *J Mol Cell Cardiol* 2002; 34:241-249.

74. Okada M, Payne TR, Zheng B *et al*. Myogenic endothelial cells purified from human skeletal muscle improve cardiac function after transplantation into infarcted myocardium. *J Am Coll Cardiol* 2008; 52:1869-1880.

75. Hierlihy AM, Seale P, Lobe CG, Rudnicki MA, Megeney LA. The post-natal heart contains a myocardial stem cell population. *FEBS Lett* 2002; 530:239-243.

76. Beltrami AP, Barlucchi L, Torella D *et al*. Adult cardiac stem cells are multipotent and support myocardial regeneration. *Cell* 2003; 114:763-776.

77. Matsuura K, Nagai T, Nishigaki N *et al*. Adult cardiac Sca-1-positive cells differentiate into beating cardiomyocytes. *J Biol Chem* 2004; 279:11384-11391.

78. Bearzi C, Rota M, Hosoda T *et al*. Human cardiac stem cells. *Proc Natl Acad Sci USA* 2007; 104:14068-14073.

79. Messina E, De AL, Frati G *et al*. Isolation and expansion of adult cardiac stem cells from human and murine heart. *Circ Res* 2004; 95:911-921.

80. Anversa P, Kajstura J, Leri A, Bolli R. Life and death of cardiac stem cells: a paradigm shift in cardiac biology. *Circulation* 2006; 113:1451-1463.

81. Fransioli J, Bailey B, Gude NA *et al*. Evolution of the c-kit-positive cell response to pathological challenge in the myocardium. *Stem Cells* 2008; 26:1315-1324.

82. Holmes C, Stanford WL. Concise review: stem cell antigen-1: expression, function, and enigma. *Stem Cells* 2007; 25:1339-1347.

83. Barile L, Messina E, Giacomello A, Marban E. Endogenous cardiac stem cells. *Prog Cardiovasc Dis* 2007; 50:31-48.

84. Pfister O, Oikonomopoulos A, Sereti KI *et al*. Role of the ATP-binding cassette transporter Abcg2 in the phenotype and function of cardiac side population cells. *Circ Res* 2008; 103:825-835.

85. Meissner K, Heydrich B, Jedlitschky G *et al*. The ATP-binding cassette transporter ABCG2 (BCRP), a marker for side population stem cells, is expressed in human heart. *J Histochem Cytochem* 2006; 54:215-221.

86. Smith RR, Barile L, Cho HC *et al*. Regenerative potential of cardiosphere-derived cells expanded from percutaneous endomyocardial biopsy specimens. *Circulation* 2007; 115:896-908.

87. Takehara N, Tsutsumi Y, Tateishi K *et al*. Controlled delivery of basic fibroblast growth factor promotes human cardiosphere-derived cell engraftment to enhance cardiac repair for chronic myocardial infarction. *J Am Coll Cardiol* 2008; 52:1858-1865.

3

Pulmonary hypertension and right heart failure: light at the end of the tunnel?

M. H. Park

INTRODUCTION

Pulmonary hypertension was first described by Romberg as 'sclerosis of the pulmonary arteries' more than 100 years ago [1]. The term primary pulmonary hypertension (PPH) was coined by Dresdale and colleagues in 1951, describing a hypertensive condition of the pulmonary vasculature [2]. Until recently, pulmonary hypertension (PH) was considered a uniformly fatal disease without effective treatment. Now termed pulmonary arterial hypertension (PAH), intense research leading to advances in understanding during the past two decades have resulted in eight Food and Drug Administration (FDA) approved therapies that have vastly improved outcome.

PATHOBIOLOGY OF PAH

PAH is defined as resting mean pulmonary arterial pressure (mPAP) > 25 mmHg and pulmonary capillary wedge pressure (PCWP) < 15 mmHg. Some definitions have also included pulmonary vascular resistance (PVR) to be elevated ≥ 2 or 3 Wood units. It is a life-threatening disease characterized by vasoconstriction, remodeling and thrombosis of pulmonary arteries, leading to progressive increase in pulmonary artery pressure (PAP) and PVR resulting in right ventricular failure and death. It is now recognized that pulmonary arterial obstruction due to vascular proliferation and remodeling is the key process of PAH pathogenesis [4]. Histological studies have shown that pulmonary vascular remodeling involves all layers of the vessel wall, characterized by intimal hyperplasia and medial hypertrophy, adventitial proliferation, formation of plexiform lesions and thrombosis *in situ*. The process by which the disease is initiated and propagated is complex and heterogeneous. Recent advances in understanding the cellular, molecular and genetic mechanisms in PAH have evolved a concept of 'multiple-hit hypothesis', which states that the disease is a result of interaction of a predisposing state and one or more stimuli [5]. Two or more 'hits' is thought to consist of a genetic abnormality or substrate, rendering an individual as susceptible. The second 'hit' may be either a systemic disorder (i.e. collagen vascular disease, human immunodeficiency virus [HIV]), an environmental trigger (i.e. hypoxia, anorexigen), or additional genetic conditions (i.e. mutation, polymorphism). Several key studies have demonstrated the importance of genetic substrate abnormalities associated with PAH, notably the mutations involving the bone morphogenetic protein receptor II

Myung H. Park, MD, FACC, Associate Professor of Medicine, Director, Pulmonary Vascular Disease Program, Division of Cardiology, University of Maryland School of Medicine, Baltimore, MD, USA.

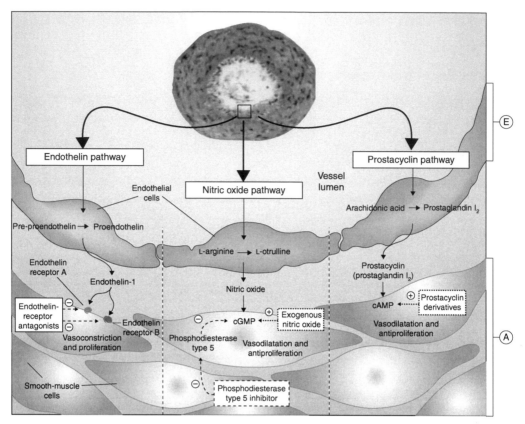

Figure 3.1 Targeting for Current of Emerging Therapies in Pulmonary Arterial Hypertension. Three major pathways involved in abnormal proliferation and contraction of the smooth muscle cells of the pulmonary artery in patients with pulmonary artery hypertension are shown. These pathways correspond to important therapeutic targets in this condition and play a role in determining which of four classes of drugs – endothelin-receptor antagonists, nitric oxide, phosphodiesterase type 5 inhibitors, and prostaglandin derivatives – will be used. At the top of the figure, a transverse section of a small pulmonary artery (<500 µm in diameter) from a patient with severe pulmonary arterial hypertension shows intimal proliferation and marked medial hypertrophy. Dysfunctional pulmonary artery endothelial cells (E) have decreased production of prostacyclin and endogenous nitric oxide, with an increased production of endothelin-1 – a condition promoting vasoconstriction and proliferation of smooth muscle cells in the pulmonary arteries (A). Current or emerging therapies interfere with specific targets in smooth muscle cells in the pulmonary arteries. In addition to their actions on smooth muscle cells, prostacyclin derivatives and nitric oxide have several other properties, including antiplatelet effects. Plus signs denote an increase in the intracellular concentration; minus signs blockage of a receptor, inhibition of an enzyme, or a decrease in the intracellular contraction; and cGMP (with permission from [8]).

(BMPR2) which promotes cellular proliferation of the pulmonary vascular smooth muscle cells [6, 7].

The endothelial injury resulting from above processes leads to an imbalance among the key neurohormonal mediators. The pulmonary artery endothelium tightly regulates the production of vasodilators (prostacyclin, nitric oxide (NO), vasoactive intestinal peptide) and vasoconstrictors (endothelin-1, thromboxane and serotonin) to maintain a low-pressured state. In PAH, an imbalance of the mediators occurs with overproduction of vasoconstricting agents and decreased level of vasodilators [8] (Figure 3.1).

Prostacyclin (prostaglandin I_2) is a metabolite of arachidonic acid, produced by both endothelial and smooth muscle cells in the vasculature. It is a potent pulmonary vasodilator acting through activation of the cyclic adenosine monophosphate (cAMP) pathway; it also strongly inhibits platelet aggregation and smooth muscle cell proliferation. Studies have demonstrated decreased production of this key mediator in patients with PAH compared with control subjects [9].

Reduction of NO synthase expression has also been demonstrated in pulmonary endothelial cells from PAH patients [10]. NO is a potent selective pulmonary vasodilator, exerting its effects through its second messenger, cyclic guanosine monophosphate (cGMP), which is degraded by phosphodiesterase (PDE). Sildenafil acts by selectively inhibiting this enzyme, promoting the accumulation of intracellular cGMP and thereby enhancing NO mediated effects [11].

Endothelin-1, a 21-amino peptide predominantly produced by endothelial cells, is a potent vasoconstrictor and a smooth muscle cell mitogen [12]. ET-1 exerts its vascular effects through activation of ET_A (located on smooth muscle cells) and ET_B receptors (located on vascular endothelial cells and smooth muscle cells). Activation of the ET_A and ET_B receptors on smooth muscle cells induces vasoconstriction and cellular proliferation and hypertrophy, whereas stimulation of ET_B receptors on endothelial cells results in production of vasodilators. ET_B receptors are also involved in the clearance of ET-1 from the circulatory system [13]. In PAH patients, plasma levels of ET-1 is increased and its level has been shown to be inversely proportional to the magnitude of the pulmonary blood flow and cardiac output [14, 15].

CLASSIFICATION AND EPIDEMIOLOGY OF PH

PH has undergone several revisions in nomenclature as well as classification scheme, reflecting advances in understanding the disease. The term PPH was replaced by idiopathic PAH (IPAH) at the Third World Symposium on Pulmonary Hypertension in 2003; furthermore, several associated conditions affecting pulmonary vascular system have been placed under PAH, recognizing that certain types of PH can be grouped together based on similar pathogenesis and responses to therapy. PH is classified into five groups with PAH designated as Group I. All the randomized clinical trials resulting in approval of eight currently available PAH therapies have been done exclusively in Group I patients which include IPAH, heritable PAH (HPAH), and PAH associated with certain systemic disorders associated with increased incidence of PAH [16] (Table 3.1).

The first comprehensive study on epidemiology and survival of PAH by the PPH Registry Group in 1987 reported that IPAH is a rare disease with an annual incidence of approximately 2 to 5 per million persons in U.S., predominantly affecting young females (female:male ratio 1.7:1; mean age 37 years) [17]. More recent epidemiologic studies show that the prevalence may be higher, up to 15 per million, and that a trend for older age range of patients being diagnosed is increasing (patients >70 years of age) [18]. Although incidence of IPAH is rare, PAH has been associated with increased incidence in patients with certain systemic disorders such as connective tissue disease (CTD), human immunodeficiency virus (HIV) and advanced liver disease. Patients with CTD comprise the largest subgroup of population affected, with rates of isolated PAH highest in patients with limited scleroderma including those with CREST (calcinosis, Raynaud's phenomenon, espophageal dysmotility, sclerodactyly, telangiectasis) syndrome [19, 20]. Patients with other CTDs including lupus, rheumatoid arthritis and mixed CTD are at increased risk as well. Patients with PAH associated with CTD have poorer survival than IPAH patients; median survival of 12 months have been reported compared to 2.6 years in IPAH patients [17, 21]. A more concerning factor is that current therapies are less effective in CTD patients compared with IPAH patients [22]. Survival in PAH has been shown to differ based on etiology of disease; patients with

Table 3.1 CLinical Classification of Pulmonary Hypertension (World Symposium, Dana Point, 2008) (with permission from [16])

1. Pulmonary arterial hypertension (PAH)
   1.1. Idiopathic PAH
   1.2. Heritable
      1.2.1. BMPR2
      1.2.2. ALK1, endoglin (with or without hereditary hemorrhagic telangiectasia)
      1.2.3. Unknown
   1.3. Drug- and toxin-induced
   1.4. Associated with
      1.4.1. Connective tissue diseases
      1.4.2. HIV infection
      1.4.3. Portal hypertension
      1.4.4. Congenital heart diseases
      1.4.5. Schistosomiasis
      1.4.6. Chronic hemolytic anemia
   1.5　Persistent pulmonary hypertension of the newborn
1′ Pulmonary veno-occlusive disease (PVOD) and/or pulmonary capillary hemangiomatosis (PCH)
2. Pulmonary hypertension owing to left heart disease
   2.1. Systolic dysfunction
   2.2. Diastolic dysfunction
   2.3. Valvular disease
3. Pulmonary hypertension owing to lung diseases and/or hypoxia
   3.1. Chronic obstructive pulmonary disease
   3.2. Interstitial lung disease
   3.3. Other pulmonary diseases with mixed restrictive and obstructive pattern
   3.4. Sleep-disordered breathing
   3.5. Alveolar hypoventilation disorders
   3.6. Chronic exposure to high altitude
   3.7. Developmental abnormalities
4. Chronic thrombo-embolic pulmonary hypertension (CTEPH))
5. Pulmonary hypertension with unclear multifactorial mechanisms
   5.1. Hematologic disorders: myeloproliferative disorders, splenectomy
   5.2. Systemic disorders: sarcoidosis, pulmonary Langerhans cell histiocytosis: lymphangioleiomyomatosis, neurofibromatosis, vasculitis
   5.3. Metabolic disorders: glycogen storage disease, Gaucher disease, thyroid disorders
   5.4. Others: tumoral obstruction, fibrosing mediastinitis, chronic renal failure on dialysis

ALK1=activin receptor-like kinase type 1; BMPR2=bone morphogenetic protein receptor type 2; HIV=human immunodeficiency virus.

congenital heart disease has the most favorable outcome and those with CTD and HIV have the worst [23] (Figure 3.2).

DIAGNOSIS AND RISK ASSESSMENT OF PAH

Evaluation for PAH encompasses four specific objectives. One is to recognize patients who are at high risk for PAH due to their associated medical conditions and genetic susceptibilities and perform screening evaluations. The second task is to have a high index of suspicion of PAH in appropriate patients to initiate diagnostic evaluation. The next steps are to determine the etiology of PH and then confirm the diagnosis with right heart catheterization.

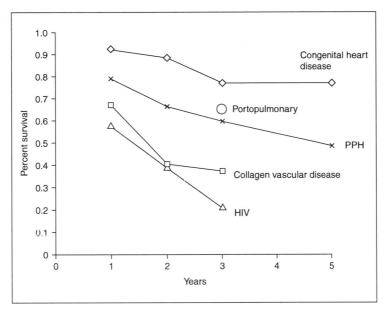

Figure 3.2 Survival with different etiologies of PAH (with permission from [23]).

SCREENING HIGH RISK POPULATION FOR PAH

High risk population for PAH include those with genetic mutation (BMPR2) or first degree relatives of patient with known mutation with HPAH. Hereditary transmission of PAH has been reported in approximately 6–10% of PAH patients where in 50–90%, BMPR2 mutations have been identified [6, 7, 24, 25]. Other groups include patients with scleroderma spectrum of diseases, patients with portal hypertension being evaluated for liver transplantation and patients with congenital heart disease with systemic-to-pulmonary shunts [19, 26–30] (Table 3.2).

STARTING EVALUATION FOR PAH

Diagnosing PAH can be challenging due to the nonspecific nature of the presenting symptoms, relative rarity of the disease and the fact that routine tests are not adequate to make the diagnosis. In the National Institutes of Health (NIH) Registry of 187 IPAH patients, the most common presenting symptoms were dyspnea followed by fatigue, chest pain, edema, presyncope or syncope [17]. Physical examination can indicate presence of PH or right ventricular (RV) failure (Table 3.3). Chest radiography findings indicative of PH include prominent hilar pulmonary arteries, peripheral hypovascularity (pruning), and RV enlargement in retrosternal space. Electrocardiogram is neither sensitive nor specific for PH; changes consistent with PH are right axis deviation, right atrial enlargement, and RV hypertrophy [30, 31].

Transthoracic Doppler echocardiography is the test of choice for screening patients suspected of PAH to obtain an estimated assessment on PAPs. Utilizing the modified Bernoulli equation $4v^2$, in which v is the velocity of the tricuspid regurgitation (TR) jet in meters per second, right ventricular systolic pressure (RVSP) is derived by adding the right atrial pressure (RAP) to the gradient (RVSP = $4v^2$ + RAP). The RAP is either a standardized value or

Table 3.2 Patient groups at high risk of PAH recommended screening with echocardiography

Patient groups	Comments
Known genetic mutations predisposing to pulmonary hypertension	BMPR2 mutation identified as the main cause of inherited PAH Accounts for at least 60% of familial cases [6, 7]
First degree relatives in a familial PAH family	Inherited as autosomal dominant trait Characterized by genetic anticipation and incomplete penetrance Phenotype may not be expressed in all generations but when expressed, it occurs at an earlier age and associated with more severe disease [24, 25]
Patients with scleroderma	Incidence of PAH up to 30% Response to approved therapy not as favorable compared with IPAH Early detection and diagnosis imperative [19–23]
Patients with portal hypertension prior to liver transplantation	Rates of PAH 1–6% Increased PAP associated with significant risk of perioperative mortality and contraindication to transplantation [26,27]
Patients with congenital systemic to pulmonary shunts	Overall have better prognosis compared with other subgroups Once cardiac dysfunction develops, prognosis guarded [28,29]

an estimated value based on the echocardiographic characteristics of the inferior vena cava, or the vertical height of the jugular venous pulse on physical examination [32]. Many studies have assessed the correlation coefficients between RVSP derived from TR jet and hemodynamics from right heart catheterizations with marked variations in results from poor to significant correlations [33–35]. Several factors attribute to the varying results: TR jets are analyzable in 39% to 86% of patients; patients with co-morbidities (obesity, pulmonary disorder) have demonstrated less correlation; the lack of accuracy of RAP estimation used; quality of the study [34, 36, 37]. Doppler echocardiography may underestimate RVSP in patients with severe PH and overestimate in patients with near normal pressures [38, 39].

Echocardiography is essential to rule out left heart disease as a cause of PAH since diagnosis of PAH mandates the absence of clinically significant left heart disease. Assessment of left ventricular (LV) size, structure and function is important to exclude LV systolic and diastolic dysfunction, enlargement and hypertrophy. Close scrutiny for diastolic abnormalities is becoming more relevant since older patients with multiple cardiac risk factors (ie. systemic hypertension) are being diagnosed with elevated pulmonary pressures [40]. Presence of left atrial enlargement, even in the absence of obvious LV dysfunction, should raise the suspicion of elevated left sided pressures and a diagnosis of pulmonary venous hypertension (PVH) rather than PAH [30]. In these patients, it is critical to obtain a reliable pulmonary capillary wedge pressure (PCWP) during right heart catheterization; if a satisfactory PCWP wave form cannot be obtained, left heart catheterization may need to be performed to accurately measure the left ventricular end diastolic pressure (LVEDP) to

Table 3.3 Physical examination suggestive of pulmonary hypertension

Physical signs indicating presence of pulmonary hypertension	
Accentuated P2	High pulmonary pressure increases force of closing of pulmonary valve
Left parasternal heave	Presence of high right ventricular pressure and hypertrophy
Right ventricular S4	
Holosystolic murmur increasing with inspiration	Tricuspid regurgitation
Increased jugular v waves	
Diastolic murmur	Pulmonary regurgitation
Phyisical signs indicating presence of right ventricular failure	
Right ventricular S3	Right ventricular dysfunction
Marked distention of jugular veins	Right ventricular dysfunction and/or tricuspid regurgitation
Hepatojugular reflux, hepatomegaly	
Peripheral edema, ascites	
Low blood pressure	Low cardiac output
Diminished pulse pressure	
Cool extremities	

definitively rule out PVH. PAH-specific therapies can worsen PVH by precipitating pulmonary edema [41].

Echocardiography is needed to assess for valvular abnormality and congenital heart disease, which can precede or coincide with diagnosis of PH. An echocardiographic contrast ('bubble') study using agitated saline solution can screen for presence of intracardiac shunting. Transesophageal echocardiography (TEE) can add more refined structural information in these cases and may better define atypically situated atrial septal defects of the sinus venosus type [42]. In addition to obtaining the estimation of pulmonary artery systolic pressure (PASP), the size and function of the right ventricle have been shown to be critical determinants in outcome in patients with PAH. The presence of dilated right ventricle with reduced systolic function is a well recognized marker of poor prognosis. Other echocardiographic feature of worse outcome for PAH is presence of right atrial enlargement, pericardial effusion and septal displacement [43] (Figure 3.3).

DETERMINING THE ETIOLOGY OF PH

The next set of evaluations in PH is directed at determining the etiology of PH. The recommended serologies are to assess for possible underlying systemic disorders which are associated with PH (CTD, liver disorder, HIV). It is imperative to fully examine pulmonary function and physiology, which include detailed pulmonary function test (PFT) as well as computed tomography (CT) scan and sleep studies as appropriate. Full evaluation for chronic thromboembolic disease in all patients is essential; the incidence of CTEPH is estimated to be 3.8% within 2 years of surviving pulmonary embolism. Young age, a large perfusion defect, and idiopathic clinical presentation are associated with a higher probability of CTEPH [44]. Screening with ventilation perfusion (VQ) scan is recommended followed by pulmonary angiography if abnormal to determine if a patient is a candidate for thromboendarectomy, a surgical intervention that can reverse PH and potentially cure the patient [45]. The 6 min walk distance test provides a baseline objective measurement which has strong correlation with prognosis and provides a method of following progress with treatment [46, 47]. Biomarker b-type natriuretic peptide (BNP) is being investigated as a marker of prognosis and therapeutic measure in PAH [48–50].

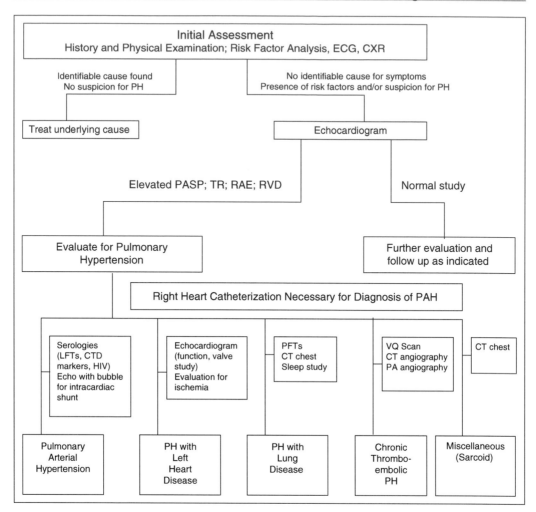

Figure 3.3 Diagnostic algorithm for evaluation of pulmonary hypertension. CT=computed tomography; CTD=connective tissue disease; CXR=chest X-ray; ECG=electrocardiogram; HIV=human immunodeficiency virus; LFT=live function test; PA=pulmonary artery; PASP=pulmonary artery systolic pressure; PFT=pulmonary function test; PH=pulmonary hypertension; RAE=right atrial enlargement; RVD=right ventricular dysfunction; TR=tricuspid regurgitation.

CONFIRMATION OF PAH: RIGHT HEART CATHETERIZATION

Right heart catheterization (RHC) is necessary to confirm PAH diagnosis, to obtain prognostic indicators and to perform acute vasodilating testing when indicated. The definition of PAH is a hemodynamically derived set of parameters which include assessment of mPAP (> 25 mmHg), PCWP (<15 mmHg) and PVR (> 3 Wood units). All three components are necessary to be diagnosed as PAH: elevation of mean PAP to demonstrate elevation of pulmonary vascular pressures; normal left sided filling pressure to exclude PVH; elevated PVR to include the effect of cardiac output. Thus factors which can elevate PAPs other than pulmonary vascular disorder, such as transmitted pressures due to increased left sided filling pressures and high output state, need to be excluded. Complete oxygen saturation measurements

Table 3.4 Agents used in acute vasodilator testing

Definition of responder	Fall in mean PAP by atleast 10mmHg to a value ≤40 mmHg Increased or unchanged cardiac output	
Commonly used agents in vasoreactivity testing	**Commonly used dose range**	**Side-effects**
Nitric oxide – inhaled	10–80 ppm	Increased left – sided filling pressure in susceptible patients
Epoprostenol – IV infusion	1–2 ng/kg/min q 10–15 min; range 5–10 ng/kg/min	Hypotension, headache, nausea, lightheadedness
Adenosine – IV infusion	50 mcg/kg/min q 2 min; range 50–250 mcg/kg/min	Dyspnea, chest pain, A-V block, hypotension

are also done as part of initial RHC when suspicious of intra cardiac shunting. Furthermore, certain hemodynamic parameters have been shown to provide important prognostic information. Several studies over the years have confirmed the finding of the PPH Registry data, which identified elevated RAP and decreased cardiac index (CI) as indicators of poor prognosis [46, 51, 52].

The purpose of acute vasodilator challenge is to identify those patients who display significant acute hemodynamic response for consideration for treatment with long-term calcium channel blocker (CCB). Before PAH-directed therapies were available, initial studies with high-dose CCB demonstrated impressive long-term survival for those few who tolerated the therapy [53]. However, for the majority of patients, treatment with high-dose CCBs was associated with clinical decompensation and mortality [54]. As more PAH-directed therapies became available, the quest to identify appropriate candidates to consider for CCBs by defining 'vasoreactivity' using short acting vasodilators has evolved. A recent analysis by the European group has demonstrated that the number of patients who remained stable long term (> 1 year) on CCB monotherapy (initially placed utilizing the previous definition of 20% reduction in PAP and PVR) was smaller than previously reported (6.8%) [55]. A comparison of the initial vasoreactivity hemodynamics between patients who remained stable on CCB alone vs. those who decompensated on CCBs has resulted in the current recommendation of a 'responder' which states that CCBs should be considered as initial therapy for: patients with IPAH in the absence of right heart failure (HF), demonstrating a favorable response to vasodilator which is defined as a fall in mPAP of at least 10mmHg to ≤ 40mmHg, with an increased or unchanged cardiac output [54, 55]. For patients with PAH associated with other underlying processes such as scleroderma or congenital heart disease, the number of patients who remained stable on CCBs long term is even less and the net benefit of vasodilator testing is at best weak if used for the sole purpose of determining candidates for CCB therapies. Some investigators have proposed that result of vasodilator challenge can provide an indirect evidence to 'RV reserve' and can be helpful in determining treatment [54].

The preferred agent of choice for acute vasodilatory testing is NO, a short acting selective pulmonary vasodilator which is administered via a face mask during the right heart catheterization. It is well tolerated with very few systemic effects; however, it is expensive and requires a member of a respiratory team to administer. Intravenous prostacyclin and intravenous adenosine can also be used; these agents can produce systemic side-effects such as hypotension, arrhythmia, as well as nausea and vomiting [56–58] (Table 3.4).

Questions regarding risks associated with performing RHC in PAH were addressed in a recent multicenter study which included 15 PAH centers over a 5-year period with >7000 procedures [59]. The overall incidence of serious adverse events was 1.1%. The most frequent complications were related to obtaining venous access; others included arrhythmia and hypotension due to vagal reactions or pulmonary vasoreactivity testing. When performed in experienced centers, the authors conclude that performing RHC in PAH patients is safe and is associated with low morbidity rates. Since PAH patients often have dilated right sided chambers which can make maneuvering the catheter difficult, it is best done under fluoroscopy. Using an ultrasound device to locate the best approach when performed from the internal jugular vein has also been helpful in making the procedure safer (Figure 3.3).

THERAPIES FOR PAH

PROSTACYCLINS

Epoprostenol
Intravenous epoprostenol, as the first therapy to be approved by the FDA in 1996, truly revolutionized the field of PAH. The landmark study which demonstrated its efficacy was an open-labeled, randomized study of 81 patients with severe IPAH comparing epoprostenol and conventional therapy with conventional therapy alone, which demonstrated not only improvement in 6-minute walk distance (6MWD) and hemodynamics, but also significant survival benefit [60]. This was followed by a study demonstrating improvements in exercise capacity, hemodynamics and functional class among patients with PAH occurring in association with the scleroderma spectrum of diseases, which broadened the approved indication for epoprostenol to include patients with CTD and PAH [61]. With long-term use, two large retrospective studies have demonstrated survival benefits among IPAH patients receiving long-term epoprostenol compared with historical control groups [46, 52].

Several challenges exist in implementing epoprostenol. Due to its short half-life (<6 min), epoprostenol must be delivered by continuous IV infusion via a tunneled catheter. Incidences of sepsis and catheter related infections are recognized risks (0.1 to 0.6 case per patient-year) and can cause significant morbidity [52, 60]. Furthermore, any interruption of the drug infusion can be potentially life threatening given its short half-life. The drug is associated with several side-effects, most of which are typical for prostacyclins (jaw pain, headache, diarrhea). Appropriate dosing can also be challenging; excessive prostacyclin can lead to a high cardiac output state and worsening of symptoms [62]. Despite the difficulties, epoprostenol remains as the therapy of choice for patients with advanced PAH (i.e. functional class IV and/or right HF, as a bridge to lung transplant) given its proven efficacy and survival benefit. Due to its complexity, it is recommended that patient requiring epoprostenol therapy be referred to centers specializing in PAH [54]. Another challenge in using epoprostenol is that it is unstable at room temperature and must be kept in ice. A temperature stable epoprostenol has recently been approved by the FDA [63] (Table 3.5).

Treprostinil
Treprostinil is a prostacyclin analogue which has longer half-life (~3–4 h). Treprostinil was first studied as a continuous subcutaneous (SC) infusion in the largest placebo-controlled PAH trial to date, enrolling 470 patients [64]. Although improvement in exercise capacity and hemodynamics were seen in patients receiving treprostinil compared with placebo, infusion site pain and erythema became major barriers (reported by 85% of the study population). It is now recognized that site pain is not dose related, and that some patients feel better after proper dose escalation that alleviates their PAH symptoms. Topical analgesics and anti-inflammatory agents have had variable success in controlling this side-effect. For those patients who can tolerate the SC infusion, this therapy provides a safer and more convenient way of receiving continuous intravenous prostacyclin treatment. Recently, two studies reported long-term results with SC treatment, demonstrating improvements in exercise capacity with survival benefits. [65].

Table 3.5 Approved PAH treatments and their common side-effects

Drug class	Name/Year approved	Route/Dose	Side-effects	Comments
Prostanoids	Epoprostenol (Flolan) 1995	Continuous IV Initiate 1–2 ng/kg/min and titrate to efficacy and side-effects	Hickman catheter infection and malfunction Side-effects related to prostacyclin*	Therapy complicated and it is recommended patients be referred to PAH treating centers for initiation and management Effective in patients with severe PAH and RHF Agent most frequently used as rescue therapy Long-term survival data available
	Epoprostenol (Veletri) 2010	Reported to be same as Flolan	Reported to be same as Flolan	Data pending
	Treprostinil (Remodulin SC) 2002	Continuous SC Initiate 1.25–2.5 ng/kg/min SC	Injection site pain Side-effects related to prostacyclin	Effective for PAH but site pain effects majority of patients Experienced centers have reported successful outcome in managing patients with site pain issues Long-term survival data available
	Treprostinil (Remodulin IV) 2004	Continuous IV Initiate 1–2 ng/kg/min IV	Hickman catheter infection and malfunction Side-effects related to prostacyclin* Leg pain	Therapy less complicated to manage than Flolan Need higher dose than Flolan for transitioning patients to achieve similar efficacy Long-term data not yet available
	Treprostinil inhaled (Tyvaso) 2009	Start 3 inhalations, 4 times a day. Titrate to target dose of 9 inhalations, 4 times a day	Cough/headache	Selective delivery of prostacyclin to lungs. Reported to enhance convenience. Ability to titrate dose. Used as combination treatment with oral therapies
	Iloprost (Ventavis) 2004	Inhaled 6–9 inhalations per day while awake 2.5 and 5.0 mcg	Cough, some jaw pain and headache	Selective delivery of prostacyclin to lungs Compliance can be an issue with need for frequent treatments Used as combination treatment with oral therapies
PDE5 Inhibitors	Sildenafil (Revatio) 2005	Oral 20 mg TID	Epistaxis, headache, flushing, diarrhea	Contraindicated with nitrates Some patients may need up titration of dose
	Tadalafil (Adcirca) 2009	Oral 40 mg QD	Headache, mylagia, flushing	Contraindicated with nitrates
ERA	Bosentan (Tracleer) 2001	Oral 62.5 and 125 mg BID	Headache, dizziness, edema	Need LFTs checked monthly Most effective in non-FC IV patients Contraindicated with cyclosporine and glyburide Decreases effectiveness of oral hormonal contraceptives Long-term observed survival data available
	Ambrosentan (Letairis) 2007	Oral 5 and 10 mg QD	Peripheral edema, nasal congestion, sinusitis	Need LFTs checked monthly; less incidence of LFT abnormality compared with other ERAs More reported incidence of edema compared with other ERAs Decreases effectiveness of oral hormonal contraceptives

*Side-effects related to prostacyclin: jaw pain, diarrhea, flushing, headache, nausea
ERA = Endothelin receptor antagonists; LFT = liver function test; QD = once a day; TID = three times a day.

Due to site pain-limiting effects of SC delivery, treprostinil was studied in intravenous (IV) route in a 12-week open-label trial of 16 patients [66]. Although a small study, it demonstrated safety and efficacy of IV infusion and it was approved by the FDA in 2004. Several potential advantages over epoprostenol are that it is potentially less dangerous from possible rebound effects in the event of infusion interruption due to its longer half-life and that it is easier to administer since it comes in a premixed system and does not need to be kept in ice packs. The TRUST study, a placebo-controlled trial evaluating intravenous treprostinil conducted in India, demonstrated improvement in 6MWD, though the study was terminated prematurely due to safety concerns [67]. Recent reports of possible increase in gram-negative infections in patients receiving IV treprostinil compared with epoprostenol is being evaluated by the manufacturer and Center for Disease Control [68]. An inhaled form of treprostinil was recently approved by the FDA [69]. Some potential advantages of inhaled treprostinil compared with inhaled iloprost (see below) are that treatment time appears to be shorter and less frequent inhalation treatments due to longer half-life of treprostinil compared with iloprost. An oral formulation of treprostinil is currently undergoing Phase III study (Table 3.5).

Iloprost

Iloprost is a prostacyclin analogue which is available as an inhaled formulation in U.S. In a multicenter randomized, placebo-controlled European study, patients treated with inhaled iloprost demonstrated improvements in exercise capacity, functional class, and hemodynamics [70]. Its half-life is approximately 20–30 min and it should be administered six to nine times a day while awake. Iloprost was generally well tolerated; coughing, headache and flushing reported as most common side-effects. The advantages of iloprost are the ability to deliver prostacyclin directly to the lungs, thereby minimizing systemic side-effects, and not requiring indwelling catheters. Compliance is the key factor with the need to adhere to frequent treatments (Table 3.5).

PHOSPHODIESTERASE-5 INHIBITOR

Sildenafil

Sildenafil was evaluated for PAH in a 12-week randomized placebo-controlled study, Sildenafil Use in Pulmonary Arterial Hypertension (SUPER) [71]. In 278 patients with PAH, treatment with sildenafil resulted in similar improvements in 6 min walk distance (6MWD) among the three doses studied (45 m, 46 m, 50 m for 20, 40, 80 mg, respectively) and sildenafil 20 mg TID was approved for treatment of PAH in 2005. However, in nearly all patients who were followed after the 12-week study period, the dose was titrated up to 80 mg TID. Noted side-effects include headache and epistaxis and the drug was overall well tolerated. Reports regarding visual disturbances have raised some concerns, especially among diabetics and patients with cardiovascular risk factors. Obtaining baseline ophthalmologic exam is followed by some practitioners although, so far, no significant reports of ophthalmologic disturbances have been reported with chronic use in PAH population (Table 3.5).

Tadalafil

Tadalafil was recently studied in a 16-week, double-blind, placebo-controlled trial among 405 PAH patients using 2.5, 10, 20, and 40 mg [72]. The 40 mg dose demonstrated a 41 meter increase in 6MWD compared with 9 meters for placebo ($P < 0.001$). There was also a delay in time to clinical worsening (defined as death, hospitalization, initiation of new PAH therapy, worsening WHO FC). A PDE5-inhibitor with a longer-half life than sildenafil, tadalafil is given once a day. Side-effects include headache, diarrhea, nausea, back pain, dizziness, dyspepsia, and flushing (Table 3.5).

ENDOTHELIN RECEPTOR ANTAGONISTS

Dual endothelin receptor antagonists – bosentan

Bosentan is a dual ET_A and ET_B receptor blocker. Its approval in 2001 marked yet another milestone in PAH treatment as the first oral therapy and as an agent targeting a different pathophysiological mechanism than epoprostenol. BREATHE-1 is a placebo-controlled study among 213 patients that demonstrated improvement in exercise capacity and functional class (FC) and decrease in the rate of clinical worsening [73]. Long-term observational findings in survival of patients treated with bosentan as first-line therapy have shown improved survival compared with expected outcome and the investigators concluded that for stable FC III patients with PAH, it is reasonable to consider bosentan as first-line therapy [74]. Another notable finding is the recent completion of EARLY study, conducted on 168 FC II PAH patients [75]. The objective was to determine efficacy and safety in treating mildly symptomatic patients. Indeed, the baseline 6MWD of this cohort was 438 meters, which is higher than all the other studies in PAH (~330–350 meters). The results demonstrated a significant decrease in PVR, which was the primary endpoint to evaluate treatment effects on vascular remodeling. There was also a significant delay in clinical worsening. This pivotal study demonstrated that PAH patients with mildly symptomatic disease benefit from early initiation of treatment.

The primary safety issue in using bosentan is its effect on the hepatic system since it is metabolized mainly through the P450 enzymes. The reported increase in transaminases more than three times upper limit of normal is about 10–12% [73]. The LFT increase is dose dependent and reversible, and all patients receiving bosentan are required to have monthly LFTs tests. Bosentan has been shown to have teratogenic effects in animals and may decrease the efficacy of hormonal contraception so women of childbearing age must be counseled to use dual contraception for birth control. Glyburide and cyclosporine A are contraindicated with bosentan due to significant interaction and potential for significant liver damage. There is no significant interaction with warfarin and bosentan. The recommended starting dose is 62.5 BID and titration to 125 mg BID in 4 weeks if patient tolerating it well with stable LFTs (Table 3.5).

Selective endothelin receptor antagonist – ambrosentan and sitaxsanten

Ambrisentan is a selective ET_A receptor antagonist that was approved by the FDA in 2007 for treatment of PAH in patients with functional class II or III symptoms to improve exercise capacity and delay clinical worsening. The two placebo-controlled randomized studies (ARIES-1 and ARIES-2) were conducted in U.S. and Europe/South America, respectively [76]. The combined studies enrolled 394 patients in a placebo-controlled, 12-week study of World Health Organization (WHO) Group I patients. The treatment resulted in a significant improvement in 6MWD and delay in clinical worsening, similar to bosentan. However, there are a couple of differences worth noting in regards to reported side-effects. First is that ambrosentan was found to cause lower incidences of LFT abnormalities (12-week incidence of aminotransferases >3 x ULN 0.8% for patients receiving ambrisentan) [76]. This was further investigated in a recently published trial where 36 patients who did not tolerate bosentan or sitaxsantan (see below) due to LFT increases were placed on ambrosentan therapy [77]. This is thought to be related to the fact that bosentan and sitaxsentan are sulfonamide-based ERAs. Edema is another side-effect of the ERA-class and was reported in mild to moderate severity in the clinical trials [76]. However, an increase in peripheral edema during the post marketing use has prompted FDA to issue a labeled warning in the package insert [78]. The mechanisms behind this observed edema is currently undergoing evaluation. There were no drug interactions found with warfarin or sildenafil [78].

Table 3.6 Results of combination therapy in PAH

Study name	Combination studied	n	Length of trial	6MWD	Other results	Comments
BREATHE-2 [82]	IV Epo ± bosentan	33	16 weeks	No improvement	Trend toward greater improvement in PVR	Only trial to date to study simultaneous initiation of two drugs Study insufficiently powered
STEP [83]	Bosentan ± inhaled iloprost	67	12 weeks	26 meters (peak^) (P=0.05) No difference at trough+	Improved FC, TTCW, post-inhalation hemo-dynamics	Combination therapy well tolerated
COMBI [84]	Bosentan ± inhaled iloprost	40	12 weeks	No improvement	No change	Trial terminated early
PACES [85]	IV Epo ± sildenafil	267	16 weeks	26 meters (P < 0.001)	Improved TTCW and hemo-dynamics	Majority of patients on 80 mg TID of sildenafil
TRIUMPH-1 [69]	Oral therapy ± inhaled treprostinil	235	12 weeks	20 meters* (peak^) (P < 0.001) 14 meters (trough+) (P=0.01)	No effect reported for TTCW, FC	

*median changes reported, changes in 6MWD are placebo corrected values; ^peak=post inhalation; +trough=pre-inhalation.
FC=functional class; PVR=pulmonary vascular resistance; TID=three times a day; TTCW=time to clinical worsening (see studies for description)

Sitaxsentan, another selective ET_A antagonist, demonstrated improvement in 6MWD in the first placebo-controlled trial; however, there were concerns relating to increases in LFTs in the higher dose (300 mg) group as well as significant interaction with warfarin [79]. The second randomized study (STRIDE-2) used lower doses of sitaxsentan (50 mg and 100 mg) along with a placebo arm with an additional group receiving open label bosentan, demonstrating similar increases in 6MWD between the 100 mg of sitaxsentan and bosentan groups [80]. Less incidence of hepatic abnormality was reported with sitaxsentan at lower doses; vigilant monitoring of international normalized ratio (INR) with warfarin dose reductions is necessary due to significant drug–drug interactions. Sitaxsentan is currently approved in Europe and Canada and undergoing further studies in U.S. (Table 3.5)

CONVENTIONAL THERAPY

Recent analysis by the European group has demonstrated that the number of patients who remained stable long term (> 1 year) on CCB was smaller than previously reported (6.8%) [55]. The current recommendation states that CCB should be considered as initial therapy for patients with IPAH in the absence of right HF, demonstrating a favorable-acute response

Table 3.7 World Health Organization classification of functional status of patients with pulmonary hypertension

Class	Description
I	Patients with PH in whom there is no limitation of physical activity. Ordinary physical activity does not cause undue dyspnea or fatigue, chest pain, or presyncope.
II	Patients with PH who have mild limitation of physical activity. There is no discomfort at rest, but normal physical activity causes increased dyspnea or fatigue, chest pain, or presyncope.
III	Patients with PH who have marked limitation of physical activity. There is no discomfort at rest, but less than ordinary activity causes undue dyspnea or fatigue, chest pain, or presyncope.
IV	Patients with PH who are unable to perform any physical activity at rest and who may have signs of right ventricular failure. Dyspnea and/or fatigue may even be present at rest and symptoms are increased by almost any physical activity.

to vasodilator which is defined as a fall in mPAP of at least 10 mmHg to ≤ 40 mmHg, with an increased or unchanged cardiac output [54, 55]. To emphasize, this recommendation is for IPAH patients only; for patients with PAH associated with other underlying processes such as scleroderma or congenital heart disease, the number of patients who benefit from CCBs long term is even less. The recommendation regarding anticoagulation is based on two small retrospective studies and from pathological studies demonstrating the importance of *in situ* microscopic thrombosis as a process propagating pulmonary arteriopathy [53, 81]. Anticoagulation is recommended for all patients with IPAH in the absence of contraindications and the recommended INR is approximately 1.5–2.5 [54]. The risk and benefit ratio must be considered especially for patients with PAH due to other systemic processes with increased risk of gastrointestinal (GI) bleeding, such as in patients with scleroderma.

COMBINATION THERAPY IN PAH

With the approval of therapies targeting different pathophyiologic pathways and routes of delivery, utilizing combination approach based on the potential for additive or synergistic effects has gained marked interest. Several completed studies demonstrate improvements in 6MWD of 20–26 meters over the 12–16 week trials [69, 82–85] (Table 3.6). Although not as robust in improvement compared with clinical trials testing monotherapy with placebo, these changes appear to be clinically beneficial since they are associated with improvement in hemodyanmics and time to clinical worsening. There are several multicenter studies currently underway to determine safety and efficacy of utilizing combination therapy, including one long-term study with a morbidity/mortality endpoint.

DETERMINING RISK AND ON-THERAPY PROGNOSIS IN PAH

Assessing risk in PAH patients is critical in determining initial choice of treatment and method of follow-up care. Several clinical parameters have been shown to correlate with long-term prognosis and to serve as a marker of response to therapy. Baseline functional classification is one such measure. A World Health Organization (WHO) functional classification, modified from New York Heart Association (NYHA) functional classification, has been adopted for PAH [86] (Table 3.7). Studies have shown more favorable prognosis for

Table 3.8 Assessing risk in PAH patients (adapted with permission from [90])

Determinants of risk*	Lower risk (Good prognosis)	Higher risk (Poor prognosis)
Clinical evidence of RV failure	No	Yes
Progression of symptoms	Gradual	Rapid
WHO Class	II, III**	IV
6MWD***	Longer (>400 meters)	Shorter (<300 meters)
Echocardiography	Normal to minimal RV dysfunction	Significant RV enlargement/ dysfunction; right atrial enlargement; pericardial effusion
Hemodynamics	Normal RAP and CI (RAP < 10 mmHg; CI > 2.5 l/min/m^2)	High RAP and low CI (RAP > 15 mmHg; CI < 2.2 l/min/ m^2)
BNP^	Normal to minimally elevated	Significantly elevated

*Most studies performed in IPAH patients. No single risk factor should be used to assess risk.
**FC III clinically encompasses a large range of disease severity. Using composite of detailed assessments of other objective characteristics critical.
***6MWD is influenced by age, gender, height and presence of other systemic conditions.
^Limited data regarding utilizing BNP on risk.
6MWD = 6 min walk distance; BNP = brain natriuretic peptide; CI = cardiac index; RAP = right atrial pressure; RV = right ventricle; WHO = World Health Organization.

Table 3.9 Goals of treatment in PAH patients

Objective assessments	Goals of therapy
WHO Fuctional Class	I or II
6MWD	>380 meters; stable to increasing
Hemodynamics	RAP < 10 mmHg and CI 2.5 l/min/m^2
BNP	Normal to near normal; decreasing

6MWD = 6 min walk distance; BNP = brain natriuretic peptide; CI = cardiac index; RAP = right atrial pressure; WHO = World Health Organization.

patients who are diagnosed earlier in the disease state. In the retrospective studies of long-term epoprostenol patients, those who presented in FC III had better outcome than those who were FC IV [46, 52]. Furthermore, patients who improved to FC I or II after 3 months of epoprostenol therapy demonstrated markedly improved survival than those who remained in FC III or IV [46] (Tables 3.8 and 3.9).

The 6MWD also correlates with prognosis. At baseline, Miyamoto and colleagues demonstrated patients who walked ≥ 332 meters had significantly better long-term survival than those who were not able to achieve that distance baseline [47]. Furthermore, Sitbon and colleagues reported among patients treated with epoprstenol, the 6MWD performed after 3 months of therapy correlated with long-term survival; specifically, patients who walked ≥ 380 meters demonstrated a significantly better outcome than the cohorts who did not [46] (Tables 3.8 and 3.9).

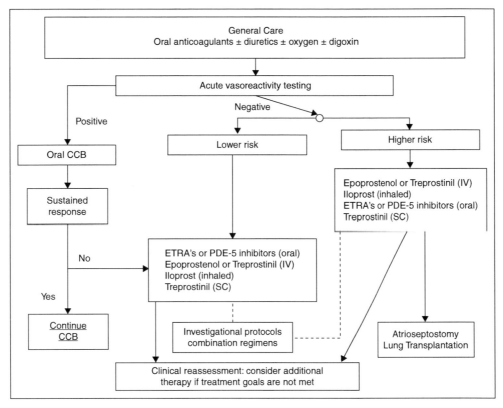

Figure 3.4 Treatment algorithm based on risk assessment (adapted with permission from [90]). CCB = calcium channel blocker; ETRA = endothelin receptor antagonist; PDE = phosphodiesterase.

Other objective parameters shown to serve as prognostic markers in PAH are hemody-namics and echocardiographic features. High RAP and low cardiac index have been the hallmark of severe disease and strong predictors of poor outcome in the PPH Registry [51]. Measurements reflecting right-sided cardiac function (right atrial and right ventricular size, Doppler parameters and indices of RV function, eccentricity index) has been shown to be reliable markers of prognosis [43, 87]. Several investigators have reported presence and severity of pericardial effusion to be significantly correlated with survival [43, 88]. Biomarkers have also been studied in PAH. Both baseline BNP and change in BNP with therapy have been shown to correlate with outcome [48–50]. Furthermore, follow-up measurements after 3 months of epoprostenol therapy indicated that changes in plasma BNP levels correlated closely with changes in hemodyhamics and demonstrated to be an independent predictor of survival [48, 49]. N-terminal prohormone brain natriuretic peptide (NT-pro BNP) has also demonstrated to have good correlation between plasma levels hemodyanmics and survival [89]. It is recommended that a composite of subjective and objective data be used to deter-mine risk of the patient which can be used to choose appropriate therapy and as a guide to determine response to treatment [90] (Table 3.8). Current recommendations include that patients in low risk category be considered for oral agent as first-line therapy; for those manifesting high risk features be started with continuous systemic prostacyclin treatments [90] (Figure 3.4). Therapy goals in PAH patients include achieving FC I or II, stable and improving 6MWD, hemodynamics demonstrating improving RV function (as determined by normal RAP and CI), and decreasing BNP levels [90] (Table 3.9).

PH AND LEFT HEART DISEASE

PH can occur in any setting where left-sided filling pressure is chronically elevated. The degree of elevation of PAP is usually proportional to the PCWP; thus optimizing therapy to normalize the left-sided filling pressure usually decreases the PAP over time. In advanced cases, normalization of filling pressures cannot be achieved and PAP remains high whereas in some patients, PAP stays elevated despite optimization of the PCWP – these conditions been coined 'PH out of proportion to left heart disease'. Consideration for use of PAH directed therapies in these clinical situations may seem plausible. However, this practice is discouraged given the potential to worsen pulmonary vascular congestion. Epoprostenol has been studied in patients with advanced systolic HF with increased mortality [91]. Similarly, using bosentan in HF population has not resulted in any benefit [92, 93]. However, a small study enrolling patients with systolic dysfunction and PH treating with bosentan reported positive results [94]. Another study of 32 patients treated with 12 weeks of sildenafil found improvement in exercise capacity and decrease in HF hospitalization [95]. Although further studies are needed to determine if any class of PAH therapy can be used for PH in the setting of left sided heart disease, initial results using sildenafil appear promising.

MANAGEMENT OF RIGHT HF AND PAH

PAH patients with right HF can present with volume overload, systemic hypotension, low output state along with renal dysfunction. Treatment needs to include assessment for other underlying sources for decompensation such as pneumonia, line infection (for patients with chronic indwelling catheters) or sources of bleeding. Managing volume can be challenging since the RV in these patients are pre-load dependent. In acute decompensated state, further volume loading of already dilated RV can worsen cardiac output [96]. Accurate assessment of filling pressures and cardiac output with right heart catheterization is often needed for proper management. Patients are often in volume overloaded state and treatment with IV diuretics becomes necessary. Hemodynamic guidance can assist in optimal diuretic dosing as well as support with inotropes or pressors. Dobutamine and dopamine have been shown to be effective in animal models. Dobutamine is generally preferred in patients with marginal blood pressure and/or renal dysfunction though tachycardia may incur in some patients. Milrinone has also been used with improvement of cardiac output and is a reasonable therapeutic choice with stable blood pressure and renal function [97].

CONCLUSION

The past decade has witnessed remarkable advances in understanding the pathobiology of PAH which has translated into discovery and approval of eight therapies. Significant improvements in quality of life and survival have been achieved. Although awareness of PAH has increased, further effort is needed for patients to be diagnosed earlier in their disease course. Several studies are currently in progress studying the effects of combination therapies in PAH which, as the data emerge from clinical trials in the next few years, can provide further guidance into evidence-based guidelines. Significant work is currently in progress studying therapies targeting different pathologic processes and new diagnostic tools are emerging to assess and follow PAH patients. With the remarkable accomplishments achieved in the last decade which have resulted in such meaningful improvement in survival and quality of life in what was considered a uniformly fatal disease, the future of PAH looks promising.

REFERENCES

1. Romberg E. Ueber sklerose der lungen arterie. *Dtsch Arch Klin Med* 1891; 48:197-206.
2. Dresdale DT, Schultz M, Michtom RJ. Primary pulmonary hypertension: I. Clinical and hemodynamic study. *Am J Med* 1951; 11:686-705.
3. Badesch DB, Champion HC, Sanchez MA *et al.* Diagnosis and assessment of pulmonary arterial hypertension. *J Am Coll Cardiol* 2009; 54:S55-S66.
4. Jeffery TK, Morrell NW. Molecular and cellular basis of pulmonary vascular remodeling in pulmonary hypertension. *Prog Cardiovasc Dis* 2002; 45:173-202.
5. Yuan JXJ, Rubin LJ. Pathogenesis of pulmonary arterial hypertension: the need for multiple hits. *Circulation* 2005; 111:534-538.
6. Lane KB, Machado RD, Pauciulo MW *et al.* Heterozygous germline mutations in BMPR2, encoding a TGF-ß receptor, cause familial primary pulmonary hypertension: the International PPH Consortium. *Nat Genet* 2000; 26:81-84.
7. Deng Z, Morse JH, Slager SL *et al.* Familial primary pulmonary hypertension (gene PPH1) is caused by mutations in the bone morphogenetic protein receptor-II gene. *Am J Hum Genet* 2000,67:e-pub.
8. Humbert M, Sitbon O, Simonneau G. Treatment of pulmonary arterial hypertension. *N Engl J Med* 2004; 351:1425-1436.
9. Christman BW, McPherson CD, Newman JH *et al.* An imbalance between the excretion of thromboxane and prostacyclin metabolites in pulmonary hypertension. *N Engl J Med* 1992; 327:70-75.
10. Giaid A, Saleh D. Reduced expression of endothelial nitric oxide synthase in the lungs of patients with pulmonary hypertension. *N Engl J Med* 1995; 333:214-221.
11. Michelaskis ED, Tymchk W, Noga M *et al.* Long term treatment with oral sildenafil is safe and improves functional capacity and hemodyanmics in patients with pulmonary arterial hypertension. *Circulation* 2003; 108:2066-2069.
12. Yanagisawa M, Kurihara H, Kimura S *et al.* A novel potent vasoconstrictor peptide produced by vascualar endothelial cells. *Nature* 1988; 332:411-415.
13. Ogawa Y, Nakao K, Arai H *et al.* Molecular cloning of a non-isopeptide-selective human endothelin receptor. *Biochem Biophys Res Commun* 1991; 178: 248-255.
14. Giad A, Yanagisawa M, Langleben D *et al.* Expression of endothelin-1 in the lungs of patients with pulmonary hypertension. *N Engl J Med* 1993; 328:1732-1739.
15. Vincent JA, Ross RD, Kassab J *et al.* Relation of elevated plasma endothelin in congenital heart disease to increased pulmonary blood flow. *Am J Cardiol* 1993; 71:1204-1207.
16. Simonneau G, Robbins IM, Beghetti M *et al.* Updated clinical classification of pulmonary hypertension. *J Am Coll Cardiol* 2009; 54;S43-S54.
17. Rich S, Dantzker DR, Ayres SM *et al.* Primary pulmonary hypertension: a national prospective study. *Ann Intern Med* 1987; 107:216-223.
18. Badesch DB, Raskob GE, Elliott CG *et al.* Pulmonary arterial hypertension: baseline characteristics from the REVEAL Registry. *Chest* 2010; 137:376-387.
19. Wigley FM, Lima JA, Mayes M *et al*: The prevalence of undiagnosed pulmonary arterial hypertension in subjects with connective tissue disease at the secondary health care level of community-based rheumagologists (the UNCOVER study). *Arthritis Rheum* 2005; 52:2125-2132.
20. Change B, Schachna L, Wigley FM *et al.* Natural history of mild-moderate pulmonary arterial hypertension and the risk factors for severe pulmonary hypertension in scleroderma. *J Rheumatol* 2006; 33:269-274.
21. Koh ET, Lee P, Gladman DD *et al.* Pulmonary hypertension in systemic sclerosis: an analysis of 17 patients. *Br J Rheumatol* 1996; 35:989-993.
22. Kuhn KP, Byrne DW, Arbogast PG *et al.* Outcome in 91 consecutive patients with pulmonary arterial hypertension receiving epoprostenol. *Am J Respir Crit Care Med* 2003; 167:580-586.
23. McLaughlin VV, Presberg KW, Doyle RL *et al.* Prognosis of pulmonary arterial hypertension: ACCP evidence-based clinical practice guidelines. *Chest* 2004; 126:78S-92S.
24. Machado R, Pauciulo MW, Thomson J *et al.* BMPRs haploinsufficiency as the inherited molecular mechanism for primary pulmolnary hypertension. *Am J Hum Genet* 2001; 68:92-102
25. Cogan JD, Vnencak-Jones CL, Phillips JA *et al.* Gross BMPR2 gene rearrangements constitute a new cause for primary pulmonary hypertension. *Genet Med* 2005; 7:169-174.
26. Colle IO, Moreau R, Godinho E *et al.* Diagnosis of portopulmonary hypertension in candidates for liver transplantation: a prospective study. *Hepatology* 2003; 37:401-409.

27. Ashfaq M, Chinnakotla S, Rogers L *et al.* The impact of treatment of portopulmonary hypertension on survival following liver transplantation. *Am J Transplant* 2007; 7:1258-1264.

28. Hopkins WE, Ochoa LL, Richardson GW *et al.* Comparison of the hemodynamics and survival of adults with severe primary pulmonary hypertension or Eisenmenger syndrome. *J Heart Lung Transplant* 1996; 15:100-105.

29. Oya H, Nagaya N, Uematsu M *et al.* Poor prognosis and related factors in adults with Eisenmenger syndrome. *Am Heart J* 2002; 143:739-744.

30. McLaughlin VV, Archer SL, Badesch DB *et al.* ACCF/AHA 2009 expert consensus document on pulmonary hypertension: a report of the American College of Cardiology Foundation Task Force on Expert Consensus Documents. *J Am Coll Cardiol* 2009; 53:1573-1619.

31. Ahearn GS, Tapson VF, Reberiz A *et al.* Electrocardiography to define clinical status in primary pulmonary hypertension and pulmonary arterial hypertension secondary to collagen vascular disease. *Chest* 2002; 122:524-527

32. Ommen SR, Nishimura RA, Hurrell DG *et al.* Assessment of right atrial pressure with two-dimensional and Doppler echocardiography: a simultaneous catheterization and echocardiographic study. *Mayo Clin Proc* 2000; 75:24-29.

33. Bossone E, Duong-Wagner TH, Paciocco G *et al.* Echocardiographic features of primary pulmonary hypertension. *J Am Soc Echocardiogr* 1999; 12:655-662.

34. Homma A, Anzueto A, Peters JI *et al.* Pulmonary artery systolic pressures estimated by echocardiogram vs cardiac catheterization in patients awaiting lung transplantation. *J Heart Lung Transplant* 2001; 20:833-839.

35. Yock PG, Popp RL. Noninvasive estimation of right ventricular systolic pressure by Doppler ultrasound in patients with tricuspid regurgitation. *Circulation* 1984; 70:657-662.

36. Murata I, Kihara H, Shinohara S *et al.* Echocardiographic evaluation of pulmonary arterial hypertension in patients with progressive systemic sclerosis and related syndromes. *Jpn Circ J* 1992; 56:983-991.

37. Hinderliter AL, Willis PW, Barst RJ *et al.* Effects of long-term infusion of prostacyclin (epoprostenol) on echocardiographic measures of right ventricular structure and function in primary pulmonary hypertension: Primary Pulmonary Hypertension Study Group. *Circulation* 1997; 95:1479-1486.

38. Brecher SJ, Gibbs JS, Fox KM *et al.* Comparison of Doppler derived hemodynamic variables and simultaneous high fidelity pressure measurements in severe pulmonary hypertension. *Br Heart J* 1994; 72:384-389.

39. Arcasoy SM, Christie JD, Ferrari VA *et al.* Echocardiographic assessment of pulmonary hypertension in patients with advanced lung disease. *Am J Respir Crit Care Med* 2003; 167:735-740.

40. Robbins IM, Newman JH, Johnson RF *et al.* Association of the metabolic syndrome with pulmonary venous hypertension. *Chest* 2009; 136:31-36.

41. Humbert M, Maitre S, Capron F *et al.* Pulmonary edema complicating continuous intravenous prostacyclin in pulmonary capillary hemangiomatosis. *Am J Respir Crit Care Med* 1998; 157:1681-1685.

42. Gorscan J, Edwards TD, Ziady GM *et al.* Transesophageal echocardiography to evaluate paitents with severe pulmonary hypertension for lung transplantation. *Ann Thorac Surg* 1995; 59:717-722.

43. Raymond RL, Hinderliter AL, Willis PW *et al.* Echocardiographic predictors of adverse outcomes in primary pulmonary hypertension. *J Am Coll Cardiol* 2002; 39:1214-1219.

44. Pengo V, Lensing A, Prins MH *et al.* Incidence of chronic thromboembolic pulmonary hypertension after pulmonary embolism. *N Engl J Med* 2004; 350:2257-2264.

45. Manecke GR Jr, Wilson WC, Auger WR *et al.* Chronic thromboembolic pulmonary hypertension and pulmonary thromboendarectomy. *Semin Cardiothorac Vasc Anesth* 2005; 9:189-204.

46. Sitbon O, Humbert M, Nunes H *et al.* Long-term intravenous epoprostenol infusion in primary pulmonary hypertension: prognostic factors and survival. *J Am Coll Cardiol* 2002; 40:780-788.

47. Miyamoto S, Nagaya N, Satoh T *et al.* Clinical correlates and prognostic significance of six-minute walk test in patients with primary pulmonary hypertension: comparison with cardiopulmonary exercise testing. *Am J Respir Crit Care Med* 2000; 161:487-492.

48. Nagaya N, Nishikimi T, Uematsu M *et al.* Plasma brain natriuretic peptide as a prognostic indicator in patients with primary pulmonary hypertension. *Circulation* 2000; 102:865-870.

49. Park MH, Scott RL, Uber PA, Ventura HO, Mehra MR. Usefulness of B-type natriuretic peptide as a predictor of treatment outcome in pulmonary arterial hypertension. *Congest Heart Fail* 2004; 10:221-225.

50. Andreassen A, Wergeland R, Simonson S *et al*. N-terminal pro-B-type natriuretic peptide as an indicator of disease severity in a heterogeneous group of patients with chronic precapillary pulmonary hypertension. *Am J Cardiol* 2006; 98:525-529.
51. D'Alonzo GE, Barst RJ, Ayres SM *et al*. Survival in patients with primary pulmonary hypertension: results from a national prospective registry. *Ann Intern Med* 1991; 115:343-349.
52. McLaughlin VV, Shillington A, Rich S. Survival in primary pulmonary hypertension: the impact of epoprostenol therapy. *Circulation* 2002; 106: 1477-1482.
53. Rich S, Kaugmann E, Levy PS. The effect of high doses of calcium-channel blockers on survival in primary pulmonary hypertension. *N Engl J Med* 1992; 327:76-81.
54. Badesch DB, Abman SH, Ahearn GS *et al*. Medical therapy for pulmonary arterial hypertension. ACCP evidence-based clinical practice guidelines. *Chest* 2004; 126:35S-62S.
55. Sitbon O, Humbert M, Jais X *et al*. Long-term response to calcium channel blockers in idiopathic pulmonary arterial hypertension. *Circulation* 2005; 111:3105-3111.
56. Sitbon O, Humbert M, Jagot JL *et al*. Inhaled nitric oxide as a screening agent for safely identifying responders to oral calcium-channel blockers in primary pulmonary hypertension. *Eur Respir J* 1998; 12:265-270.
57. Groves BM, Badesch DB, Turkevich D *et al*. Correlation of acute prostacyclin response in primary (unexplained) pulmonary hypertension with efficacy of treatment with calcium channel blockers and survival. In:Weir K, ed. *Ion Flux in Pulmonary Vascular Control*. New York, NY: Plenum Press, 1993, pp 317-330.
58. Schrader BJ, Inbar S, Kaufmann L *et al*. Comparison of the effects of adenosine and nifedipine in pulmonary hypertension. *J Am Coll Cardiol* 1992; 19:1060-1064.
59. Hoeper MM, Lee SH, Voswinckel R *et al*. Complications of right heart catheterization procedures in patients with pulmonary hypertension in experienced centers. *J Am Coll Cardiol* 2006; 48:2546-2552.
60. Barst RJ, Rubin LJ, Long WA *et al*. A comparison of continuous intravenous epoprostenol (prostacyclin) with conventional therapy for primary pulmonary hypertension. The Primary Pulmonary Hypertension Study Group. *N Engl J Med* 1996; 334:296-302.
61. Badesch DB, Tapson VF, McGoon MD *et al*. Continuous intravenous epoprostenol for pulmonary hypertension due to the scleroderma spectrum of disease: a randomized, controlled trial. *Ann Intern Med* 2000; 132:425-434.
62. Rich S, McLaughlin VV. Effects of chronic prostacyclin therapy on cardiac output and symptoms in primary pulmonary hypertension. *J Am Coll Cardiol* 1999; 34:1184-1187.
63. http://www.veletri.com
64. Simonneau G, Barst RJ, Galie N *et al*. Continuous subcutaneous infusion of treprostinil, a prostacyclin analogue, in patients with pulmonary arterial hypertension: a double-blind, randomized, placebo-controlled trial. *Am J Respir Crit Care Med* 2002; 165:800-804.
65. Lang I, Gomez-Sanchez M, Kneussl M *et al*. Efficacy of long-term subcutaneous treprostinil sodium therapy in pulmonary hypertension. *Chest* 2006; 129:1636-1643.
66. Barst RJ, Galie N, Naeije R *et al*. Long-term outcome in pulmonary arterial hypertension patients treated with subcutaneous treprostinil. *Eur Respir J* 2006; 28:1195-1203.
67. Hiremath J, Thanikachalam S, Parikh K *et al*. Exercise improvement and plasma biomarker changes with intravenous treprostinil therapy for pulmonary arterial hypertension: a placebo-controlled trial. *J Heart Lung Transplant* 2010; 29:137-149.
68. Centers for Disease Control Report. Bloodstream infections among patients treated with intravenous epoprostenol or intravenous treprostinil for pulmonary hypertension – Seven Sites, United States, 2003-2006; MMWR, March 2, 2007.
69. McLaughlin VV, Benza RL, Rubin LJ *et al*. Addition of inhaled treprostinil to oral therapy for pulmonary arterial hypertension: a randomized controlled clinical trial. *J Am Coll Cardiol* 2010; 55:1915-1922.
70. Olschewski H, Simonneau G, Galie N *et al*. Inhaled iloprost for severe pulmonary hypertension. *N Engl J Med* 2002; 347:322-329.
71. Galie N, Ghofrani HA, Torbicki A *et al*. Sildenafil Use in Pulmonary Arterial Hypertension (SUPER) Study Group. Sildenafil citrate therapy for pulmonary arterial hypertension. *N Engl J Med* 2005; 353:2148-2157.
72. Galie N, Brundage BH, Ghofrani HA *et al*. Tadalafil therapy for pulmonary arterial hypertension. *Circulation* 2009; 119:2894-2903.

73. Rubin LJ, Badesch DB, Barst RJ *et al.* Bosentan therapy for pulmonary arterial hypertension. *N Engl J Med* 2002; 346:896-903.

74. McLaughlin VV, Sitbon O, Badesch DB *et al.* Survival with first-line bosentan in patients with primary pulmonary hypertension. *Eur Respir J* 2005; 25:244-249.

75. Galie N, Rubin LJ, Hoeper MM *et al.* Treatment of patients with mildly symptomatic pulmonary arterial hypertension with bosentan (EARLY study): a double-blind, randomized controlled trial. *Lancet* 2008; 317:2093-2100.

76. Galie N, Olschewski H, Oudiz R *et al.* Ambrosentan for the treatment of pulmonary arterial hypertension. Results of the ambrosentan in pulmonary arterial hypertension, randomized, double-blind, placebo-controlled, multicenter, efficacy (ARIES) study 1 and 2. *Circulation* 2008; 117:3010-3019.

77. McGoon M, Frost AE, Oudiz RJ *et al.* Ambrosentan therapy in patients with pulmonary arterial hypertension who discontinued bosentan or sitaxsentan due to liver function test abnormalities. *Chest* 2008; published online.

78. Highlights of prescribing information Letairis http://www.gilead.com/pdf/letairis_pi.pdf.

79. Bartst RJ, Langleben D, Frost A *et al.* Sitaxsentan therapy for pulmonary arterial hypertension. *Am J Respir Crit Care Med* 2004; 169:441-447.

80. Barst RJ, Langleben D, Badesch D *et al.* Treatment of pulmonary arterial hypertension with the selective endothelin-A receptor antagonist sitaxsentan. *J Am Coll Cardiol* 2006; 47:2049-2056.

81. Fuster V, Steele PM, Edwards WD *et al.* Primary pulmonary hypertension: natural history and the importance of thrombosis. *Circulation* 1984; 70:580-587.

82. Humber M, Barst RJ, Robbins IM *et al.* Combination of bosentan with epoprostenol in pulmonary arterial hypertension: BREATHE-2. *Eur Respir J* 2004; 24:353-359.

83. McLaughlinVV, Oudiz RJ, Frost A *et al.* Randomized study of adding inhaled iloprost to existing bosentan in pulmonary arterial hypertension. *Am J Respir Crit Care Med* 2006; 174:1257-1263.

84. Hoeper MM, Leuchte H, Halank M *et al.* Combining inhaled iloprost with bosentan in patients with idiopathic pulmonary arterial hypertension. *Eur Respir J* 2006; 28:691-694.

85. Simonneau G, Rubin LJ, Galie N *et al.* Addition of sildenafil to long-term intravenous epoprostenol therapy in patients with pulmonary arterial hypertension: a randomized trial. *Ann Intern Med* 2008; 149:521-530.

86. Rubin LJ. Introduction. Diagnosis and management of pulmonary arterial hypertension: ACCP evidence-based clinical practice guidelines. *Chest* 2004; 126:7S-10S.

87. Eysmann S, Palevsky H, Reichek N *et al.* Two-dimensional and Doppler-echocardiographic and cardiac catherization correlates of survival in primary pulmonary hypertension. *Circulation* 1989; 80:353-360.

88. Hinderliter A, Willis P 4th, Long W *et al.* Frequency and prognostic significance of pericardial effusion in primary pulmonary hypertension. PPH Study Group. *Am J Cardiol* 1999; 84:481-484.

89. Andreassen A, Wergeland R, Simonson S *et al.* N-terminal pro-B-type natriuretic peptide as an indicator of disease severity in a heterogeneous group of patients with chronic precapillary pulmonary hypertension. *Am J Cardiol* 2006; 98:525-529.

90. McLaughlin VV, McGoon MD. Pulmonary arterial hypertension. *Circulation* 2006; 114:1417-1431.

91. Califf RM, Adams KF, McKenna WJ *et al.* A randomized controlled trial of epoprostenol therapy for severe congestive heart failure: The Flolan International Randomized Survival Trial (FIRST). *Am Heart J* 1997; 134:44-54.

92. Mylona P, Cleland JG. Update of REACH-1 and MERIT-HF clinical trials in heart failure. *Eur J Heart Fail* 1999; 1:197-200.

93. Teerlink JR. Recent heart failure trials of neurohormonal modulation (OVERTURE and ENABLE): approaching the asymptote of efficacy? *J Card Fail* 2002; 8:124-127.

94. Perez-Villa F, Cuppoletti A, Rossel V *et al.* Initial experience with bosentan therapy in patients considered ineligible for heart transplantation because of severe pulmonary hypertension. *Clin Transplant* 2006; 20:239-244.

95. Lewis GD, Shah R, Shahzad K *et al.* Sildenafil improves exercise capacity and quality of life in patients with systolic heart failure and secondary pulmonary hypetension. *Circulation* 2007; 116:1555-1562.

96. Belenkie I, Dani R, Smith ER *et al.* Effects of volume loading during experimental acute pulmonary embolism. *Circulation* 1989; 80:178-188.

97. Molloy DW, Lee KY, Jones D *et al.* Effects of noradrenaline and isoproterenol on cardiopulmonary function in a canine model of acute pulmonary hypertension. *Chest* 1985; 88:432-435.

4

Will pharmacogenomics and pharmacogenetics transform heart failure therapy?

D. M. McNamara

'Variability is the law of life, ...and no two individuals react alike and behave alike under the abnormal conditions which we know as disease'
Sir William Osler, The Principles and Practice of Medicine [1]

'It is easy to get a thousand prescriptions but hard to get one single remedy.'
Chinese Proverb

OVERVIEW

Much of the variability in clinical response is based on genomic variation. *Pharmacogenetics* refers to the interaction of genetic variation at a single gene locus with the impact of drug intervention in terms of efficacy, metabolism and side-effects. Pharmacogenetic studies to date have primarily focused on a single gene locus known to be central to a drug's therapeutic response. Investigation of renin angiotensin and sympathetic activation suggest significant genetic variation does influence the therapeutic impact of angiotensin-converting-enzyme (ACE) inhibitors and beta blockade, and will one day allow clinicians to target subjects who receive the greatest benefit.

While for many drugs a variation in a single gene encoding an enzyme or receptor critical to its action will influence therapy, it is increasing recognized that variations at multiple loci usually act in concert to influence a given pharmacologic effect. The interaction of multiple sites on the human genome with drug action is referred to as *pharmacogenomics*. The use of pharmacogenomics as a clinical tool will require incorporation of multiple genomic drivers into a single clinical paradigm. The technique of Genome-Wide Association Studies (GWAS) uses large cohorts to investigate the contribution of the entire genome to a specific clinical risk assessment. GWAS will be the foundation of next wave in pharmacogenomics analysis and has the potential to provide a reliable prediction of an individual's expected benefit from a specific drug therapy. The day is coming when most clinical decisions, from the addition of beta blockers, to the implantation of an implantable cardioverter defibrillator (ICD) will be assisted by a genomic assessment of the risk/benefic ratio.

Dennis M. McNamara, MD, Professor of Medicine, Director, Heart Failure/Transplantation Program, Cardiovascular Institute, University of Pittsburgh Medical Center, Pittsburgh, PA, USA.

INTRODUCTION

Advances in medical therapy have markedly improved heart failure (HF) outcomes over the past two decades. Angiotensin-converting-enzyme (ACE) inhibitors [2], beta receptor antagonists (beta blockers) [3, 4] and aldosterone receptor antagonists [5, 6] all improve survival for subjects with systolic dysfunction. Recently the addition of isosorbide dinitrate and hydralazine (ISD-HYD) in fixed combination has been shown to improve survival in African-Americans with systolic HF [7]. As a result of data from clinical trials, evidence-based medicine must advocate polypharmacy [8]. Current guidelines would recommend that in order to optimize survival an African-American with class 3 HF from ischemic heart disease should be treated with seven drugs: an ACE inhibitor, beta blocker, aldosterone receptor antagonist, hydralazine and nitrates, aspirin and a statin. Give this same patient issues with fluid retention or diabetes, and his list of daily medications can easily grow and exceed ten or more. This growth in complexity of the medical regime comes at a cost: increased expense, unwanted side-effects, and a marked decrease in patient compliance. Pharmacogenomics will one day be used to develop personalized genomic 'signatures' which accurately predict drug efficacy, and allow targeting of medical therapeutics. The ability to tailor drug therapy to the individual patient rather than the 'cohort' will reduce polypharmacy, improve efficiency, and lower costs. Pharmacogenomics will transform HF therapy.

CLINICAL TRIALS, GUIDELINES, AND INDIVIDUAL BENEFIT

Clinical trials have been the driving force for improvements in medical therapy of HF over the past three decades. The addition of ACE inhibitors and beta blockers to the treatment of symptomatic HF has led to significant reductions in the annual mortality rate [9]. While these advances in medical therapy have improved outcomes in *populations* with heart failure, the response in *individual* patients is more difficult to delineate. For example, treatment with beta blockers in Metoprolol CR/XL Randomized Intervention Trial in Congestive Heart Failure (MERIT-HF) led to a marked improvement in survival compared with subjects treated with placebo [10], with a decline in mortality rate from 18% on placebo to 12% on therapy at the end of 18 months. However this also means that over 80% of individuals on placebo were alive and well at the end of the study in the absence of any beta blocker therapy. Will these 'placebo survivors' still benefit from beta blockers? In addition, despite receiving therapy with beta blockade, 12% of the treatment group still died. These 'treatment failures' may have been candidates for alternative therapies if they could be identified pre-mortem. The ability to better predict these outcomes based on genomics would allow clinicians to more efficiently target beta blocker therapy to those subjects who benefit.

GENOMIC VARIATION

There is significant diversity in the genome and over the last decade investigations have been focused on the influence of genetic variability on clinical outcomes and therapeutic efficacy. Genetic variation or polymorphisms generally consist of either single nucleotide polymorphisms (SNPs) or insertions (or deletions) of sections of DNA. These polymorphisms affect the function of the gene product in two ways: alter the amount of protein produced or alter the functional activity of the protein itself. Deletions which occur in the coding region (which encodes the amino acid sequence) frequently result in a truncated, less functional protein. SNPs in the coding region can alter the amino acid sequence and influence enzymatic or receptor function. Insertions/deletions or SNPs in non-coding regions will not alter the amino acid sequence of the protein, however, such polymorphisms may alter the *amount of protein produced* if they affect transcriptional activity or message (mRNA [ribonucleic acid]) stability. SNPs in the coding region which do not alter amino acid sequence are functionally 'silent' and unlikely to affect gene function or regulation, however, they may still serve as markers linked (that is likely to be co-inherited) to more functionally significant polymorphisms in relatively close proximity.

PHARMACOGENOMICS OF HF

NEUROHORMONAL INHIBITORS AND THE ACE D/I POLYMORPHISM

Renin angiotensin activation plays a central role in HF progression [11], and pharmacologic inhibition of the ACE by ACE inhibitors reliably improves survival in populations with HF [12, 13]. The degree of ACE activation and rate of HF progression vary significantly among individual patients, and a significant portion of this is derived from genetic variation at the ACE gene locus [14]. The ACE deletion/insertion (D/I) polymorphism is a model for how genetic variation of a central mediator enzyme can affect HF outcomes and influence the impact of pharmacologic therapy. This polymorphism is based on the presence or absence of a 287 base pair segment or 'insertion' in a regulatory region of intron 16, and has been studied extensively in cardiovascular disease. In most populations, the D allele is slightly more prevalent than the I allele, and on average 30% of subjects are homozygous for the D allele (ACE DD genotype) 50% are heterozygous (ACE DI), and 20% are homozygous for the I allele (ACE-II). The D/I polymorphism in a non-coding region does not change the ACE enzyme amino acid sequence, but by improving translation into protein, the D allele is consistently linked to higher ACE activity and angiotensin II levels [15] and, as a result, greater left ventricular remodeling after myocardial infarction [16, 17].

Given the linkage of the D allele with greater ACE activity, subjects with this allele should have poorer HF outcomes. Indeed, the D allele has been associated with poorer HF survival in three prospective studies involving nearly 2000 subjects, including cohorts with non-ischemic cardiomyopathy [18], post myocardial infarction [19] and in a mixed population of subjects referred to a tertiary sub-specialty clinic [20, 21]. In a prospective genetic outcomes analysis from the University of Pittsburgh (GRACE, Genetic Risk Assessment of Cardiac Events) the adverse impact of the ACE deletion for subjects with HF was eliminated by treatment with beta blockers [21] (Figure 4.1). Selective antagonists and non-selective antagonists are equally effective [22], and the pharmacogenetic interaction of the ACE D allele and beta blockers appears to be mediated by the β_1 receptor. Control of renin release in the kidney by adrenergic stimulation is also through β_1 receptors [23], and blockade of this receptor reduces plasma renin. This is an important aspect of the antihypertensive action of beta blockade and appears to be the likely mechanism for this pharmacogenetic interaction as well.

A significant pharmacogenetic interaction also exits for the ACE D/I polymorphism and the impact of ACE inhibitors. The impact of ACE inhibitors on blood pressure is affected by ACE D genotype [24, 25]. ACE DD subjects have a greater tendency toward 'ACE inhibitor escape' or a failure of ACE inhibitor treatment to suppress neurohormonal activation [26, 27]. In analysis from GRACE, high-dose ACE inhibitors did diminish the adverse impact of the D allele [21] (Figure 4.2). For both ACE inhibitor dose and beta blockers, analysis of reduction in relative risk demonstrated that the benefit of therapy was greatest in ACE DD patients, diminished in heterozygotes, and minimal in ACE-II homozygotes.

While overall neurohormonal blockade is beneficial for HF subjects, determining the optimal degree and nature of inhibition is complex [28], and recent attempts to improve survival by increasing neurohormonal blockade have been unsuccessful. The ATLAS trial compared survival in subjects treated with high-doses of the ACE inhibitor Lisinopril (mean daily dose greater than 30 mg) with a cohort treated with low dose (mean daily dose approximately 3 mg) and failed to demonstrate significant improvement, though a modest trend was evident with high-dose (8% risk reduction) [29]. The combination of therapy with ACE

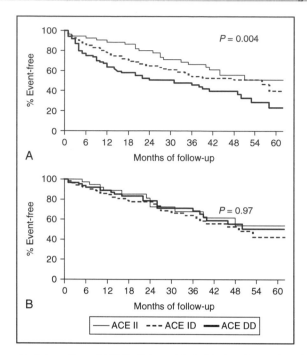

Figure 4.1 Pharmacogenetic interaction of ACE D allele and beta blockers in a cohort in subjects from the GRACE study. (A) Transplant-free survival by ACE genotype for subjects with systolic heart failure not treated with beta blockers ($n=277$). ACE D allele associated with poor outcome ($P=0.004$) (B) Transplant-free survival by ACE genotype for subjects treated with beta blocker ($n=202$) demonstrates the impact of the ACE D allele is no longer evident ($P=0.97$) (with permission from [21]).

inhibitors and angiotensin receptor blockers (ARBs) in Valsartan Heart Failure Trial (Val-Heft) also failed to improve survival [30]. While these trials demonstrated no benefit for maximal inhibition in a *population* with HF, it is likely that selected *individuals* may benefit. Genetic testing of the ACE gene locus was not performed in these trials but would have allowed investigators to target the one-third of HF subjects (those with the ACE DD geno-type) who get the greatest benefit from either high-dose ACE inhibitors or a combination of ACE inhibitors and ARBs. By eliminating those patients less likely to benefit, a 'pharmaco-genetically targeted' ATLAS trial for example, would potentially demonstrate a much greater impact of high-dose ACE inhibitors in ACE DD subjects.

BETA RECEPTOR POLYMORPHISMS AND BETA BLOCKER THERAPY

The therapeutic impact of beta blockers in HF reflects not only their impact through β_1 receptors inhibiting renin release, but their direct effects on myocardial β_1 and β_2 receptors [31–33]. Two β_1 and three β_2 receptor polymorphisms influence receptor function or down regulation *in vitro* (Table 4.1) and have been reported to influence therapeutic efficacy in subjects with hypertension, asthma and HF [34]. The β_2 Gly27Gln and Glu16Arg polymor-phisms are in the extracellular region and influence receptor down regulation (Figure 4.3B). In contrast the Ile164Thr polymorphism is in the core region and the Ile164 variant is less responsive to agonist stimulation [35], and is linked to poorer exercise capacity [36] and prognosis in HF cohorts [37]. The low frequency of the adverse allele, only 1–3% of the

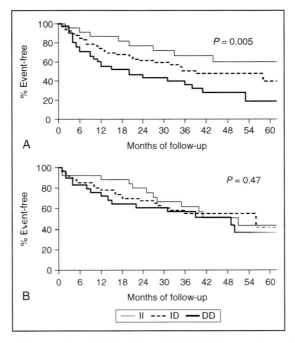

Figure 4.2 Pharmacogenetic interaction of ACE D allele and ACE inhibitor dose in a cohort in GRACE. (A) Transplant-free survival by ACE genotype for subjects with systolic heart failure on low dose ACE inhibitors and no beta blockers (*n*=130). ACE D allele associated with markedly poor outcome (*P*=0.005) (B) Transplant-free survival by ACE genotype for subjects treated with high-dose ACE inhibitors and no beta bloackers (*n*=117) demonstrates the impact of the ACE D allele is diminished (*P*=0.47) (with permission from [21]).

Table 4.1 Frequency and functional significance of common beta adrenergic receptor polymorphisms (with permission from [34])

Codon	Region	Polymorphism	Allele frequency	Function in vitro
β_1				
389	Cytoplasmic	Arg/Gly	0.70/0.30	Arg=gain of function ($\uparrow$cAMP)
49	Extracellular	Ser/Gly	0.85/0.15	Gly=enhanced downregulation
β_2				
16	Extracellular	Arg/Gly	0.40/0.60	Gly=enhanced downregulation
27	Extracellular	Gln/Glu	0.55/0.45	Glu=resistance to downregulation
164	Transmembrane Domain #4	Thr/Ile	0.95/0.05	Ile=loss of function $\downarrow$ agonist binding, $\downarrow$ cAMP

Arg=arginine; cAMP=cyclic adenosine monophosphate; Gln=glutamine; Glu=glutamate; Gly=glycine; Ile=isoleucine; Ser=serine; Thr=threonine.

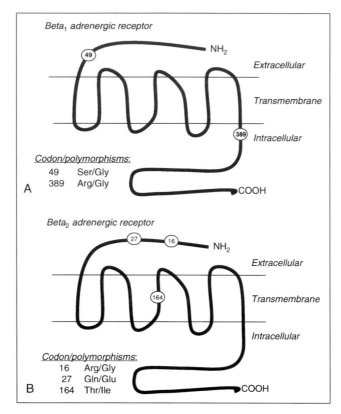

Figure 4.3 (A) Structure of the β₁ Adrenergic Receptor: Common Polymorphisms: Ser=serine, Gly=glycine, Arg=arginine, NH₂=amino terminus, COOH=carboxyl terminus. (B) Structure of the β₂ Adrenergic Receptor: Common Polymorphisms: Arg=arginine, Gly=glycine, Gln=glutamine, Glu=glutamate, Thr=threonine, Ile=Isoleucine, NH₂=amino terminus, COOH=carboxyl terminus (with permission from [34]).

population is heterozygous for Ile164, has thus far limited pharmacogenetic investigations.

For β₁, the Gly49Ser is also in the extracellular region (Figure 4.3A) and influences receptor down regulation. The Gly49 variant has enhanced receptor down regulation compared to Ser49 [38, 39] and this appears to influence HF survival [40]. The strongest evidence for pharmacogenetic interactions with beta blockade in HF exists for the β₁ Arg389Gly polymorphism. This polymorphism is in the intracellular region and influences the production of cAMP in response to catecholamine stimulation. The Arg variant is more active in response to agonist stimulation *in vitro* and is more prevalent than the Gly389, with approximately 50% of white subjects being homozygous for Arg389. In the genetic substudy of the Beta Blocker Evaluation of Survival Trial (BEST) study, a large NHLBI sponsored trial of beta blocker therapy with bucindolol [41], the therapeutic efficacy of beta blockade was marked among Arg389Arg homozygotes, but less evident among subjects with at least a single Gly389 allele [42] (Figure 4.4).

This influence of the Arg389 allele on beta blocker effectiveness was not evident in an earlier investigation from the MERIT trial with metoprolol succinate in class III HF [43], and this genetic analysis found that beta blockers were equally effective regardless of Arg389 genotype. While the contrast between genetic analysis of BEST and MERIT may reflect dif-

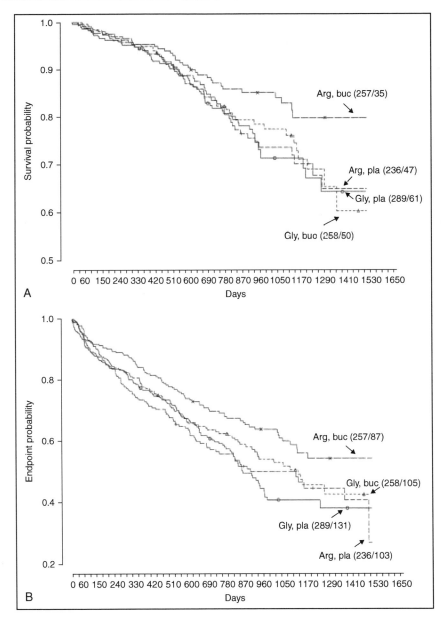

Figure 4.4 Kaplan–Meier analysis from BEST stratified by treatment and β_1AR genotype. (A) Survival: bucindolol improved survival for Arg389Arg (HR=0.62, P=0.03), but not in β_1-Gly-389 carriers (HR=0.90, P=0.57). (B) Combined endpoint: bucindolol improved free from HF hospitalization: for Arg289Arg homozygotes (HR=0.66, P=0.004), to a greater degree than evident in β_1-Gly-389 carriers (HR=0.87, P=0.25).

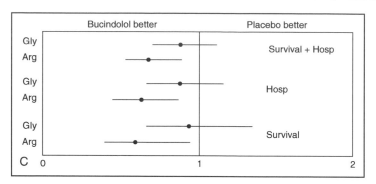

Figure 4.4 Kaplan–Meier analysis from BEST stratified by treatment and β₁AR genotype. (C) Hazard ratios and confidence intervals by bucindolol and placebo is shown for survival, hospitalization and combined endpoint in genotype subsets (with permission from [42]).

ferences in the receptor sensitivities of the two agents, the differences in the two outcomes may reflect differences in 'genetic background' or the prevalence of polymorphisms in other areas of the genome which modify the impact of Arg389, particularly since MERIT was a European investigation and BEST was performed in the United States. Variation in alpha adrenergic receptors is one important modifier that appears to influence the effect of the beta receptor variants. The alpha 2c receptor has a common deletion allele missing four amino acids [44] which affects the reuptake of catecholamines by the presynaptic cell [45, 46] and magnifies the effect of the Arg389 receptor. The coinheritance of Arg389 and alpha 2C increases the risk of HF in African-Americans [47]. In a study of the impact of metoprolol on left ventricular ejection fraction (LVEF), co-inheritance of the alpha2C deletion and Arg389Arg genotype predicted the greatest therapeutic impact of beta blockade [48]. Recent similar analysis from BEST [49] suggests predictive models of beta blocker response need to incorporate both loci.

RACE, GENOMICS, AND HF THERAPY

The clinical trials which formed the foundation of HF treatment guidelines were performed in predominantly white cohorts, however, the effectiveness of HF therapeutics appears to be distinctly different in blacks [50, 51]. Analysis by racial subset of the V-HeFT investigations suggests the efficacy of ACE inhibitors was greater among whites, while the combination of ISDN-HYD appeared more effective in the black subset [52–54]. This observation led to African American Heart Failure trial (A-HeFT) [55] which demonstrated the addition of ISDN-HYD to standard HF treatment improved survival in a cohort of self designated African-Americans with systolic HF [7]. Food and Drug Administration (FDA) approval of a fixed combination of ISDN-HYD specifically in blacks was the first such drug approved for a specific racial/ethnic cohort and remains controversial [56, 57]. Race, however, is likely a poor surrogate marker for genomic differences which influence drug efficacy, and the search for more specific genetic biomarkers continues [58].

Common polymorphisms in genes which control vascular tone have been investigated for their role in the development of essential hypertension. Hypertension is much more prevalent in blacks and significant racial differences in the prevalence of genomic variants are evident for endothelial nitric oxide synthase (NOS3), aldosterone synthase, and alpha and beta adrenergic receptors. In addition to their role in hypertension, these genetic loci also play central roles in HF pathogenesis and therapeutics. The role of genetic polymor-

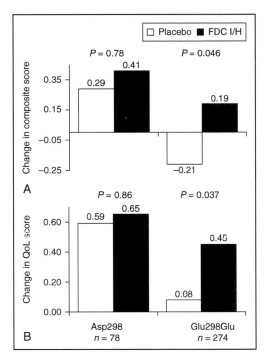

Figure 4.5 Interaction of NOS3 Glu298Asp polymorphisms on the impact of therapy with FDC I/H on outcomes. (A) Effect on composite score: treatment associated with improvement in the Glu298Glu homozygotes ($n=274$, $P=0.046$), but not in subjects with the Asp298 allele ($n=78$, $P=0.78$). (B) Effect on change in QoL: Significant improvement in the change of QoL score at 6 months from baseline in Glu298Glu subjects ($P=0.037$) but not with the Asp298 (with permission from [65]). FDC I/H=fixed-dose combination of isosorbide dinitrate/hydralazine; QoL=quality of Life.

phisms in HF in African-Americans was investigated in the genetic substudy of the A-HeFT trial (Genetic Risk in African Americans with Heart Failure, GRAHF). This genetic outcomes analysis was designed to determine whether genetic alleles would predict benefit from treatment with ISDN-HYD. As the prevalence of several polymorphisms of NOS3, the primary source of vascular nitric oxide (NO) production [59], differs markedly in black and white cohorts [60, 61], this locus emerged as a prime candidate for a genetic modifier of therapeutic efficacy. A polymorphism exists in exon 7 of NOS3 which results in the substitution of Glutamic acid for Aspartic acid at codon 298. The Asp298 variant is a reported risk factor for hypertension [62], coronary disease [63], and poor HF survival [64]. The Glu298 variant is far more prevalent in black cohorts. For the primary endpoint in A-HeFT, a composite score of survival, HF hospitalization and quality of life, subjects in GRAHF with the Glu298Glu genotype received significant benefit from therapy, while subjects with the Asp298 variant did not [65] (Figure 4.5). Further investigation is required to determine whether NOS3 genotype can effectively target NO donor therapy.

Racial differences also exist in the genomics of aldosterone synthesis. Aldosterone plays a significant role in hypertension and HF [66], and aldosterone synthase is the rate limiting enzyme in aldosterone production. A polymorphism in the promoter region (-344 T/C) in a steroid binding sequence appears to affect transcription [67] with the -344C allele associated with increased aldosterone production and hypertension [68, 69]. In GRAHF, the C allele linked to higher aldosterone production was also linked to poorer outcomes [70]

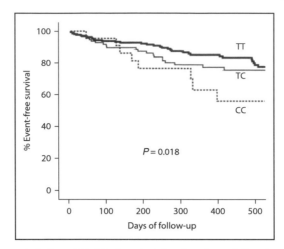

Figure 4.6 Kaplan–Meier analysis from A-HeFT of survival free from heart failure hospitalization; impact of Aldosterone synthase (CYP11B2) promoter genotype. The −344C allele linked to increase aldosterone associated with poorer event free survival (P=0.018) (with permission from [70]).

(Figure 4.6). This polymorphism also appears to influence left ventricular remodeling in HF [71, 72], and this appears to be the mechanism of the adverse impact of the −344C allele in GRAHF. A remodeling substudy of A-HeFT investigated the influence of therapy on left ventricular ejection fraction after 6 months, and the −344C allele was associated with lower ejection fraction for subjects on placebo but not for those treated with the ISD-HYD [70, 73] (Figure 4.7). Surprisingly, while treatment with ISDN-HYD eliminated the impact of −344C allele on remodeling, treatment with aldosterone receptor antagonists had no effect [73] (Figure 4.8). In terms of the utility of the aldosterone promoter polymorphism for targeting treatment, determination of who will obtain the most benefit from an NO donor will require analysis of several key genomic loci.

GWAS AND THE FUTURE

To date, most studies of pharmacogenetic interaction have been small genetic outcome studies, with no more than 1000 subjects in the larger multi center cohorts, and frequently less than 500 subjects in single center studies. These investigations generally have been limited to a single candidate 'gene of interest', and are of insufficient power to investigate gene–gene interactions. This prevents the evaluation of genomic modifiers of 'targeting' alleles. Given the conflicting results of many single gene studies and the absence of any prospective validation studies, there is no variant or polymorphism yet approved for use in targeting therapeutics. The hope of most investigators is that a broader approach which encompasses the entire genome and simultaneously incorporates several genetic drivers and their background modifiers will be necessary prior to the successful application of genomically tailored therapeutics.

Recent advance in technology have made large scale mapping of the human genome more efficient and affordable, as the realization that most human DNA is 'inherited' in large blocks or haplotypes has led to the development of high density genomic 'maps' [74]. This has facilitated Genome-Wide Association Studies (GWAS) where the frequency of variants or markers across the entire genome is assessed in large cohorts with a disorder under investigation and compared to a large control group. This technology has been

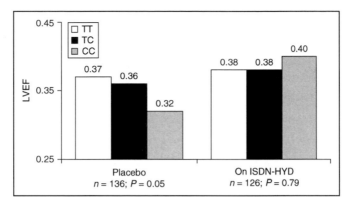

Figure 4.7 LVEF at 6 months in A-HeFT: comparison by treatment group, placebo or ISDN-HYD (fixed combination of isosorbide dinitrate and hydralazine) of the impact of aldosterone promoter genotype. The −344C allele associated with lower LVEF at six months for subjects on placebo ($P=0.05$) but not on ISDN-HYD ($P=0.79$) (with permission from [73]).

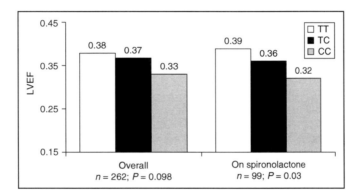

Figure 4.8 A-HeFT: impact of aldosterone promoter genotype on LVEF at 6 months overall and in subjects treated with aldosterone receptor antagonist (sprironolactone). The −344C allele associated with a trend toward lower LVEF at six months overall ($P=0.098$) which was more pronounced for subjects on spironolactone ($P=0.03$) (with permission from [73]).

applied to common complex polygenic diseases such as coronary disease [75], hyperlipidemia [76], and diabetes [77], and has led to an explosion of new information about novel genes contributing to these complex disorders. GWAS technology has thus far only been applied to risk factor analysis and not yet to pharmacogenomics, mostly because they require very large cohorts (generally several thousand in both the control and comparison groups) not yet available for outcomes analysis. Once appropriate sized cohorts are obtained (e.g. 2000 subjects who improve their LVEF and NYHA class on beta blockers, compared 2000 who do poorly on therapy) GWAS would allow the identification of all genomic loci which influence and mediate any therapeutic response. Such analysis will be the beginning of converting genomics into a reliable clinical tool for efficiently targeting therapeutics.

SUMMARY

Genetic variation of key HF mediators alters the impact of therapeutics acting on that pathway. Subjects genetically predisposed to greater renin-angiotensin activation by the presence of the ACE deletion allele obtain greater benefit from therapies (beta blockers and high-dose ACE inhibitors) designed to blunt this response. In addition, subjects with the more active β_1 389Arg variant appear to obtain more clinical benefit when that receptor is blocked, than subjects with the less active 389Gly variant. Significant genetic differences in the NO pathway exist between white and black HF cohorts, and may underlie the apparent enhanced response in African-Americans to treatment with ISDN-HYD.

All these examples demonstrate the potential power of pharmacogenomics to target treatments and transform HF therapy.

Given the potential power of this transformation, why is it still in the future and not yet a clinical reality? Despite these findings in single gene studies over the last decade, disagreement between pharmacogenetic analysis in clinical trials such as BEST and MERIT, and the lack of prospective validation studies have prevented pharmacogenomics from entering into clinical use in tailoring HF therapeutics. Much of the difficulties in replication reflect the limitations of single gene analysis in complex processes such as beta blocker response which are clearly polygenic. Large scale prospective studies including GWAS hold much promise and will allow identification of all key genomic drivers necessary to reliable predict clinical response. In the words of an editorial early in this decade, pharmacogenomics is still '*not ready for prime time but getting there*' [78]. Given the accelerated pace of recent investigations, it is likely that genomic predictions will soon become a part tailoring HF therapeutics.

REFERENCES

1. Osler W. *The Principles and Practice of Medicine*. D. Appleton and Co., New York, 1892.
2. Braunwald E. ACE inhibitors – a cornerstone of the treatment of heart failure. *N Engl J Med* 1991; 325:351-353.
3. Packer M, Bristow MR, Cohn JN, *et al*. The effect of carvedilol on morbidity and mortality in patients with chronic heart failure. *N Engl J Med* 1996; 334:1349-1355.
4. MERIT-HF Study group. Effect of Metoprolol CR/XL in chronic heart failure: Metoprolol CR/XL Randomized Intervention Trial in Congestive Heart Failure (MERIT-HF). *Lancet* 1999; 353:2001-2007.
5. Pitt B, Zannad F, Remme WJ, Cody R *et al*. The effect of spironolactone on morbidity and mortality in patients with severe heart failure. Randomized Aldactone Evaluation Study Investigators. *N Engl J Med* 1999; 341:709-717.
6. Pitt B, Remme W, Zannad F, Neaton J *et al*. Eplerenone Post-Acute Myocardial Infarction Heart Failure Efficacy and Survival Study Investigators. Eplerenone, a selective aldosterone blocker, in patients with left ventricular dysfunction after myocardial infarction. *N Engl J Med* 2003; 348:1309-1321.
7. Taylor AL, Ziesche S, Yancy C *et al*. Combination of isosorbide dinitrate and hydralazine in blacks with heart failure. *N Engl J Med* 2004; 351:2049-2057.
8. Parmley WW. How many medicines do patients with heart failure need? *Circulation* 2001; 103:1611-1612.
9. McMurray JJ. Major beta blocker mortality trials in chronic heart failure: a critical review. *Heart* 1999; (suppl 4):IV14-IV22.
10. Hjalmarson A, Goldstein S, Fagerberg B *et al*. The effects of controlled release metoprolol on total mortality, hospitalizations and well-being in patients with heart failure (MERIT-HF). *JAMA* 2000; 283:1295-1302.
11. Packer M. The neurohormonal hypothesis: a theory to explain the mechanism of disease progression in heart failure. *J Am Coll Cardiol* 1992; 20:248-254.
12. Pfeffer MA. Angiotensin-converting enzyme inhibition in congestive heart failure: benefit and perspective. *Am Heart J* 1993; 126:789-793.
13. Greenberg BH. Effects of angiotensin converting enzyme inhibitors on remodeling in clinical trials. *J Card Fail* 2002; (6 Suppl):S486-S490.

14. Rigat B, Hubert C, Alhenc-Gelas F, Cambien F, Corvol P, Soubrier F. An insertion/deletion polymorphism in the angiotensin I-converting enzyme gene accounting for half the variance of serum enzyme levels. *J Clin Invest* 1990; 86:1343-1346.

15. Tiret L, Rigat B, Visvikis S *et al*. Evidence, from combined segregation and linkage analysis, that a variant of the angiotensin I-converting enzyme (ACE) gene controls plasma ACE levels. *Am J Hum Genet* 1992; 51:197-205.

16. Nagashima J, Musha H, So T, Kunishima T, Nobuoka S, Murayama M. Effect of angiotensin-converting enzyme gene polymorphism on left ventricular remodeling after anteroseptal infarction. *Clin Cardiol* 1999; 22:587-590.

17. Ulgen MS, Ozturk O, Alan S *et al*. The relationship between angiotensin-converting enzyme (insertion/deletion) gene polymorphism and left ventricular remodeling in acute myocardial infarction. *Coron Artery Dis* 2007; 18:153-157.

18. Andersson B, Sylven C. The DD genotype of the angiotensin-converting enzyme gene is associated with increased mortality in idiopathic heart failure. *J Am Coll Cardiol* 1996; 28:162-167.

19. Palmer BR, Pilbrow AP, Yandle TG *et al*. Angiotensin-converting enzyme gene polymorphism interacts with left ventricular ejection fraction and brain natriuretic peptide levels to predict mortality after myocardial infarction. *J Am Coll Cardiol* 2003; 41:729-736.

20. McNamara DM, Holubkov R, Janosko K *et al*. Pharmacogenetic interactions between beta blocker therapy and the angiotensin converting enzyme deletion polymorphism in patients with congestive heart failure. *Circulation* 2001; 103:1644-1648.

21. McNamara DM, Holubkov R, Postava L *et al*. Phamacogenetic interactions between ACE inhibitor therapy and the angiotensin-converting enzyme deletion polymorphism in patients with congestive heart failure. *J Am Coll Cardiol* 2004; 44:2019-2026.

22. Ishizawar D, Teuteberg JJ, Cadaret LM, Mathier MA, McNamara DM. Impact of B selectivity on the pharmacogenetic interaction of the ACE D/I polymorphisms and b blockers. *Clin Transl Sci* 2008; 1:151-154.

23. Oates HF, Stoker LM, Monaghan JC, Stokes GS. The beta-adrenergic receptor controlling renin release. *Arch Int Pharmacodyn Ther* 1978; 234:205-213.

24. Ueda S, Meredith PA, Morton JJ *et al*. ACE (I/D) genotype as a predictor of the magnitude and duration of the response to an ACE inhibitor drug (enalaprilat) in humans. *Circulation* 1998; 98:2148-2153.

25. Bhatnagar V, O'Connor DT, Schork NJ *et al*. Angiotensin-converting enzyme gene polymorphism predicts the time-course of blood pressure response to angiotensin converting enzyme inhibition in the AASK trial. *J Hypertens* 2007; 25:2082-2092.

26. Tang WHW, Vagelos RH, Yee YG *et al*. Impact of angiotensin-converting enzyme gene polymorphism on neurohormonal responses to high- versus low-dose enalapril in advanced heart failure. *Am Heart J* 2004; 148:889-894.

27. Cicoira J, Zanolla L, Rossi A *et al*. Failure of aldosterone suppression despite angiotensin-converting enzyme (ACE) inhibitor administration in chronic heart failure is associated with ACE DD genotype. *J Am Coll Cardiol* 2001; 37:1808-1812.

28. Mehra MR, Uber PA, Francis GS. Heart failure therapy at a crossroad: are there limits to the neurohormonal model? *Am Coll Cardiol* 2003; 41:1606-1610.

29. Packer M, Poole-Wilson PA, Armstrong PW *et al*. Comparative effects of low and high doses of the angiotensin-converting enzyme inhibitor, lisinopril, on morbidity and mortality in chronic heart failure. *Circulation* 1999; 100:2312-2318.

30. Cohn JN, Tognoni G; Valsartan Heart Failure Trial Investigators. A randomized trial of the angiotensin-receptor blocker valsartan in chronic heart failure. *N Engl J Med* 2001; 345:1667-1675.

31. Feldman DS, Carnes CA, Abraham WT *et al*. Mechanisms of disease β-adrenergic receptors – alternations in signal transduction and pharmacogenomics in heart failure. *Cardio Med* 2005; 2:475-483.

32. Brodde OE. β_1 and β_2 adrenoceptor polymorphisms: functional importance, impact on cardiovascular diseases and drug responses. *Pharmacol Ther* 2008; 117:1-29.

33. Muthumala A, Drenos F, Elliott PM *et al*. Role of β adrenergic receptor polymorphisms in heart failure: systematic review and meta-analysis. *Eur J Heart Fail* 2008; 10:3-13.

34. McNamara DM, MacGowan GA, London B. Clinical importance of beta receptor polymorphisms in cardiovascular disease. *Am J Pharamcogenomics* 2001; 2:73-78.

35. Brodde OE, Buscher R, Tellkamp R *et al*. Blunted cardiac responses to receptor activation in subjects with Thr164Ile β_2-adrenoceptors. *Circulation* 2001; 103:1048-1050.

36. Wagoner LE, Craft LL, Singh B et al. Polymorphisms of the [beta]$_2$-adrenergic receptor determine exercise capacity in patients with heart failure. Circ Res 2000; 86:834-840.

37. Liggett SB, Wagoner LE, Craft LL et al. The Ile164 β$_2$-adrenergic receptor polymorphism adversely affects the outcome of congestive heart failure. J Clin Invest 1998; 102:1534-1539.

38. Levin MC, Marullo S, Muntaner O et al. The myocardium-protective Gly-49 variant of the β$_1$-adrenergic receptor exhibits constitutive activity and increased desensitization and down-regulation. J Biol Chem 2002; 277:30429-30435.

39. Rathz DA, Brown KM, Kramer LA, Liggett SB. Amino acid 49 polymorphisms of the human [beta]$_1$-adrenergic receptor affect agonist-promoted trafficking. J Cardiovasc Pharmacol 2002; 39:155-160.

40. Börjesson M, Magnusson Y, Hjalmarson A et al. A novel polymorphism in the gene coding for the beta (1)-adrenergic receptor associated with survival in patients with heart failure. Eur Heart J 2000; 21:1853-1858.

41. The BEST Investigators. A trial of the beta blocker bucindolol in patients with advanced chronic heart failure. New Engl J Med 2001; 344:1659-1667.

42. Liggett SB, Mialet-Perez J, Thaneemit-Chen S et al. A polymorphism within a conserved β$_1$-adrenergic receptor motif alters cardiac function and β-blocker response in human heart failure. Proc Natl Acad Sci USA 2006; 103:11288-11293.

43. White H, deBoer RA, Maqbool A et al. An evaluation of the beta-1 adrenergic receptor Arg389Gly polymorphism in individuals with heart failure: a MERIT-HF sub-study. Eur J Heart Fail 2003; 5:463-468.

44. Small KM, Forbes SL, Rahman FF et al. A four amino acid deletion polymorphism in the third intracellular loop of the human α$_{2C}$-adrenergic receptor confers impaired coupling to multiple effectors. J Biol Chem 2000; 275:23059-23064.

45. Small KM, Mialet-Perez J, Seman CA et al. Polymorphisms of cardiac presynaptic α$_{2C}$ adrenergic receptors: diverse intragenic variability with haplotype-specific function effects. PNAS 2004; 101:13020-13025.

46. Gerson MC, Wagoner LE, McGuire N, Liggett SB. Activity of the uptake-1 norepinephrine transporter as measured by I-123 MIBG in heart failure patients with a loss-of-function polymorphism of the presynaptic α$_{2C}$-adrenergic receptor. J Nucl Cardiol 2003; 10:583-589.

47. Small KM, Wagoner LE, Levin AM et al. Synergistic polymorphisms of beta1- and alpha2C-adrenergic receptors and the risk of congestive heart failure. N Engl J Med 2002; 347:1135-1142.

48. Lobmeyer MT, Gong Y, Terra SG et al. Synergistic polymorphisms of β$_1$ and α$_{2c}$-adrenergic receptors and the influence on left ventricular ejection fraction response to β–blocker therapy in heart failure. Pharma Geno 2007; 17:277-282.

49. O'Connor CM, Anand I, Fiuzat M et al. Additive effects of beta-1 389 Arg/Gly and alpha-2c 322-325 wild-type/del genotype combinations on adjudicated hospitalizations and death in the Beta Blocker Evaluation of Survival Trial (BEST). Heart Fail Soc Am 2008. Toronto, ON: Scientific Meeting, September 2008.

50. Taylor JS, Ellis GR. Racial differences in responses to drug treatment: implications for pharmacotherapy of heart failure. Am J Cardiovasc Drugs 2002; 2:389-399.

51. Exner DV, Dries DL, Domanski MJ, Cohn JN. Lesser response to angiotensin-converting-enzyme inhibitor therapy in black as compared with white patients with left ventricular dysfunction. N Engl J Med 2001; 344:1351-1357.

52. Cohn JN, Archibald DG, Ziesche S et al. Effect of vasodilator therapy on mortality in chronic congestive heart failure. Results of a Veterans Administration Cooperative Study. N Engl J Med 1986; 314:1547-1552.

53. Cohn JN, Johnson G, Ziesche S et al. A comparison of enalapril with hydralazine-isosorbide dinitrate in the treatment of chronic congestive heart failure. N Engl J Med 1991; 325:303-310.

54. Carson P, Ziesche S, Johnson G, Cohn JN. Racial differences in response to therapy for heart failure: analysis of the vasodilator-heart failure trials. Vasodilator-Heart Failure Trial Study Group. J Card Fail 1999; 5:178-187.

55. Taylor AL. The African-American Heart Failure Trial (A-HeFT): rationale and methodology. J Card Fail 2003; 9(5 suppl Nitric Oxide):S216-S219.

56. Cohn J. The use of race and ethnicity in medicine: lessons from the African-American heart failure trial. J Law Med Ethics 2006; Fall:552-553.

57. Kahn J. Race, pharmacogenomics, and marketing: putting BiDil in context. Am J Bioethics 2006; 6:5, W1-W5.

58. Cooper RS, Kaufman JS, Ward R. Race and genomics. *N Engl J Med* 2003; 348:1166-1175.
59. Hare JM. Nitroso-redox balance in the cardiovascular system. *N Engl J Med* 2004; 351:2112-2114.
60. Tanus-Santos JE, Desai M, Flockhart DA. Effects of ethnicity on the distribution of clinically relevant endothelial nitric oxide variants. *Pharmacogenetics* 2001; 11:719-725.
61. Marroni AS, Metzger IF, Souza-Costa DC *et al*. Consistent interethnic difference in the distribution of clinically relevant endothelial nitric oxide synthase genetic polymorphisms. *Nitric Oxide* 2005; 12:177-182.
62. Jáchymová M, Horký K, Bultas J *et al*. Association of the Glu298Asp polymorphism in the endothelial nitric oxide synthase gene with essential hypertension resistant to conventional therapy. *Biochem Biophys Res Commun* 2001; 284:426-430.
63. Hingorani AD, Liang CF, Fatibene J *et al*. A common variant of the endothelial nitric oxide synthase (Glu^{298}→Asp) is a major risk factor for coronary artery disease in the UK. *Circulation* 1999; 100:1515.
64. McNamara DM, Holubkov R, Postava L *et al*. The Asp^{298} variant of endothelial nitric oxide synthase: Effect on survival for patients with congestive heart failure. *Circulation* 2003; 107:1598-1602.
65. McNamara DM, Tam SW, Sabolinski ML *et al*. Endothelial nitric oxide synthase (NOS3) polymorphisms in African Americans with heart failure: results from the A-HeFT trial. *J Card Fail* 2009; 15:191-198
66. Weber KT. Aldosterone in congestive heart failure. *N Engl J Med* 2001; 345:1689-1698.
67. White PC, Hautanen A, Kupari M. Aldosterone synthase (CYP11B2) polymorphisms and cardiovascular function. *J Steroid Biochem Mol Biol* 1999; 69:409-412.
68. Pojoga L, Gautier S, Blanc H *et al*. Genetic determination of plasma aldosterone levels in essential hypertension. *Am J Hypertens* 1998; 11:856-860.
69. Davies E, Holloway CD, Ingram MC *et al*. Aldosterone excretion rate and blood pressure in essential hypertension are related to polymorphic differences in the aldosterone synthase gene CYP11B2. *Hypertension* 1999; 33:703-707.
70. McNamara DM, Tam SW, Sabolinski ML *et al*. Aldosterone synthase promoter polymorphism predicts outcome in African Americans with heart failure. *J Am Coll Cardiol* 2006; 48:1277-1282.
71. Tiago AD, Badenhorst D, Skudicky D *et al*. An aldosterone synthase gene variant is associated with improvement in left ventricular ejection fraction in dilated cardiomyopathy. *Cardiovasc Res* 2002; 54:584-589.
72. Biolo A, Chao T, Duhaney TA, Kotlyar E *et al*. Usefulness of the aldosterone synthase gene polymorphism C-344-T to predict cardiac remodeling in African-Americans versus non-African-Americans with chronic systolic heart failure. *Am J Cardiol* 2007; 100:285-290.
73. McNamara DM. Emerging role of pharmacogenomics in heart failure. *Curr Opin Cardiol* 2008; 23:261-268.
74. Altshuler D, Brooks LD, Chakravarti A *et al*. A haplotype map of the human genome. *Nature* 2005; 437:1299-1320.
75. O'Donnell CJ, Cupples LA, D'Agostino RB *et al*. Genome-wide association study for subclinical atherosclerosis in major arterial territories in the NHLBI's Framingham Heart Study. *BMC Med Genet* 2007; 8(suppl 1):S4.
76. Kathiresan S, Manning AK, Demissie S *et al*. A genome-wide association study for blood lipid phenotypes in the Framingham Heart Study. *BMC Med Genet* 2007; 8(suppl 1):S17.
77. Rampersaud E, Damcott CM, Fu M *et al*. Identification of novel candidate genes for type 2 diabetes from a genome-wide association scan in the Old Order Amish: evidence for replication from diabetes-related quantitative traits and from independent populations. *Diabetes* 2007; 56:3053-3062.
78. Roden DM, Brown NJ. Preprescription genotyping: not yet ready for prime time, but getting there. *Circulation* 2001; 103:1608-1610.

5

Anticoagulation in heart failure: are we missing an important target?

F. Brandimarte, L. De Luca, M. R. Mehra, G. S. Filippatos, K. Dickstein, A. Ambrosy, M. Gheorghiade

INTRODUCTION

Heart failure (HF) remains a major public health issue and has reached epidemic proportions despite the combination of primary preventive measures and improved disease management [1]. The age-adjusted incidence of HF has remained stable over the past 20 years [2, 3]. It affects 1–2% of the adult population and 6–10% of those who are over the age of 65 years [4]. Admissions to hospitals because of HF continue to rise partly because of an ageing population but also because of increased survival after acute myocardial infarction and decreased sudden cardiac death.

In spite of an initial improvement in signs and symptoms of HF, patients admitted with acute HF syndromes (AHFS), defined as gradual or rapid change in HF signs and symptoms resulting in a need for urgent therapy, appear to be a distinct population at particularly high risk with very high post-discharge event rates [5–11]. It is now clear that co-morbidities such as CAD, diabetes mellitus, history of hypertension, atrial fibrillation (AF) and renal abnormalities are frequently observed and make AHFS population complex and heterogeneous.

There is increasing evidence that chronic HF is associated with a hypercoagulable state, secondary to platelet activation and endothelial dysfunction (Figure 5.1). Thromboembolism (TE), the direct consequence of these abnormalities, is rarely observed in HF, appears to be 'silent' in a significant number of cases and consequently is often not diagnosed. Although the mechanistic link that thromboembolic events precede, involve or follow major adverse

Filippo Brandimarte, MD, Cardiologist, Department of Cardiovascular Diseases, San Giovanni – Addolorata Community Hospital, Rome, Italy.

Leonardo De Luca, MD, PhD, FACC, Department of Cardiovascular Sciences, Laboratory of Interventional Cardiology, European Hospital, Rome, Italy.

Mandeep R. Mehra, MBBS, FACC, FACP, Herbert Berger Professor of Medicine and Head of Cardiology, University of Maryland School of Medicine, Baltimore, MD, USA.

Gerasimos S. Filippatos, MD, FACC, FCCP, FESC, Head, Heart Failure Unit, Department of Cardiology, Athens University Hospital Attikon, Athens, Greece.

Kenneth Dickstein, MD, PhD, University of Bergen, Stavanger University Hospital, Stavanger, Rogaland, Norway.

Andrew Ambrosy, BS, Center for Cardiovascular Innovation, Northwestern University, Feinberg School of Medicine, Chicago, IL, USA.

Mihai Gheorghiade, MD, FACC, Professor of Medicine and Surgery, Director of Experimental Therapeutics, Center of Cardiovascular Innovation, Northwestern University Feinberg School of Medicine, Co-Director, Cardiovascular Center for Drug Development, Duke University, Chicago, IL, USA.

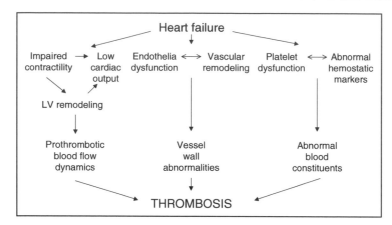

Figure 5.1 Thrombogenesis in heart failure.

cardiac events in patients with HF remains speculative, it appears reasonable that these events might play a role in determining worsening HF by causing myocardial ischemia and contributing to the high in-hospital and post discharge mortality by increasing the rate of sudden death [12–20]. The impact of these phenomena in AHFS patient population remains to be clarified.

Thus, a theoretical rationale for the use of antithrombotic therapy in HF has emerged. Unfortunately, as will be discussed later, data to support this hypothesis are still inconclusive and based on retrospective analyses. In addition, the conclusions drawn from many studies are limited by the inclusion of patients with AF, a well-known cause of TE. Lastly, anticoagulation is not without risk for serious side-effects including major hemorrhage, the incidence of which ranges from 2 to 7% per year, being the highest in the elderly population [21].

This chapter will describe in detail the mechanisms that may lead to the hypercoagulable state in HF, illustrate the incidence and the consequences of TE in this setting, and finally discuss the results of the available and ongoing trials on anticoagulation therapy in an effort to provide a rationale for designing clinical trials that may help to implement a safe and effective anticoagulant therapy in HF both in the acute and chronic setting.

HF AS A PREDISPOSITION TO THROMBOEMBOLIC EVENTS

Patients with HF are at increased risk for arterial and venous thrombosis. The pathophysiology of thrombogenesis can be summarized with the original Virchow's triad: 1. abnormal blood flow, 2. abnormalities in the vessel wall and 3. abnormalities in the blood constituents (increased platelet activity, activation of coagulation cascade). All three components frequently coexist in HF patients and correlate with the severity of left ventricular systolic dysfunction (LVD). Thus, it appears that structural and hematological abnormalities, atrial arrhythmias and endothelial dysfunction are likely to be the pathophysiological substrates that predispose HF patients to TE (Table 5.1) [19].

STRUCTURAL ABNORMALITIES

Left ventricle
Dilated cardiac chambers and decreased cardiac output due to diffuse or localized poor contractility, contribute to pooling and stasis of blood visualized by echocardiography

Table 5.1 Heart failure as a prothrombotic state

Abnormalities	Mechanism responsible for TE
Structural	
1. LV (Dilatation and poor contractility due to cardiomyopathies or ischemic disease)	Stasis, arterial thrombus formation, embolization
2. LA (Dilatation due to hypertention)	Stasis, arterial thrombus formation
3. RV and RA (IPH, device such as PM and ICD)	Venous thrombus formation, embolization (rare)
4. Coronary thrombosis (ACS)	Plaque rupture, arterial thrombus formation, embolization
5. Aortic plaque (> 4 mm or complicated)	Plaque rupture, arterial thrombus formation, embolization
6. Other (DVT due to prolonged immobilization, COPD etc.)	Stasis, venous thrombus formation, embolization
Hematological	
1. Platelets (↑Beta-thromboglobulin, ↑P-selectin, ↑PECAM-1 and ↑Osteonectin)	Arterial thrombus formation, embolization
2. Coagulation cascade (↑ TAT and ↑ FPA)	Arterial and venous thrombus formation, embolization
3. Fibrynolitic pathway (↑D-dimer, ↑PAI-1 and ↑TNF)	Arterial and venous thrombus formation, embolization
Hemoconcentration (high-dose diuretics, or rarely polycythemia vera)	Stasis, arterial and venous thrombus formation
Atrial arrhythmias (AFib or AFlu)	Stasis, arterial thrombus formation
Endothelial dysfunction (↓NO, ↑ Endothelin, ↑RAS)	Vasoconstriction, arterial and venous thrombus formation

ACS = acute coronary syndrome; Afib = atrial fibrillation; Aflu = atrial flutter; COPD = chronic obstructive pulmonary disease; DVT = deep vein thrombosis; FPA = plasma fibrinopeptide A; ICD = implantable cardioverter defibrillator; IPH = idiopathic pulmonary hypertension; LA = left atrium; LV = left ventricle; NO = nitric oxide; PAI-1 = plasminogen activator inhibitor-1; PECAM-1 = platelet/endothelial cell adhesion molecule-1; PM = pacemaker; RA = right atrium; RAS = renin-angiotensin system; RV = right ventricle; TAT = thrombin–antithrombin complex; TE = thromboembolism; TNF = tumor necrosis factor.

appearing as spontaneous echo contrast or 'smoke' in dilated atria or ventricles. Both echocardiography and autopsy studies suggest that the majority of left ventricular (LV) thrombi are often localized at the LV apex, suggesting that decreased or absent apical blood flow in this region may represent an additional risk factor [22–26].

In addition, patients with ischemic cardiomyopathies may have endocardial abnormalities in the ischemic or infarcted regions of the ventricle which provide a thrombogenic surface for clot formation absent or different in the idiopathic etiology. Conversely, factors such as mitral regurgitation, by increasing intracavity flow velocities, may provide a protective effect against the development of thrombus [27–30].

The etiology of HF has not been shown to significantly modify the incidence of the development of mural thrombi. Gottdiener *et al.* [31] studied 96 patients with an average follow-up of 2 years and found that 38 patients (40%) developed mural thrombus. The presence of thrombus was not different for patients with HF of ischemic etiology compared with those with idiopathic dilated cardiomyopathy. Interestingly, the embolic events were not related to the presence or absence of LV thrombus. Quinones *et al.* demonstrated the presence of mural thrombus in 22 of 112 patients (20%) with LVD. Consistently, the presence of mural thrombus did not correlate with the etiology of HF [23].

Although the presence of mural thrombi is high in autopsy studies (reaching 75% in some series), the clinical incidence of thromboembolic events is relatively low [32]. Indeed, several studies have failed to find a correlation between the presence of mural thrombus and increased embolic events [32, 34]. Three different studies, all non-randomized, suggest that this is probably due to differences in the thrombus morphology. In fact, large, protruding and mobile thrombi are more likely to embolize than small flat thrombi (reported in the majority of studies) because they expose a larger surface area to flowing blood. In addition, regional wall motion abnormalities, often seen in ischemic cardiomyopathies, are considered less likely to develop thrombi susceptible to embolization, compared to the global hypokinesis frequently observed in the dilated cardiomyopathy, suggesting a possible role of the contractile status of the underlying LV wall to the incidence of the embolization phenomena [26, 35, 36].

Left atrium

Left atrial (LA) enlargement is frequently observed in HF patients with hypertension and/or mitral valve disease. Atrial enlargement is also the most frequent abnormality contributing to the development of atrial arrhythmias and is known to impair atrial contractility and consequently facilitate stasis. In fact, the available data suggest that LA appendage (particularly when enlarged and/or low flow velocities at the trans esophageal echocardiogram are present) is the most common site of thrombi and source of TE, especially in patients with AF [37–39].

Right cardiac chambers

Right heart chambers are rarely source of thrombi, except for patients with idiopathic pulmonary hypertension [40]. However, the widespread use of electrical device with endocavitary electrodes in HF patients raised the possibility of TE coming from access site or from right atrium and ventricle. Numerous reports of venous complications such as stenosis, occlusions, and superior vena cava syndrome have been published particularly in patients who need system revision or upgrade of pacemaker or implantable cardioverter defibrillator system [41]. A small trial conducted by van Rooden and colleagues on 145 consecutive patients with permanent pacemaker leads documented thrombosis in 23% of cases using Doppler ultrasound technique. Thrombosis did not cause any signs or symptoms in 31 patients but resulted in overt clinical symptoms in three patients. The absence of anticoagulant therapy, use of hormone therapy, and a personal history of venous thrombosis were associated with an increased risk of thrombosis [42]. Unfortunately, even after 40 years of experience the incidence of device-related TE remains unclear and the real impact of these phenomena in the HF population largely unknown.

Coronary arteries

It is reasonable to speculate that in patients with HF secondary to CAD (the underlying etiology in more than 70% of cases of HF), ongoing silent or symptomatic ischemic events may contribute to progression of HF, thus, indirectly, increasing the risk of TE. In a subanalysis of the ATLAS trial, autopsy results of 171 patients have shown an unexpected, high prevalence of acute coronary findings (defined as coronary thrombus, ruptured plaque or myocardial infarction), particularly in patients with CAD who died suddenly (Figure 5.2) [13].

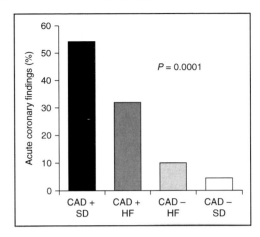

Figure 5.2 Relation of acute coronary findings to mode of death and presence of CAD is shown (168 patients). + Indicates presence of; −, absence of. CAD patients with sudden death (SD) had highest prevalence of acute coronary findings (with permission from [13]).

Accordingly, in a more recent analysis of the Optimal Trial in Myocardial Infarction with the Angiotensin II Antagonist Losartan (OPTIMAAL), among 180 deaths for which autopsies were available, acute myocardial infarction (MI) was found in 102 cases while clinically the adjudicated MIs were only 29. In addition, acute MI (defined as recent coronary thrombus) was found at autopsy in 55% (37 of 67) of the deaths that had been classified as due to an arrhythmia and in 81% (21 of 26) of the deaths classified as due to progressive HF (Figure 5.3) [43].

These data support the hypothesis that coronary thrombosis (the more common pathophysiological substrate for acute MI) occurs more frequently than it is generally believed, and may explain, in addition to ventricular arrhythmias, the high incidence of sudden deaths in this patient population.

Aorta

Aortic plaques, as part of the systemic process of arterial atherosclerosis, are a relevant cause of cerebrovascular and systemic embolizations. An analysis conducted by Tunick *et al.* [44] on 519 patients with severe aortic plaque assessed by trans esophageal echocardiography, revealed that an embolic event occurred in 21% of patients.

The results of a subanalysis of the Stroke Prevention and Atrial Fibrillation (SPAF) III also documented that among 382 patients with AF who underwent trans esophageal echocardiography, aortic plaque was diagnosed in 63% of the cases. Patients with complex plaques (incorporating any combination of mobile, pedunculated, or ulcerated morphologies, or whenever plaque thickness > 4 mm) experienced a significant higher death and embolic rate compared to patients without aortic plaques (16.8%/patients/year vs. 9.3%/patients/year and 26.2%/patients/year vs. 5.9%/patients/year respectively) [45].

Venous system

HF is known to significantly increase also the risk of venous TE. In critically ill patients, in addition to the previously mentioned device related TE, chronic obstructive pulmonary disease and immobilization due to prolonged hospital stay are often observed and play an

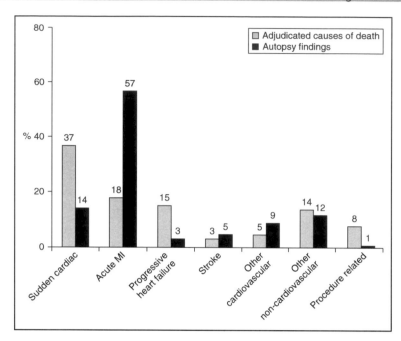

Figure 5.3 Causes of death in all autopsied patients (*n* = 180) before and after the result of autopsy was used to determine cause of death in the OPTIMAAL trial (with permission from [43]).

important role in the development of venous TE [46]. In addition, once venous TE develops, HF signs and symptoms may hide its detection.

A recent study conducted by Piazza *et al.* [47] showed that patients with HF had an increased frequency of co-morbid conditions such as neurologic disease including stroke, acute lung disease including pneumonia, and ACS contributing to a higher medical acuity than in patients without HF. Furthermore, patients with HF were more likely to have venous TE risk factors of immobilization, acute infection, chronic obstructive pulmonary disease and extremity discomfort than patients without HF.

HEMATOLOGICAL ABNORMALITIES

Platelet abnormalities

Studies conducted in the late 1970s reported that patients with HF had significantly more circulating platelet aggregates and reduced platelet survival when compared with healthy controls [48]. Since that time several markers of platelet activity outlined below have been found to be increased in HF patients. These data may help to better understand the potential processes beneath the pathogenesis and natural progression of HF.

Beta-thromboglobulin, P-selectin, platelet/endothelial cell adhesion molecule-1, and osteonectin are molecules expressed on platelets that participate in platelet activation and aggregation, are specific markers of platelet activity, and have been shown to be elevated in HF patients and correlate [49–65]. With the only exception of osteonectin, all of them appear to correlate with the degree of LVD [66].

Although it is still unclear the real impact of these molecules in the pathogenesis of thrombus formation, they may contribute to the prothrombotic state observed in HF patients.

Activation of coagulation cascade

Plasma fibrinopeptide A (FPA) and thrombin–antithrombin III (TAT) complex levels are highly sensitive markers for thrombin activity *in vivo*. Measures of thrombin activity in HF patients have been variable. Jafri *et al.* [49] showed that TAT complexes were significantly increased in HF patients while there was no significant difference in the concentration of fibrinopeptide A. In contrast, Yamamoto *et al.* [67] found that both plasma levels of FPA and TAT complexes in patients with HF were significantly higher compared to those in normal subjects. In interpreting these contradictory results, it should be noted that the first study involved patients with ischemic and non-ischemic HF, whereas the latter only evaluated patients with non-ischemic HF due to hypertrophic or dilated disease. Sbarouni *et al.* [50] found no significant differences in FPA levels in patients with dilated cardiomyopathy versus patients with ischemic HF.

Thus, it appears that not only LV enlargement but also LA stretching, both frequently observed in all these patients, may be potential triggers for activation of coagulation cascade.

Activation of fibrinolytic pathway

Increased markers of fibrinolytic activity have been reported in patients with HF. D-dimer, a fibrin degradation product, has been found to be significantly elevated in HF patients, regardless of etiology [49, 50, 67]. However, no definitive results can be drawn based on D-dimer levels since this marker has low specificity.

High levels of plasminogen activator inhibitor-1 (PAI-1) are also observed in patients with LVD. This may be due to the fact that angiotensin II (which is elevated in HF patients) can stimulate the expression of PAI-1 in endothelial and smooth muscle cells and tip the fibrinolytic balance towards a prothrombotic state [68–70].

It has been demonstrated by several studies that in HF there is a predominant production of pro-inflammatory cytokines secreted by Th1 lymphocytes. Among them, tumor necrosis factor (TNF), a proinflammatory cytokine, may be involved in the disturbance of the procoagulant–fibrinolytic balance leading to possible microvascular thrombosis. Elevated levels of TNF have been identified in patients with HF and its synthesis is stimulated by high levels of cathecolamines and angiotensin II [71–75]. Although the exact role of cytokines in these phenomena is still unclear, it seems that they may be considered potential contributors to myocyte injury and consequently progression of HF.

Hemoconcentration

Hemoconcentration, leading to a consequent increase in hematocrit, is mainly due to inappropriately high doses of diuretics as part of the fluid removal strategy in patients with HF and infrequently due to coexisting diseases, such as polycythemia vera, which may increase blood viscosity and the probability of thrombus formation [76, 77].

ATRIAL ARRHYTHMIAS

As mentioned before, AF and/or atrial flutter are a common comorbidity in patients with HF. Although the Vasodilator Heart Failure Trials (V-HeFT) failed to identify AF as an independent risk factor for thromboembolic events, it may clearly account for some of the excess risk of stroke in HF [78]. In addition, AF *per se* is associated with LA enlargement and abnormalities in hemostasis that may lead to thrombus formation within the LA and possibly cause strokes and/or pulmonary emboli if there is an anatomical condition such as atrial septal defects that permits communication between right and left chambers of the heart [79].

ENDOTHELIAL DYSFUNCTION

The endothelium is now considered the largest organ in the human body rather than simply a cellular layer at direct contact to blood stream. In fact, it is clear that it modulates vascular tone and contributes to the balance between anticoagulant and procoagulant factors [80, 81].

Endothelial dysfunction, considered as a consequence of coronary arteriosclerosis, is often present in HF patients particularly in those with an ischemic etiology [82]. Nitric oxide (NO) is a potent vasodilator secreted by the endothelium. *In vivo* studies have shown that HF patients have impaired production of NO in response to stimuli. This impairment may be further exacerbated by angiotensine II's stimulation of superoxide radical production that results in rapid degradation of free NO molecules. The lack of NO results also in an increased platelet activity and monocyte adhesion to the endothelial surface. In turn, activated platelets are known to release prothrombotic mediators [83].

Endothelin is a potent, endothelial cell derived, venous and arterial vasoconstrictor peptide involved in the regulation of vascular tone. It has been found to be elevated in HF and correlates with the severity of LVD. This imbalance between vasodilator and vasoconstrictor in favor of the latter, contribute to the increased peripheral resistances which are characteristic of severe HF [83–87].

Another specific marker of endothelial damage or dysfunction is the von Willebrand factor (vWf), a mediator of platelet adhesion at sites of vascular injury. Lip *et al.* [88] demonstrated that patients with LVD had elevated plasma levels of vWF. The importance of this marker in the pathophysiology of LVD is underscored by data coming from a study by Thompson *et al.* [89]. This study showed that in 3043 patients with significant CAD high levels of vWF were associated with an increased incidence of MI. In addition, Sbarouni *et al.* [50] found a significant correlation between endothelin and vWF in patients with HF, although the precise relation between these two markers is not known.

Lastly, activation of the renin-angiotensin system (RAS) has been well described in HF patients as part of the compensatory response to hemodynamic derangements. As a potential neurohormonal mediator of endothelial dysfunction, angiotensin II promotes the release of endothelin from endothelial cells and, as discussed above, indirectly contributes to the increased NO degradation. Furthermore, angiotensin II directly enhances platelet aggregability [90, 91].

CLINICAL MANIFESTATIONS OF TE IN HF

Although early observational studies reported a frequency of thromboembolic events as high as 50% [92–95], more recently, the clinical incidence of TE in patients with HF is estimated at approximately 2% per year (Table 5.2) [21, 78, 96–100]. However, referral bias, bias in allocating warfarin to patients, lack of standardized monitor of anticoagulation, underreporting or misclassification of the diagnoses, sampling error due to small study populations, the retrospective nature of some studies, high prevalence of rheumatic heart disease or, more importantly, AF may all account for differences between the studies.

Because of such a low event rate and probably because of technical difficulties in the diagnosis, no prospective clinical trials have been designed to date to clarify the impact of TE in HF patients. Even more challenging is to establish the clinical role of different thromboembolic events in this patient population (e.g. strokes, pulmonary emboli, deep vein and coronary thrombosis).

STROKE

Retrospective data from multiple large trials reveal that stroke is an important contributor to HF mortality [101, 102].

Table 5.2 Incidence of thromboembolic events in reported in selected heart failure trials (with permission from [21])

Trial	n	Follow-up (years)	AF (%)	CVA (% per year)	Pulm TE (% per year)	Peripheral TE (% per year)
V-HeFT-I [78]	632	2.3	15	1.8	0.3	0.3
Consensus [96]	253	0.5	50	4.6	NR	NR
V-HeFT-II [78]	804	2.6	15	1.8	0.3	0.08
SOLVD [98]	6797	3.3	6	1.2	0.3	0.3
CIBIS-II [99]	2647	1.3	1.4	NR	NR	NR
SCD-HeFT [97]	2114	4	0	2.64	0.3	0.3

AF=atrial fibrillation; CIBIS=Cardiac Insufficiency Bisoprolol Study; CVA=cerebrovascular accident; NR=not reported; peripheral TE=peripheral thromboembolism; pulm TE=pulmonary thromboembolism; SCD-HeFT=Sudden Cardiac Death in Heart Failure Trial; SOLVD=Studies of Left Ventricular Dysfunction; V-HeFT=Veterans Affairs Vasodilator-Heart Failure.

Several trials involving patients with post-MI LVD with and without HF have indirectly demonstrated increased incidence of stroke. For example, in the Survival and Ventricular Enlargement (SAVE) trial, which included patients with LVD after MI, the incidence of stroke was 1.5/100 patient-years. Risk was increased in patients who were older and who had a lower LVEF, with an 18% risk of stroke for every 5% decrease in LVEF [22]. A comparable incidence of stroke was quoted in the Acute Infarction Ramipril Efficacy (AIRE) trial, in a similar patient population [103]. The Cooperative North Scandinavian Enalapril Survival Study (CONSENSUS-I) demonstrated an annual rate of fatal cerebrovascular events of 2.3%, likely due to the higher percentage of patients with New York Heart Association (NYHA) class IV and AF included [96]. The Prospective Randomized Milrinone Survival Evaluation (PROMISE) trial, enrolling 1088 patients with severe chronic HF (NYHA class III or IV) and advanced LVD, showed an incidence of stroke of 3.5 per 100 patient-year follow-up [104]. The Veterans Affairs Vasodilator-Heart Failure (V-HeFT) I and II trials conducted in a similar patient population (n = 1436) documented an incidence of stroke of 1.8 per 100 patient-year after a follow up of approximately 2.5 months [78].

Precious data come from a recent analysis of the Sudden Cardiac Death in Heart Failure Trial (SCD-HeFT) since only patients with moderate HF in sinus rhythm were included. Among 2114 patients, stroke was observed in 2.6% of the population [97].

In spite of these data, the real impact of strokes in the HF patient population may be underestimated, since there is increasing evidence that silent stokes are not rare, particularly in patients with poor LV systolic function. A study conducted by Siachos et al. [14] showed that among 168 neurologically asymptomatic patients with chronic HF who were being evaluated for heart transplantation, the prevalence of silent ischemic stroke, assessed by magnetic resonance imaging or computed tomography without contrast, was as high as 34%.

PULMONARY EMBOLI

HF is known to increase the risk of pulmonary emboli (PE) [31, 105, 106]. However, the impact of PE on outcomes in this patient population is still unclear. This is probably due to the fact that such events are frequently silent and to the lack of sensitivity and specificity of the current available diagnostic tools. In addition, even when symptoms are manifest (e.g. acute dyspnea) they are often non-specific and make the diagnosis of PE a real challenge, particularly in the setting of acute and chronic HF.

Data based on certificates coming from United States Census Bureau reveal that among 755807 adults with HF who died over the 19-year period of study (1980 to 1998), PE was the cause of death in 3–10% of the cases [46]. In the Registro Informatizado de la Enfermedad TromboEmbólica (RIETE) registry, patients with HF ($n = 422$) had an incidence of fatal PE as high as 6.6% [18]. Darze *et al.* [107] found the incidence of PE to be 9.1% in 198 patients admitted for worsening HF. The presence of PE was also associated with a longer hospital stay (37.5±71.6 days vs. 15.4±15.0 days, $P = 0.001$) and a higher incidence of death or re-hospitalization at 3 months (72.2% vs. 43.9%, $P = 0.02$). PE remained an independent predictor of death or re-hospitalization at 3 months ($P = 0.038$). A retrospective analysis of the Studies of Left Ventricular Dysfunction (SOLVD) trial revealed that PE represented 16% of all TE events, 38% of which were fatal [98]. In the SCD-HeFT trial, the incidence of PE was 0.3%, much lower compared to all other trials suggesting the important role of atrial arrhythmias in the development of TE [97].

Once diagnosed, mortality from PE in patients with HF is higher than the general population. In the International Cooperative Pulmonary Embolism Registry (ICOPER) enrolling 2454 patients with acute PE both in Europe and North America, the overall mortality was 15% and approximately 45% of the deaths were attributed to PE. In addition, congestive HF was identified as a significant prognostic factor [108].

Thus, it appears that PE is an important contributor to overall mortality in HF patients and may contribute to the progression of this syndrome. Furthermore, given the fact that PE is always misdiagnosed, data may significantly underestimate its magnitude.

DEEP VEIN THROMBOSIS

Deep vein thrombosis (DVT) is one of the most important causes of PE, especially in patients with HF and impaired LV function [109]. In an analysis of the National Hospital Discharge Survey (NHDS), among patients hospitalized for HF, DVT was diagnosed in 1.03% and venous TE in 1.63%, while in patients not admitted with HF values were 0.85% and 1.11%, respectively [15].

CORONARY THROMBOSIS

Coronary thrombosis has been recognized to be an important pathophysiological substrate in patients with HF and CAD.

Data coming from ATLAS and OPTIMAAL trials suggest the hypothesis that coronary thrombosis (commonly silent and consequently misdiagnosed) may be considered another potential mechanism, in addition to arrhythmias, that may explain the high rate of sudden death in HF patients [13, 16].

Furthermore, patients admitted with AHFS are likely to be at higher risk for coronary events since the prothrombotic state might be more evident because of the further activation of neurohormones observed in this patient population. In fact, data coming from the European Heart Failure Survey II enrolling 3580 patients showed that ACS were an important precipitating factor of AHFS hospitalizations and were observed in up to 30% of the cases [110]. Accordingly, in a recent analysis of the Organized Program to Initiate Lifesaving Treatment in Hospitalized Patients With Heart Failure (OPTIMIZE-HF) registry, ACS/ischemia was identified as a frequent precipitating factor for hospital admission for HF and associated with increased risk of mortality at 60 to 90 days after discharge [111].

EFFICACY AND SAFETY OF ANTICOAGULATION IN HF

Given the evidence suggesting that a hypercoagulable state exists in HF patients, it is reasonable that anticoagulant therapy could be beneficial for these patients. Although anticoagulation in patients with HF has been investigated for over 50 years, no placebo-controlled prospective trials are available to date. Accordingly, data on the effectiveness of anticoagulation derive mainly from retrospective studies in patients with HF who were treated with anticoagulant agents (mostly warfarin) for AF, a previous TE event or known LV thrombus. In addition, most of the analyses available were performed in a non-randomized manner, including patients with AF (a well-established risk for TE), and without guidelines for target international normalized ratio range.

Early studies analyzed the efficacy of anticoagulant therapy mainly in patients with idiopathic dilated cardiomyopathy and showed trends for benefit with warfarin therapy. In the study by Fuster *et al.* [112], there were 19 embolic events over 103 patients who were not treated with anticoagulant agents (3.5 events/100 patient-years), whereas none of the 32 patients who received warfarin (101 patient-years) had an embolic complication. Natterson *et al.* [113] documented arterial embolization in five (4%) of 142 patients not receiving warfarin and in 1 (1%) of 82 patients receiving anticoagulation. Among the nine patients who had a cerebral TE in the study by Katz *et al.* [114], five were receiving long-term anticoagulation; notably, three of these patients had LV thrombus documented by two-dimensional echocardiography, and one had AF.

Retrospective analysis of most recent larger trials, which included patients with both ischemic and idiopathic dilated cardiomyopathy, failed to show protective effect of anticoagulation in this setting (Table 5.3). In V-HeFT I study, there was no significant difference in the incidence of TE events with or without antithrombotic therapy (2.7 events per 100 patient-years vs. 2.9 events per 100 patient-years, respectively). Surprisingly, in the V-HeFT II trial, the incidence of TE events was higher in the warfarin group than in those without treatment (4.9 events per 100 patient-years vs. 2.1 events per 100 patient-years, $P = 0.01$) [78].

The SAVE trial reported an 81% risk reduction of stroke among patients receiving anticoagulants. Furthermore, although not confirmed by other HF studies, the trial reported that use of aspirin alone reduced the relative risk of stroke by 56% making the efficacy of warfarin questionable [22]. In addition, it should be emphasized that in these trials anticoagulation therapy was not randomized and its intensity was not controlled.

A retrospective analysis from SOLVD trial, enrolling patients in sinus rhythm at the time of randomization, showed that anticoagulant therapy was associated with a significant reduction in all-cause mortality (adjusted hazard ratio [HR] 0.76; 95% confidence interval [CI] 0.65–0.89; $P = 0.0006$] and death or hospitalization for HF (HR 0.82, 95% CI 0.72–0.93, $P = 0.0002$) in patients both with ischemic and non-ischemic etiology. However, long-term warfarin was not associated with a reduction in the total number of fatal and non-fatal TE events [98].

The Warfarin and Antiplatelet Therapy in Chronic Heart Failure (WATCH) trial randomized 1587 HF patients to anticoagulation (target international normalized ratio [INR] 2.5) or antiplatelet therapy (blinded aspirin 162 mg or clopidogrel 75 mg) and found no significant difference in the composite endpoint of death/MI/stroke between the three groups (20.5% vs. 21% vs. 19.8% for aspirin, clopidogrel and warfarin, respectively). However, patients on warfarin had less hospitalization (16.1% vs. 22.2% vs. 18.3%, $P = 0.01$) for HF but significantly higher bleeding events than the antiplatelet groups (major bleeding 5.56% vs. 3.6% vs. 2.48% with warfarin, aspirin and clopidogrel, respectively, $P < 0.01$). Notably, the trial was designed without a placebo arm and was terminated early because of poor recruitment making these data still inconclusive (Table 5.3) [115].

The Warfarin/Aspirin Study in Heart Failure (WASH) study randomized 279 chronic systolic HF patients to no antithrombotic treatment, aspirin (300 mg) and warfarin (target INR 2.5), and there was no difference in the primary endpoints of death, non-fatal MI or non-fatal stroke between the three arms (26%, 32% and 26% in patients on placebo, aspirin and warfarin, respectively). Again, patients on warfarin had fewer hospitalizations for HF

Table 5.3 Selected randomized clinical trials of warfarin and antiplatelet agents (with permission from [21])

Trial	n	Intervention	Outcomes	Comment
WASH [116]	279	Warfarin (INR: 2.5) vs. ASA (300 mg)	Death, MI Stroke	Underpowered, signal of increased heart failure hospitalizations in ASA group
WATCH [115]	1587	Warfarin vs. ASA (162.5 mg) vs. Clopidogrel (75 mg)	All-cause mortality, MI, CVA, ischemic events, thromboembolic events	Underpowered, signal of increased heart failure hospitalizations in ASA group
HELAS [118]	197	Ischemic: ASA or warfarin; nonischemic: warfarin or placebo	Stroke, embolization, infarction, hospitalization, exacerbation of heart failure, all-cause death	Underpowered

ASA = acylsalicylic acid; CVA = cerebrovascular accident; HELAS = Heart failure Long-term Antithrombotic Study; INR = International Normalized Ratio; MI = myocardial infarction; WASH = Warfarin/Aspirin Study in Heart Failure; WATCH = Warfarin and Antiplatelet Therapy in Chronic Heart Failure.

than those on aspirin (48%, 47% and 64% patients without antithrombotic treatment, aspirin and warfarin, respectively, $P = 0.044$) and the incidence of minor hemorrhages was greater in the aspirin and warfarin groups compared with that without antithrombotic treatment group (13%, 17%, and 5%, respectively, $P = 0.033$) (Table 5.3) [116].

These data raise some important considerations. First, there is a weak trend in favor of a lower mortality with warfarin compared with aspirin (at least on an intention to treat analysis). Second, although the incidence of bleeding was relatively low, it was more frequent in patients receiving warfarin. Lastly, the lower rate of HF hospitalizations with warfarin may be due to the fact that aspirin may have an adverse effect in this patient population.

The Eighth American College of Chest Physicians Consensus Conference on Antithrombotic Therapy has estimated the annual risk of bleeding to be 2% for major bleedings and 0.8% for fatal bleedings, making routine use of anticoagulant therapy for the prevention of TE events in all HF patients equivocal at this point. The intensity of anticoagulation (particularly above INR 3), elevated blood pressure, previous cerebral ischemia, combined therapy of antiplatelet and antithrombotic agents and possibly old age are associated with increased bleeding risk. Furthermore, hepatic congestion in HF patients may interfere with warfarin metabolism increasing the risk of bleeding and complicating the control of therapeutic levels of anticoagulation [117].

In order to clarify the role of anticoagulation in patients with HF, the results of the Heart failure Long-term Antithrombotic Study (HELAS) have been recently become available. This study enrolled patients with NYHA class II–IV HF with a LVEF <35%. Those with an ischemic etiology were randomized to warfarin (INR = 2.0–3.0) or aspirin (325 mg), whereas those with non-ischemic cardiomyopathy were randomized to warfarin (INR = 2.0–3.0) or placebo. Composite endpoints include death, MI, peripheral or pulmonary embolism and non-fatal cardiogenic stroke. Although this trial suffered from enrollment problems and was terminated early, no difference was observed between aspirin and warfarin in the ischemic cardiomyopathy group, although there was a trend toward benefit of warfarin versus placebo in the nonischemic cardiomyopathy group (8.9 events per 100 patient-years in warfarin group versus 14.8 events per 100 patient-years in the placebo group) (Table 5.3) [118].

The Warfarin vs. Aspirin in Reduced Cardiac Ejection Fraction (WARCEF) trial is underway and aims to recruit 2860 patients with LVEF < 30% randomized to aspirin (325 mg) and warfarin (INR = 2.5–3.0). Primary endpoints include death, recurrent stroke and intracranial hemorrhage. Data coming from this large cohort of patients will be particularly interesting to guide the antithrombotic strategy in HF patients [119].

The current American College of Cardiology/American Heart Association (ACC/AHA) guidelines for the management of chronic HF only recognize AF or a history of TE as indications for anticoagulation (Class of Recommendation IIb, level of evidence B). The European Society of Cardiology (ESC) guidelines for acute and chronic HF recognize also a mobile LV thrombus, in addition to AF and a previous episode of TE, as a firm indication to anticoagulant therapy (Class of Recommendation I, level of evidence A). [120, 121]

FUTURE THERAPEUTIC DIRECTIONS

In an effort to improve safety and stability of anticoagulation, several compounds have been developed. Enoxaparin, a low molecular weight heparin, has been tested in 1102 acutely ill (including AHFS patients), immobilized general medical patients in the Medical Patients With Enoxaparin Trial (MEDENOX) [122]. This prospective, double-blind, randomized, placebo-controlled study was designed to evaluate the efficacy of two dosage regimens (20 mg and 40 mg) of enoxaparin or placebo for prevention of venous TE. The risk of venous TE was significantly reduced in patients with HF, as well as in patients with other medical illnesses, including respiratory failure, infectious disease, or rheumatic disorders only at the higher dose (5.5% vs. 14.9%, $P < 0.001$), a benefit that was maintained at 3-month follow-up. Adverse effects did not significantly differ between the placebo group and enoxaparin group.

Ximelagatran, a direct thrombin inhibitor, has been compared with warfarin in patients with non-valvular atrial fibrillation (SPORTIF) III and V trials enrolling 7329 patients. The event rates in SPORTIF III were 1.64 vs. 2.30%, corresponding to a difference of −0.66% (95% CI −1.4, 0.13) and in SPORTIF V were 1.61 vs. 1.16%, corresponding to a difference of +0.45% (95% CI −0.13, 1.03) [123]. Because of a documented liver toxicity, the compound was not approved by the Food and Drug Administration (FDA) and is no longer being developed.

Recently, a selective factor Xa inhibitor, rivaroxaban, has been developed in an effort to reduce TE in HF patients. This compound appears to meet the criteria for an ideal compound in this setting. In fact, it is an oral agent and its efficacy is not altered by food. Also, it provides stable anticoagulation, thus there no need for close monitoring [124]. Data from short-term phase II trials demonstrate that rivaroxaban 10 mg once a day provided an anticoagulation as effective as enoxaparin in the prevention of DVT after major orthopedic surgery without being associated with excessive bleeding [125–128].

In order to evaluate its impact in patients with both acute and chronic HF, a phase 1 trial has been designed and will start recruitment soon. It is expected to enroll patients with HF already receiving standard medical therapy. In the chronic HF arm, patients will be randomized to rivaroxaban 20 mg once a day for 6 days and placebo. The acute group will be randomized to the same dose of rivaroxaban and to enoxaparin 40 mg once a day. The results of this trial are needed to establish the importance of TE in the setting of both chronic HF and AHFS.

CONCLUSIONS

Attention to overt and covert arterio-venous TE in HF represents an important diagnostic and therapeutic target. The basis of this contention is supported by a growing literature with evidence of complex hemostatic abnormalities in patients with HF, which form the pathophysiological substrate for TE. Although the mechanistic role of covert TE in HF decompensation and progression remains poorly studied, it is conceivable that the high morbidity and mortality in this patient population is at least partially attributable to this phenomenon.

Although theoretically anticoagulation should benefit this patient population, with early studies supporting this hypothesis, retrospective analyses based on recent large clinical trials have failed to demonstrate a reduction in the incidence of TE. However, there are limitations to the available data, including the lack of randomization, inconsistent guidelines regarding the intensity of anticoagulation, and the failure to adjust for potential cofounders such as age and AF. In addition, since systemic congestion and low cardiac output may impair hepatic and renal function respectively, in the absence of close monitoring, patients with HF may be at increased risk for serious bleeding. As newer antithrombotic agents with greater safety and efficacy become available, there will be a potential therapeutic imperative to use anticoagulation in HF patients. This will mandate the design and conduct of large clinical trials in an effort to further reduce morbidity and mortality in this traditionally high-risk population.

REFERENCES

1. American Heart Association. Heart Disease and Stroke Statistics 2008 Update. Dallas, TX: American Heart Association, 2008.
2. Levy D, Kenchaiah S, Larson MG et al. Long-term trends in the incidence of and survival with heart failure. N Engl J Med 2002; 347:1397-1402.
3. Roger VL, Weston SA, Redfield MM, Hellermann-Homan JP, Killian J, Yawn BP. Trends in heart failure incidence and survival in a community-based population. JAMA 2004; 292:344-350.
4. McMurray JJ, Pfeffer MC. Heart failure. Lancet 2005; 365:1877-1889.
5. Gheorghiade M, Zannad F, Sopko G et al. International Working Group on Acute Heart Failure Syndromes. Acute heart failure syndromes: current state and framework for future research. Circulation 2005; 112:3958-3968.
6. Adams KF, Fonarow GC, Emerman CL et al. Characteristics and outcomes of patients hospitalized for heart failure in the United States: rationale, design, and preliminary observations from the first 100 000 cases in the Acute Decompensated Heart Failure National Registry (ADHERE). Am Heart J 2005; 149:209-216.
7. Yancy CW, Lopatin M, Stevenson LW et al. Clinical presentation, management, and in-hospital outcomes of patients admitted with acute decompensated heart failure with preserved systolic function: a report from the Acute Decompensated Heart Failure National Registry (ADHERE) Database. J Am Coll Cardiol 2006; 47:76-84.
8. Fonarow GC, Abraham WT, Albert NM et al. Organized Program to Initiate Lifesaving Treatment in Hospitalized Patients with Heart Failure (OPTIMIZE-HF): rationale and design. Am Heart J 2004; 148:43-51.
9. Cleland JG, Swedberg K, Follath F et al. For the Study Group on Diagnosis of the Working Group on Heart Failure of the European Society of Cardiology. The EuroHeart Failure Survey programme: a survey on the quality of care among patients with heart failure in Europe. Part 1: patient characteristics and diagnosis. Eur Heart J 2003; 24:442-463.
10. Tavazzi L, Maggioni AP, Lucci D et al. Nationwide survey on acute heart failure in cardiology ward services in Italy. Eur Heart J 2006; 27:1207-1215.
11. Zannad F, Mebazaa A, Juilliere Y et al. For the EFICA [Etude Française de l'Insuffisance Cardiaque Aiguë] Investigators. Clinical profile, contemporary management and one-year mortality in patients with severe acute heart failure syndromes: the EFICA study. Eur J Heart Fail 2006; 8:697-705.
12. Gheorghiade M, Gattis Stough W, Adams KF Jr, Jaffe AS, Hasselblad V, O'Connor CM. The Pilot Randomized Study of Nesiritide Versus Dobutamine in Heart Failure (PRESERVD-HF). Am J Cardiol 2005; 96:18G-25G.

13. Uretsky BF, Thygesen K, Armstrong PW *et al*. Acute coronary findings at autopsy in heart failure patients with sudden death: results from the assessment of treatment with lisinopril and survival (ATLAS) trial. *Circulation* 2000; 102:611-616.

14. Siachos T, Vanbakel A, Feldman DS, Uber W, Simpson KN, Pereira NL. Silent strokes in patients with heart failure. *J Card Fail* 2005; 11:485-489.

15. Beemath A, Stein PD, Skaf E, Al Sibae MR, Alesh I. Risk of venous thromboembolism in patients hospitalized with heart failure. *Am J Cardiol* 2006; 98:793-795.

16. Orn S, Cleland JG, Romo M, Kjekshus J, Dickstein K. Recurrent infarction causes the most deaths following myocardial infarction with left ventricular dysfunction. *Am J Med* 2005; 118:752-758.

17. Gheorghiade M, Sopko G, De Luca L *et al*. Navigating the crossroads of coronary artery disease and heart failure. *Circulation* 2006; 114:1202-1213.

18. Monreal M, Muñoz-Torrero JF, Naraine VS *et al*. RIETE Investigators. Pulmonary embolism in patients with chronic obstructive pulmonary disease or congestive heart failure. *Am J Med* 2006; 119:851-858.

19. Lip GYH, Gibbs CR. Does heart failure confer a hypercoagulable state? *J Am Coll Cardiol* 1999; 33:1424-1426.

20. Solomon SD, Zelenkofske S, McMurray JJ *et al*. For the Valsartan in Acute Myocardial Infarction Trial (VALIANT) Investigators. Sudden death in patients with myocardial infarction and left ventricular dysfunction, heart failure, or both. *N Engl J Med* 2005; 352:2581-2588.

21. Ahnert AM, Freudenberger RS. What do we know about anticoagulation in patients with heart failure? *Curr Opin Cardiol* 2008; 23:228-232.

22. Loh E, Sutton MS, Wun CC *et al*. Ventricular dysfunction and the risk of stroke after myocardial infarction. *N Engl J Med* 1997; 336:251-257.

23. Quinones MA, Nelson JG, Winters WL *et al*. Clinical spectrum of left ventricular mural thrombi in a large cardiac population: assessment by two-dimensional echocardiography. *Am J Cardiol* 1980; 45:435 (abstr).

24. Reeder GS, Tajik AJ, Seward JB. Left ventricular mural thrombus two-dimensional echocardiographic diagnosis. *Mayo Clin Proc* 1981; 56:82-86.

25. Yokota Y, Kawanishi H, Hayakawa M *et al*. Cardiac thrombus in dilated cardiomyopathy: relationship between left ventricular pathophysiology and left ventricular thrombus. *Jpn Heart J* 1989; 30:1-11.

26. Falk RH, Foster E, Coats MH. Ventricular thrombi and thromboembolism in dilated cardiomyopathy: a prospective follow-up study. *Am Heart J* 1992; 123:136-142.

27. Meltzer RS, Visser CA, Fuster V. Intracardiac thrombi and systemic embolization. *Ann Intern Med* 1986; 104:689-698.

28. Ciaccheri M, Castelli G, Cecchi F *et al*. Lack of correlation between intracavitary thrombosis detected by cross sectional echocardiography and systemic emboli in patients with dilated cardiomyopathy. *Br Heart J* 1989; 62:26-29.

29. Falk RH. A plea for a clinical trial of anticoagulation in dilated cardiomyopathy. *Am J Cardiol* 1990; 65:914-915.

30. Blondheim DS, Jacobs LE, Kotler MN, Costacurta GA, Parry WR. Dilated cardiomyopathy with mitral regurgitation: decreased survival despite a low frequency of left ventricular thrombus. *Am Heart J* 1991; 122:763-771.

31. Gottdiener JS, Gay JA, VanVoorhees L *et al*. Frequency and embolic potential of left ventricular thrombus in dilated cardiomyopathy: assessment by 2-dimensional echocardiography. *Am J Cardiol* 1983; 52:1281-1285.

32. Roberts WC, Siegel RJ, McManus BM. Idiopathic dilated cardiomyopathy: analysis of 152 necropsy patients. *Am J Cardiol* 1987; 60:1340-1355.

33. Massumi RA, Rios JC, Gooch AS *et al*. Primary myocardial disease: report of fifty cases and review of the subject. *Circulation* 1965; 31:19-41.

34. Tobin R, Slutsky RA, Higgins CB. Serial echocardiograms in patients with congestive cardiomyopathies: lack of evidence for thrombus formation. *Clin Cardiol* 1984; 7:99-101.

35. Cabin HS, Roberts WC. Left ventricular aneurysm, intraaneurysmal thrombus and systemic embolus in coronary heart disease. *Chest* 1980; 77:586-590.

36. Katz SD. Left ventricular thrombus and the incidence of thromboembolism in patients with congestive heart failure: can clinical factors identify patients at increased risk? *J Cardiovasc Risk* 1995; 2:97-102.

37. Hart RG, Halperin JL, Pearce LA *et al*. Stroke Prevention in Atrial Fibrillation Investigators. Lessons from the Stroke Prevention in Atrial Fibrillation trials. *Ann Intern Med* 2003; 138:831-838.

38. Blackehear JL, Odell JA. Appendage obliteration to reduce stroke in cardiac surgical patients with atrial fibrillation. *Ann Thorac Surg* 1996; 61:755-759.

39. Fountain RB, Holmes DR, Chandrasekaran K *et al*. The PROTECT AF (WATCHMAN Left Atrial Appendage System for Embolic PROTECTion in Patients with Atrial Fibrillation) trial. *Am Heart J* 2006; 151:956-961.

40. Friedman R, Mears JG, Barst RJ. Continuous infusion of prostacyclin normalizes plasma markers of endothelial cell injury and platelet aggregation in primary pulmonary hypertension. *Circulation* 1997; 96:2782-2784.

41. Lip GY, Kamath S. Do electrophysiological interventions confer a prothrombotic state? *Pacing Clin Electrophysiol* 2001; 24:1-4.

42. van Rooden CJ, Molhoek SG, Rosendaal FR, Schalij MJ, Meinders AE, Huisman MV. Incidence and risk factors of early venous thrombosis associated with permanent pacemaker leads. *J Cardiovasc Electrophysiol* 2004; 15:1258-1262.

43. Orn S, Cleland JG, Romo M, Kjekshus J, Dickstein K. Recurrent infarction causes the most deaths following myocardial infarction with left ventricular dysfunction. *Am J Med* 2005; 118:752-758.

44. Tunick PA, Nayar AC, Goodkin GM *et al*. NYU Atheroma Group. Effect of treatment on the incidence of stroke and other emboli in 519 patients with severe thoracic aortic plaque. *Am J Cardiol* 2002; 90:1320-1325.

45. Blackshear JL, Zabalgoitia M, Pennock G *et al*. Warfarin safety and efficacy in patients with thoracic aortic plaque and atrial fibrillation. SPAF TEE Investigators. Stroke Prevention and Atrial Fibrillation. Transesophageal echocardiography. *Am J Cardiol* 1999; 83:453-455.

46. Beemath A, Skaf E, Stein PD. Pulmonary embolism as a cause of death in adults who died with heart failure. *Am J Cardiol* 2006; 98:1073-1075.

47. Piazza G, Seddighzadeh A, Goldhaber SZ. Heart failure in patients with deep vein thrombosis. *Am J Cardiol* 2008; 101:1056-1059.

48. Mehta J, Mehta P. Platelet function studies in heart disease. VI. Enhanced platelet aggregate formation activity in congestive heart failure: inhibition by sodium nitroprusside. *Circulation* 1979; 60:497-503.

49. Jafri SM, Ozawa T, Mammen E, Levine TB, Johnson C, Goldstein S. Platelet function, thrombin and fibrinolytic activity in patients with heart failure. *Eur Heart J* 1993; 14:205-212.

50. Sbarouni E, Bradshaw A, Andreotti F, Tuddenham E, Oakley CM, Cleland JG. Relationship between hemostatic abnormalities and neuroendocrine activity in heart failure. *Am Heart J* 1994; 127:607-612.

51. Jafri SM, Riddle JM, Raman SB, Goldstein S. Altered platelet function in patients with severe congestive heart failure. *Henry Ford Hosp Med J* 1986; 34:156-159.

52. Andreassen AK, Nordoy I, Simonsen S *et al*. Levels of circulating adhesion molecules in congestive heart failure and after heart transplantation. *Am J Cardiol* 1998; 81:604-608.

53. Devaux B, Scholz D, Hirche A, Klovekorn WP, Schaper J. Upregulation of cell adhesion molecules and the presence of low grade inflammation in human chronic heart failure. *Eur Heart J* 1997; 18:470-479.

54. Gershlick AH. Are there markers of the blood–vessel wall interaction and of thrombus formation that can be used clinically? *Circulation* 1990; 81:I28–I34.

55. Hsu-Lin SC, Berman CL, Furie BC, August D, Furie B. A platelet membrane protein expressed during platelet activation. *J Biol Chem* 1984; 259:9121-9126.

56. Boukerche H, Ruchaud Sparagano MH, Rouen C, Brochier J, Kaplan C, Mcgregor JL. A monoclonal antibody directed against a granule membrane glycoprotein (GMP-140/PADGEM, P-selectin, CD62P) inhibits ristocetin-induced platelet aggregation. *Br J Haematol* 1996; 92:442-451.

57. Frenette PS, Johnson RC, Hynes RO, Wagner DD. Platelets roll on stimulated endothelium in vivo: an interaction mediated by endothelial P-selectin. *Proc Natl Acad Sci USA* 1995; 92:7450-7454.

58. Kuijper PHM, Torres HIG, Vanderlinden JAM *et al*. Platelet-dependent primary hemostasis promotes selectin-and integrin-mediated neutrophil adhesion to damaged endothelium under flow conditions. *Blood* 1996; 87:3271-3281.

59. Diacovo TG, Puri KD, Warnock RA, Springer TA, Vonandrian UH. Platelet-mediated lymphocyte delivery to high endothelial venules. *Science* 1996; 273:252-255.

60. O'Connor CM, Gurbel PA, Serebruany VL. Usefulness of soluble and surface-bound P-selectin in detecting heightened platelet activity in patients with congestive heart failure. *Am J Cardiol* 1999; 83:1345-1349.

61. Newman PJ, Berndt MC, Gorsky J, White GC, Paddock LS, Muller WA. PECAM-1 (CD 31) cloning and relation to adhesion molecules of the immunoglobulin gene superfamily. *Science* 1990; 247:1219-1223.

62. Muller WA, Berman ME, Newman PJ, DeLisser HM, Albelda SM. A heterophylic adhesion mechanisms for platelet/endothelial adhesion molecule 1 (CD 31). *J Exp Med* 1992; 175:1401-1404.
63. Lasters P, Almendro N, Bellon T, Lopez-Guerrero JA, Eritia R, Bernabeu C. Functional regulation of platelet/endothelial cell adhesion molecule-1 by TGF-b1 in promonocytic U-937 cells. *J Immunol* 1994; 153:4206-4218.
64. Cramer EM, Berger G, Berndt MC. Platelet alpha-granule and plasma membrane share two new components: CD9 and PECAM-1. *Blood* 1994; 84:1722-1730.
65. Serebruany VL, Murugesan SR, Pothula A *et al*. Increased soluble platelet/endothelial cellular adhesion molecule-1 and osteonectin levels in patients with severe congestive heart failure. Independence of disease etiology, and antecedent aspirin therapy. *Eur J Heart Fail* 1999; 1:243-249.
66. Breton-Gorius J, Clezardin P, Guichard J *et al*. Localization of platelet osteonectin at the internal face of the alpha-granule membranes in platelets and megakaryocytes. *Blood* 1992; 79:936-941.
67. Yamamoto K, Ikeda U, Furuhashi K, Irokawa M, Nakayama T, Shimada K. The coagulation system is activated in idiopathic cardiomyopathy. *J Am Coll Cardiol* 1995; 25:1634-1640.
68. Hamsten A, de Faire U, Walldius G *et al*. Plasminogen activator inhibitor in plasma: risk factor for recurrent myocardial infarction. *Lancet* 1987; 2:3-9.
69. Smith D, Gilbert M, Owen WG. Tissue plasminogen activator release in vivo in response to vasoactive agents. *Blood* 1985; 66:835-839.
70. Brown NJ, Vaughan DE. Role of angiotensin II in coagulation and fibrinolysis. *Heart Fail Rev* 1999; 3:193-198.
71. van der Poll T, Levi M, Buller HR *et al*. Fibrinolytic response to tumor necrosis factor in healthy subjects. *J Exp Med* 1991; 174:729-732.
72. van der Poll T, Buller HR, ten Cate H *et al*. Activation of coagulation after administration of tumor necrosis factor to normal subjects. *N Engl J Med* 1990; 322:1622-1627.
73. Oral H, Kapadia S, Nakano M *et al*. Tumor necrosis factor-alpha and the failing human heart. *Clin Cardiol* 1995; 18:IV20–IV27.
74. Levine B, Kalman J, Mayer L, Fillit HM, Packer M. Elevated circulating levels of tumor necrosis factor in severe chronic heart failure. *N Engl J Med* 1990; 323:236-241.
75. Seta Y, Shan K, Bozkurt B, Oral H, Mann DL. Basic mechanisms in heart failure: the cytokine hypothesis. *J Card Fail* 1996; 2:243-249.
76. Boyle A, Sobotka PA. Redefining the therapeutic objective in decompensated heart failure: hemoconcentration as a surrogate for plasma refill rate. *J Card Fail* 2006; 12:247-249.
77. De Stefano V, Za T, Rossi E *et al*. GIMEMA CMD-Working Party. Recurrent thrombosis in patients with polycythemia vera and essential thrombocythemia: incidence, risk factors, and effect of treatments. *Haematologica* 2008; 93:372-380.
78. Dunkman WB, Johnson GR, Carson PE *et al*. Incidence of thromboembolic events in congestive heart failure. The V-HeFT VA Cooperative Studies Group. *Circulation* 1993; 87:VI94–VI101.
79. Kumagai K, Fukunami M, Ohmori M, Kitabatake A, Kamada T, Hoki N. Increased intracardiovascular clotting in patients with chronic atrial fibrillation. *J Am Coll Cardiol* 1990; 16:377-380.
80. Harrison DG. Endothelial dysfunction in atherosclerosis. *Basic Res Cardiol* 1994; 89:87-102.
81. Levin ER. Endothelins. *N Engl J Med* 1995; 333:356-363.
82. Bauersachs J, Widder JD. Endothelial dysfunction in heart failure. *Pharmacol Res* 2008; 60:119-126.
83. Kubo SH, Rector TS, Bank AJ, Williams RE, Heifetz SM. Endothelium-dependent vasodilatation is attenuated in patients with heart failure. *Circulation* 1991; 84:1589-1596.
84. Yanagisawa M, Kurihara H, Kimura S *et al*. A novel potent vasoconstrictor peptide produced by vascular endothelial cells. *Nature* 1988; 332:411-415.
85. Wei CM, Lerman A, Rodeheffer RJ *et al*. Endothelin in human congestive heart failure. *Circulation* 1994; 89:1580-1586.
86. Rodeheffer RJ, Lerman A, Heublein DM, Burnett JC Jr. Increased plasma concentrations of endothelin in congestive heart failure in humans. *Mayo Clin Proc* 1992; 67:719-724.
87. Margulies KB, Hildebrand FL Jr, Lerman A, Perrella MA, Burnett JC Jr. Increased endothelin in experimental heart failure. *Circulation* 1990; 82:2226-2230.
88. Lip GYH, Lowe GDO, Metcalfe MJ, Rumley A, Dunn FG. Effects of warfarin therapy on plasma fibrinogen, von Willebrand Factor and fibrin d-dimer in left ventricular dysfunction secondary to coronary artery disease with and without aneurysms. *Am J Cardiol* 1995; 76:453-458.

89. Thompson SG, Kienast J, Pyke SD, Haverkate F, van de Loo JC. Hemostatic factors and the risk of myocardial infarction or sudden death in patients with angina pectoris. European Concerted Action on Thrombosis and Disabilities Angina Pectoris Study Group. *N Engl J Med* 1995; 332:635-641.
90. Holtz J. Pathophysiology of heart failure and the renin–angiotensin system. *Basic Res Cardiol* 1993; 88:183-201.
91. Brown NJ, Vaughan DE. Role of angiotensin II in coagulation and fibrinolysis. *Heart Fail Rev* 1999; 3:193-198.
92. Fuster V, Gersh BJ, Giuliani ER, Tajik AJ, Brandenbury RO, Frye RL. The natural history of idiopathic dilated cardiomyopathy. *Am J Cardiol* 1981; 47:525-531.
93. Gottdiener JS, Gay JA, Van Voorhees L, DiBianco R, Fletcher RD. Frequency and embolic potential of left ventricular thrombus in dilated cardiomyopathy. Assessment by 2-dimensional echocardiography. *Am J Cardiol* 1983; 52:1281-1285.
94. Diaz RA, Obasohan A, Oakley CM. Prediction of outcome in dilated cardiomyopathy. *Br Heart J* 1987; 58:393-399.
95. Ciaccheri M, Castelli G, Cecchi F *et al*. Lack of correlation between intracavity thrombus detected by cross-sectional echocardiography and systemic emboli in patients with dilated cardiomyopathy. *Br Heart J* 1989; 62:26-29.
96. The CONSENSUS Trial Study Group. Effects of enalapril on mortality in severe congestive heart failure. Results of the Cooperative North Scandinavian Enalapril Survival Study (CONSENSUS). *N Engl J Med* 1987; 316:1429-1435.
97. Freudenberger RS, Hellkamp AS, Halperin JL *et al*. SCD-HeFT Investigators. Risk of thromboembolism in heart failure: an analysis from the Sudden Cardiac Death in Heart Failure Trial (SCD-HeFT). *Circulation* 2007; 115:2637-2641.
98. Dries DL, Rosenberg YD, Waclawiw MA, Domanski MJ. Ejection fraction and risk of thromboembolic events in patients with systolic dysfunction and sinus rhythm: evidence for gender differences in the studies of left ventricular dysfunction trials. *J Am Coll Cardiol* 1997; 29:1074-1080.
99. The Cardiac Insufficiency Bisoprolol Study II (CIBIS-II): a randomised trial. *Lancet* 1999; 353:9-13.
100. Cioffi G, Pozzoli M, Forni G *et al*. Systemic thromboembolism in chronic heart failure. A prospective study in 406 patients. *Eur Heart J* 1996; 17:1381-1389.
101. Witt BJ, Gami AS, Ballman KV *et al*. The incidence of ischemic stroke in chronic heart failure: a meta-analysis. *J Card Fail* 2007; 13:489-496.
102. Appelros P. Heart failure and stroke. *Stroke* 2006; 37:1637.
103. Effect of ramipril on mortality and morbidity of survivors of acute myocardial infarction with clinical evidence of heart failure. The Acute Infarction Ramipril Efficacy (AIRE) Study Investigators. *Lancet* 1993; 342:821-828.
104. Packer M, Carver JR, Rodeheffer RJ *et al*.Effect of oral milrinone on mortality in severe chronic heart failure. The PROMISE Study Research Group. *N Engl J Med* 1991; 325:1468-1475.
105. Pulido T, Aranda A, Zevallos MA *et al*. Pulmonary embolism as a cause of death in patients with heart disease: an autopsy study. *Chest* 2006; 129:1282-1287.
106. Goldhaber SZ, Savage DD, Garrison RJ *et al*. Risk factors for pulmonary embolism. The Framingham Study. *Am J Med* 1983; 74:1023-1028.
107. Darze ES, Latado AL, Guimarães AG *et al*. Acute pulmonary embolism is an independent predictor of adverse events in severe decompensated heart failure patients. *Chest* 2007; 131:1838-1843.
108. Goldhaber SZ, Visani L, De Rosa M. Acute pulmonary embolism: clinical outcomes in the International Cooperative Pulmonary Embolism Registry (ICOPER) *Lancet* 1999; 353:1386-1389.
109. Howell MD, Geraci JM, Knowlton AA. Congestive heart failure and outpatient risk of venous thromboembolism: a retrospective, case control study. *J Clin Epidemiol* 2001; 54:810-816.
110. Nieminen MS, Brutsaert D, Dickstein K *et al*. EuroHeart Survey Investigators; Heart Failure Association, European Society of Cardiology. EuroHeart Failure Survey II (EHFS II): a survey on hospitalized acute heart failure patients: description of population. *Eur Heart J* 2006; 27:2725-2736.
111. Fonarow GC, Abraham WT, Albert NM *et al*. OPTIMIZE-HF Investigators and Hospitals. Factors identified as precipitating hospital admissions for heart failure and clinical outcomes: findings from OPTIMIZE-HF. *Arch Intern Med* 2008; 168:847-854.
112. Fuster V, Gersh BJ, Guiliani ER, Tajik AJ, Brandenburg RO, Frye RL. The natural history of idiopathic dilated cardiomyopathy. *Am J Cardiol* 1981; 47:525-531.
113. Natterson PD, Stevenson WG, Saxon LA, Middlekauff HR, Stevenson LW. Risk of arterial embolization in 224 patients awaiting cardiac transplantation. *Am Heart J* 1995; 129:564-570.

114. Katz SD, Marantz PR, Biasucci L *et al.* Low incidence of stroke in patients with heart failure: a prospective study. *Am Heart J* 1993; 126:141-146.
115. Cleland JG, Ghosh J, Freemantle N *et al.* Clinical trials update and cumulative meta-analyses from the American College of Cardiology: WATCH, SCDHeFT, DINAMIT, CASINO, INSPIRE, STRATUS-US, RIO-Lipids and cardiac resynchronisation therapy in heart failure. *Eur J Heart Fail* 2004; 6:501-508.
116. Cleland JG, Findlay I, Jafri S *et al.* The Warfarin/Aspirin Study in Heart failure (WASH): a randomized trial comparing antithrombotic strategies for patients with heart failure. *Am Heart J* 2004; 148:157-164.
117. Hirsh J, Guyatt G, Albers GW, Harrington R, Schünemann HJ. American College of Chest Physicians. Executive summary: American College of Chest Physicians Evidence-Based Clinical Practice Guidelines, 8th edition. *Chest* 2008; 133:71S-109S.
118. Cokkinos DV, Haralabopoulos GC, Kostis JB, Toutouzas PK. HELAS investigators. Efficacy of antithrombotic therapy in chronic heart failure: the HELAS study. *Eur J Heart Fail* 2006; 8:428-432.
119. Pullicino P, Thompson JL, Barton B, Levin B, Graham S, Freudenberger RS. WARCEF Investigators. Warfarin versus aspirin in patients with reduced cardiac ejection fraction (WARCEF): rationale, objectives, and design. *J Card Fail* 2006; 12:39-46.
120. Hunt SA, Abraham WT, Chin MH *et al.* American College of Cardiology; American Heart Association Task Force on Practice Guidelines; American College of Chest Physicians; International Society for Heart and Lung Transplantation; Heart Rhythm Society. ACC/AHA 2005 Guideline Update for the Diagnosis and Management of Chronic Heart Failure in the Adult: a report of the American College of Cardiology/American Heart Association Task Force on Practice Guidelines (Writing Committee to Update the 2001 Guidelines for the Evaluation and Management of Heart Failure): developed in collaboration with the American College of Chest Physicians and the International Society for Heart and Lung Transplantation: endorsed by the Heart Rhythm Society. *Circulation* 2005; 112:e154-e235.
121. Task Force for Diagnosis and Treatment of Acute and Chronic Heart Failure 2008 of European Society of Cardiology, Dickstein K, Cohen-Solal A, Filippatos G *et al.* ESC Guidelines for the diagnosis and treatment of acute and chronic heart failure 2008: the Task Force for the Diagnosis and Treatment of Acute and Chronic Heart Failure 2008 of the European Society of Cardiology. Developed in collaboration with the Heart Failure Association of the ESC (HFA) and endorsed by the European Society of Intensive Care Medicine (ESICM). *Eur Heart J* 2008; 29:2388-2442.
122. Alikhan R, Cohen AT, Combe S *et al.* MEDENOX Study. Risk factors for venous thromboembolism in hospitalized patients with acute medical illness: analysis of the MEDENOX Study. *Arch Intern Med* 2004; 164:963-968.
123. Ford GA, Choy AM, Deedwania P *et al.* SPORTIF III, V Investigators. Direct thrombin inhibition and stroke prevention in elderly patients with atrial fibrillation: experience from the SPORTIF III and V Trials. *Stroke* 2007; 38:2965-2971.
124. Agnelli G, Gallus A, Goldhaber SZ *et al.* ODIXa-DVT Study Investigators. Treatment of proximal deep-vein thrombosis with the oral direct factor Xa inhibitor rivaroxaban (BAY 59-7939): the ODIXa-DVT (Oral Direct Factor Xa Inhibitor BAY 59-7939 in Patients With Acute Symptomatic Deep-Vein Thrombosis) study. *Circulation* 2007; 116:180-187.
125. Eriksson BI, Borris LC, Friedman RJ *et al.* RECORD1 Study Group. Rivaroxaban versus enoxaparin for thromboprophylaxis after hip arthroplasty. *N Engl J Med* 2008; 358:2765-2775.
126. Kakkar AK, Brenner B, Dahl OE *et al.* for the RECORD2 Investigators. Extended duration rivaroxaban versus short-term enoxaparin for the prevention of venous thromboembolism after total hip arthroplasty: a double-blind, randomised controlled trial. *Lancet* 2008; 372:31-39.
127. Lassen MR, Ageno W, Borris LC *et al.* RECORD3 Investigators. Rivaroxaban versus enoxaparin for thromboprophylaxis after total knee arthroplasty. *N Engl J Med* 2008; 358:2776-2786.
128. Mueck W, Eriksson BI, Bauer KA *et al.* Population pharmacokinetics and pharmacodynamics of rivaroxaban – an oral, direct factor Xa inhibitor – in patients undergoing major orthopaedic surgery. *Clin Pharmacokinet* 2008; 47:203-216.

6

Has the death knell been sounded for oral and intravenous vasodilators in decompensated heart failure?

J. G. Prempeh, J. R. Teerlink

INTRODUCTION

In the past few decades, we have seen significant advances in therapeutics and treatment strategies that have had a dramatically positive effect on the morbidity and mortality of chronic heart failure patients. However, until recently and despite exceedingly high in-hospital mortality and re-hospitalization rates, acute heart failure (AHF) had been largely ignored. The number of hospital admissions for heart failure (HF) has increased to over 1.1 million in 2006, a 26% increase in the last decade, and it is estimated that the total hospitalization cost of HF in the US will be greater than $20 billion [1]. The multiple recent studies with novel agents for AHF attest to the rapidly growing interest in this field [2–10]. Data obtained through these trials have provided new insights [11] and put forth the new paradigm of AHF as a vascular disorder that can be managed with vasodilators [12]. This chapter will discuss the underlying principle of AHF as a vascular disorder, the rationale of vasodilators in the treatment of AHF, currently available vasodilators and future therapies and directions.

THE PARADIGM: AHF AS A VASCULAR DISORDER

The term AHF is somewhat misleading when one reviews the data from patients admitted to the hospital with this diagnosis. AHF is has been defined as the rapid or gradual onset of signs and symptoms of HF that result in the urgent need for medical care [13]. While some may have acute onset of signs and symptoms, most cases tend to be more gradual, resulting from increases in peripheral or pulmonary edema and the vascular responses to fluid accumulation. Tsuyuki *et al.* [14] prospectively examined factors involved in HF exacerbations and found that the most frequent precipitant was non-compliance with salt restriction in diet, occurring in 22% of patients, while 10% had inappropriate reductions in their congestive heart failure (CHF) therapy. Patients who presented with acute onset of signs and symptoms were usually due to another type of vascular abnormality, such as an acute coronary syndrome. In a subgroup analysis of the Organized Program to Initiate Lifesaving Treatment in Hospitalized Patients With Heart Failure (OPTIMIZE-HF) cohort,

James G. Prempeh, MD, Clinical Research Fellow, Section of Cardiology, San Francisco Veterans Affairs Medical Center, School of Medicine, University of California, San Francisco, CA, USA.

John R. Teerlink, MD, FACC, FAHA, FESC, Professor of Medicine (UCSF), Director, Heart Failure (SFVAMC), Director, Clinical Echocardiography (SFVAMC), Section of Cardiology, San Francisco Veterans Affairs Medical Center, School of Medicine, University of California, San Francisco, CA, USA.

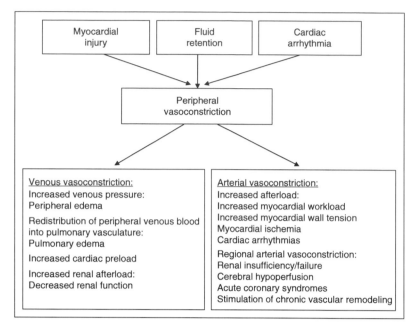

Figure 6.1 The central role of vasoconstriction in the pathogenesis of acute heart failure.

pneumonia or other respiratory process, myocardial ischemia and arrhythmias were important precipitants [15].

Although symptoms may be initiated by some degree of left ventricular systolic dysfunction, more than half of the patients with AHF tend to have preserved ejection fractions. The central abnormality in AHF may be viewed as pathologic vasoconstriction (Figure 6.1). Peripheral venoconstriction moves blood centrally, thereby increasing pulmonary venous congestion and edema, resulting in the symptoms of dyspnea and fatigue. Perhaps equally important, the central redistribution of venous volume increases central venous pressure, increasing the 'afterload' on the kidney, causing reduced renal function [16, 17]. Elevations in peripheral venous pressures also directly result in the peripheral edema that often represents the most obvious sign of AHF. Peripheral arterial vasoconstriction leads to increased afterload, elevated LV filling pressures, increased post-capillary pulmonary venous pressures, all of which contribute to worsening of pulmonary edema and dyspnea. Increased afterload results in elevated ventricular wall stress and increased myocardial ischemia, which can initiate cardiac arrhythmias. Moreover, systemic vasoconstriction contributes to poor organ perfusion, decreasing blood flow to the kidney, brain, and gut, resulting in renal failure and symptoms of fatigue, confusion, anorexia, and abdominal discomfort.

Furthermore, most currently available therapies in the treatment of AHF directly affect the vasculature instead of the heart itself. Diuretics, vasodilators and positive inotropes with vasodilatory properties have been the mainstay in the treatment of AHF for decades. The main effect of these agents is to reduce central venous pressures through diuresis and direct vasodilating properties, even with diuretics [18], rather than any direct effect on the heart.

This new model of AHF as a *vascular disorder* has important implications for the clinical development of new AHF therapies [19]. For acute symptom resolution, the new therapy must be an effective vasodilator, relieving the elevated venous pressures that lead to congestion and dyspnea, and reducing the abnormally high afterload that results in organ hypop-

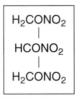

$$H_2CONO_2$$
$$|$$
$$HCONO_2$$
$$|$$
$$H_2CONO_2$$

Figure 6.2 Structural formula of nitroglycerin.

erfusion and increased cardiac wall stress with the attendant increases in ischemia and arrhythmias. Yet, the new therapy must also target the underlying mediators of these vascular abnormalities to prevent acute and chronic damage. New therapies for AHF need to improve clinical outcomes and a vasodilating agent that can antagonize vascular and end-organ damage has the potential to have both short-term and long-term benefits for patients.

CURRENTLY AVAILABLE VASODILATORS

The recently published guidelines from the European Society of Cardiology state that 'vasodilators are recommended at an early stage for AHF patients without symptomatic hypotension, SBP < 90 mmHg or serious obstructive valvular disease.' (Class of recommendation I, level of evidence B) [20]. Currently, there are three available, Food and Drug Administration (FDA) approved vasodilators that function under the general principle of increasing intracellular cyclic guanosine monophosphate (cGMP), but each has unique characteristics.

NITROGLYCERIN

Since the first medical uses of nitroglycerin in the late 1800s, organic nitrates have been used in the treatment of cardiovascular disease and are one of the oldest therapies for AHF. Nitroglycerin is 1,2,3-propanetriol trinitrate, an organic nitrate with an empiric formula of $C_3H_5N_3O_9$ and a molecular weight of 227.09 (Figure 6.2). Nitroglycerin works by relaxation of smooth muscle, producing a vasodilator effect on the peripheral veins and arteries. At low doses, these nitrates dilate veins, producing a rapid decrease in pulmonary venous and ventricular filling pressures (thus reducing preload) and improvement in pulmonary congestion, dyspnea, and myocardial oxygen demand. At higher doses and in the presence of vasoconstriction, nitrates dilate arteries (reducing afterload), improving collateral flow to ischemic regions.

In spite of, or perhaps due to its long history of being used as a vasodilator in AHF, nitrates have not been evaluated in large, blinded randomized studies. Smaller studies have shown nitrates to improve certain features of the AHF syndrome. Cotter et al. [21] demonstrated that high-dose early administration of intravenous nitrates is favorable in improving arterial oxygenation and possibly avoiding some consequences of AHF (myocardial infarction [MI], and the need for mechanical ventilation), compared to furosemide alone or non-invasive ventilation [22]. The Vasodilatation in the Management of Acute Congestive Heart Failure (VMAC) study showed that low doses of nitrates improve some aspects of dyspnea during the first two h of administration [7], while a single center report from that same trial by Elkayam et al. [23] suggested that nitroglycerin was not comparable to nesiritide during the initial 12–24h of therapy (Figure 6.3 A), even if the nitroglycerin dose was aggressively up-titrated. However, this study also demonstrated that in the context of this aggressive up-titration, tolerance to the nitrate effect developed and the hemodynamic effects were eventually attenuated (Figure 6.3 B). The effects of nitrates on end-organ damage (renal impairment, MI, cardiac arrest) or on intermediate- and long-term outcomes (re-admission and death) have not been examined. Some investigators have recently raised the concern

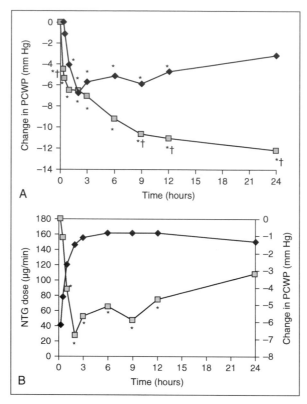

Figure 6.3 High-dose nitroglycerin and nesiritide in a single site from the VAMC trial. (A) Change in PCWP from baseline during 24 h of intravenous infusion of nitroglycerin and nesiritide. *Squares*, nesiritide; *diamonds*, nitroglycerin. *$P < 0.05$ versus baseline; †$P < 0.02$ versus nitroglycerin. (B) Nitroglycerin (NTG) dose and change in PCWP during treatment with NTG. *Squares*, change in PCWP; *diamonds*, nitroglycerin dose. *$P < 0.05$ versus baseline (adapted with permission from [23]). PCWP = pulmonary capillary wedge pressure.

that therapies that produce an accumulation of reactive oxygen species, such as tolerance-inducing doses of nitroglycerin, may lead to plasma volume expansion, neurohormonal activation, and increased sensitivity to vasoconstrictors with rebound angina and ischemia[24]. The role of these theoretical and potentially deleterious effects in the acute administration of nitrates is unknown.

Clinical experience seems to support the role of nitrates in providing fast symptom relief. These agents are widely used in Europe with apparent beneficial effect [25], although their use is less frequent in the United States for unclear reasons [26]. However, the efficacy of nitroglycerin is limited by the tolerance that many patients develop after 24 h. Side-effects include headaches and symptomatic hypotension, which typically resolve within minutes of stopping treatment.

SODIUM NITROPRUSSIDE

Sodium nitroprusside (SNP) is another vasodilator, available as a parenteral agent. It is a dianion, $[Fe(CN)^5NO]^2$, and the iron moiety is an octahedral surrounded by five cyanide

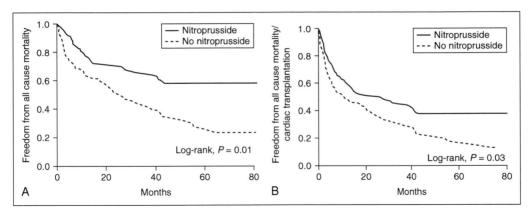

Figure 6.4 Kaplan–Meier curves of all cause mortality (A) and the combined endpoint of all-cause mortality and cardiac transplant (B) between patients who did and did not receive intravenous SNP during hospitalization (adapted with permission from [28]).

ligands and one nitric oxide (NO) ligand. SNP rapidly metabolizes to cyanide and nitric oxide, which causes peripheral vasodilation by direct action on both venous and arteriolar smooth muscle, thus reducing peripheral resistance. This vasodilation increases cardiac output by decreasing afterload and reduces aortic and left ventricular impedance. SNP is easily titratable due to a very short half-life (seconds to a few minutes). Intravenous administration is often monitored with an intraarterial line in a critical care setting, although careful, frequent blood pressure cuff measurement may be a reasonable alternative to invasive monitoring.

There are currently no randomized studies of SNP in patients with AHF [2], but several studies have shown significant improvements in hemodynamics, associated with increases in diuresis, natriuresis and decreased neurohormonal activation [27]. Mullens *et al.* [28] recently reviewed the clinical course of 175 consecutive patients admitted for acutely decompensated HF and found that although given to patients with a worse hemodynamic profile at baseline, intravenous SNP was associated with greater hemodynamic improvement and lower rates of inotropic support or worsening renal function during hospitalization and with lower rates of all-cause mortality after discharge (Figure 6.4).

However, despite these apparent beneficial effects in treating AHF, especially in the setting of elevated blood pressure, SNP is significantly underutilized; it is used in less than 1% of AHF patients in Europe and US [25, 26]. Concerns about SNP stem from rare but documented evidence of thiocyanate toxicity usually related to prolonged use, high-doses or in the setting of renal failure (GI and CNS symptoms), as well as concerns about neurohormonal activation and rebound vasoconstriction after abrupt withdrawal of SNP in patients with severe AHF [29, 30].

NESIRITIDE

Nesiritide is the most recent FDA-approved vasodilator therapy for AHF. Nesiritide is a recombinant human B-type natriuretic peptide (BNP) that binds to a membrane-bound receptor coupled to guanylate cyclase on vascular smooth muscle and endothelial cells, increasing intracellular cGMP, resulting in smooth muscle cell relaxation. This relaxation causes potent vasodilation in veins and arteries and leads to dose-dependent reductions in pulmonary capillary wedge pressure and systemic vascular resistance. Nesiritide is indicated for patients with clear evidence of volume overload and although it has a relatively short half-life (18 min), prolonged hypotension has been noted, especially in patients with volume depletion [7]. It should not be administered for the indication of replacing diuretics, enhancing diuresis, protecting renal function, or improving survival.

Early studies by Mills *et al.* [31] and Colucci *et al.* [32] demonstrated that the aforementioned effects of nesiritide were accompanied by increases in cardiac output and improvement in dyspnea. The Vasodilation in the Management of Acute Congestive Heart Failure (VMAC) study also demonstrated an improvement in dyspnea in the first 3 h of administering nesiritide as compared to placebo [7]. Moreover, in the previously mentioned single center VMAC substudy by Elkayam comparing nesiritide to high-dose nitroglycerin [23], nesiritide was shown to cause an earlier decrease in pulmonary capillary wedge pressure (<15 min) which was sustained for 24 h without the need for up-titration. On the other hand, nitroglycerin required aggressive up-titration and, gradually, the decrease in pulmonary capillary wedge pressure was minimized due to early development of tolerance.

In spite of the short-term improvement in dyspnea, other outcomes of the use of nesiritide, such as persistent dyspnea improvement, possible harmful end-organs effects, hospital readmission rates or mortality, have yet to be fully studied and Drs. Sackner-Bernstein and Aaronson, as well as others, have raised concerns about worsening renal function and increased risk of death after treatment with nesiritide in patients with AHF [33–36]. The Acute Study of Clinical Effectiveness of Nesiritide in Decompensated Heart Failure (ASCEND-HF) is a prospective, multicenter, randomized, double-blinded, placebo-controlled trial which is enrolling 7000 patients to address some of the concerns mentioned above [37].

INVESTIGATIONAL THERAPIES AND FUTURE DIRECTIONS

In addition to the currently approved and available therapies, there are several other investigational vasodilators that are being studied which may improve symptoms and clinical outcome of patients while providing a better understanding of AHF as a whole.

ENDOTHELIN RECEPTOR ANTAGONISTS (TEZOSENTAN)

In the last decade, there has been growing interest in the significance of endothelin in HF. Endothelin is the most potent known vasoconstrictor, produced predominantly by cardiovascular tissues in response to stress, as well as in the brain and kidneys. Endothelin-1 (ET-1) is a 21 amino-acid peptide first isolated in 1988, [38] with a structure homologous to sarafotoxins, potent toxins from the venom of *Atractaspis engaddensis* or the Israeli burrowing asp. The first report of pathologically elevated ET-1 concentrations was in patients with AHF due to cardiogenic shock [39], and multiple subsequent studies showed markedly increased endothelin levels in acute and chronic HF which also correlated with the extent of pulmonary hypertension [40], severity of symptoms and ventricular dysfunction [41], and mortality [42]. ET-1 may be involved in many aspects of the pathogenesis of HF [43], including direct vasoconstriction of arteries (increasing afterload) and veins (central redistribution of volume with commensurate venous hypertension), potentiating vasoconstriction of other neurohormones like angiotensin, and exacerbating peripheral and pulmonary edema by affecting capillary hemodynamics and increasing vascular permeability. Endothelin causes an increase in capillary pressure resulting in net transcapillary fluid filtration and increased interstitial edema. ET-1's potent vasoconstricting effects are mediated by ET_A and ET_B receptors on vascular smooth muscle cells and as such, tezosentan, a short-acting, intravenous dual (ET_A and ET_B) receptor-competitive antagonist, was developed. In patients with HF, tezosentan reduces systemic vascular resistance and pulmonary capillary wedge pressure, while increasing cardiac output in a dose-dependent manner [44–46].

The clinical development program confirmed the hemodynamic efficacy of tezosentan, including the Randomized Intervention of TeZosentan (RITZ) studies [47–50]. Unfortunately, the initial dose selected for these Phase III trials did not significantly improve dyspnea in patients admitted for AHF and caused hypotension and renal insufficiency. The subsequent Value of Endothelin Receptor Inhibition with Tezosentan in Acute Heart Failure Studies (VERITAS) [5, 51] was an international trial that enrolled 1435 patients hospitalized for AHF with dyspnea who were randomized to treatment with a much lower dose of tezosentan or placebo in addition to standard care. Despite decreasing pulmonary capillary wedge pressure and systemic vascular resistance in the small subset of patients with invasive monitoring, tezosentan did not improve dyspnea or reduce worsening of HF or death in these patients.

Given the excellent scientific rationale, pre-clinical data, and hemodynamic benefits of tezosentan, it is unclear why these effects of tezosentan did not translate into favorable clinical outcomes. Many explanations have been advanced, including the possibility that tezosentan may not actually work, that the instruments to measure dyspnea in these and trials of other agents were insensitive or confounded, or that the presence of invasive hemodynamic monitoring in other trials biased the evaluation of dyspnea. However, we believe the most likely reason is that the patient population enrolled in VERITAS was not sufficiently targeted or objectively defined to optimize the risk:benefit ratio. The failure of tezosentan in these clinical trials was felt by many to be the death knell for novel vasodilators in AHF.

OTHER NATRIURETIC PEPTIDES (ULARITIDE AND CD-NP)

Ularitide is a synthetic version of urodilatin, a member of the family of atrial natriuretic peptides (ANP) that are produced in renal tubular cells and regulate renal sodium and water excretion [52]. As with BNP, concentrations of urodilatin are also elevated in HF [53]. Ularitide has potentially unique vasodilatory, natriuretic and diuretic effects that make it a promising agent in managing AHF. Early studies demonstrated its preload and afterload reducing and diuretic effects [54, 55], and in a Phase II randomized, double-blind, ascending dose, placebo-controlled trial, Mitrovic and his colleagues found that within 6 h of administering the drug, there was a significant decrease in pulmonary capillary wedge pressure and systemic vascular resistance associated with an increased cardiac index and improvement in dyspnea score [56]. A subsequent 221 patient randomized, parallel group, placebo-controlled study, confirmed these beneficial hemodynamic effects [57]. The most frequent adverse effect of ularitide in these studies was hypotension. The effect of ularitide on clinical outcomes and mortality has yet to be studied in larger prospective, randomized trials.

A series of novel natriuretic peptides have been engineered with the intent of targeting specific pharmacologic effects [58]. C-type natriuretic peptide (CNP) is structurally homologous to other natriuretic peptides such as ANP and BNP, but appears to induce less hypotension than either of them while unloading the heart due to venodilation. *Dendroaspis* natriuretic peptide (DNP), on the other hand, is a potent natriuretic and diuretic peptide but can induce significant hypotension and functions via a separate receptor than CNP. Thus, Dr. Burnett *et al.* engineered a novel chimeric peptide, CD-NP, by fusing the 22-amino acid CNP, for venodilation, with the 15-amino acid linear C-terminus of DNP, for renal effects (Figure 6.5). Studies in animals demonstrated that CD-NP produced greater natriuresis and diuresis, enhanced glomerular filtration rate, unloaded the heart, inhibited renin production, and was less hypotensive when compared to BNP. CD-NP was also noted to inhibit cardiac fibroblast proliferation *in vitro* [59]. The hemodynamic effects, clinical efficacy, tolerability, and safety of CD-NP are currently being evaluated in other trials of patients with AHF.

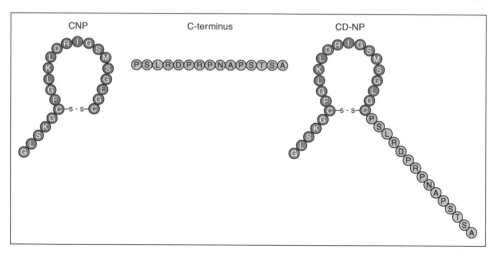

Figure 6.5 Design of CD-NP (adapted with permission from [59]).

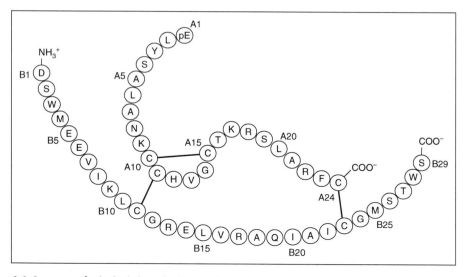

Figure 6.6 Structure of relaxin (adapted with permission from [60]).

RELAXIN

Relaxin [60] is a 6-kDa peptide made up of 53 amino acids (Figure 6.6) that is present in low basal concentrations in both men and women, although production dramatically increases during pregnancy. In humans, relaxin appears to play a central role in the hemodynamic and renovascular adaptations that occur during pregnancy, including decreasing systemic vascular resistance and increasing renal blood flow and function. Relaxin binds to the LGR7 receptor, present in the renal and systemic vasculature, to initiate its action. It has several mechanisms of action including effects on nitric oxide, ANP, the endothelin type B receptor, and possibly increasing arterial compliance. One open-label, ascending dose study in 16 patients with stable HF demonstrated relaxin-induced decreases in pulmonary capillary wedge pressure and systemic vascular resistance, associated with increases in cardiac index [61]. A subsequent randomized, double-blind, placebo-controlled, dose-finding study (Pre-RELAX-AHF) in 234 patients admitted for AHF with objective evidence of congestion, normal to elevated systolic blood pressure (SBP > 125 mmHg) and mild-to-moderate renal insufficiency suggested improvement in multiple endpoints, including dyspnea improvement, signs of HF, hospital length of stay, and re-hospitalization for heart or renal failure or death [10]. In this study, the 30 mcg/kg/d dose of relaxin appeared to not only provide the greatest efficacy, but also had no evidence of adverse renal effects and no significant hypotension (Table 6.1). The Phase III study, RELAX-AHF, is being performed to confirm these findings and demonstrate the safety and efficacy of relaxin in patients with AHF.

SOLUBLE GUANYLATE CYCLASE ACTIVATORS (CINACIGUAT)

NO is the major effector molecule of vascular tone. NO binds to the ferrous heme iron of soluble guanylate cyclase which activates the enzyme and leads to conversion of guanosine triphosphate (GTP) to cGMP, which leads to vasodilatation [62]. As a NO and heme-independent soluble G protein activator, Cinaciguat (BAY 58-2667) has a novel and unique mechanism of action compared to conventional nitrovasodilators (Figure 6.7).

Boerrigter et al. [63] studied cinaciguat in dogs with tachycardia pacing-induced severe HF. The peptide was shown to cause a dose-dependent reduction in mean arterial, right atrial, pulmonary artery, and pulmonary capillary wedge pressure, with increases in the cardiac output and renal blood flow. However, there were no changes in glomerular filtration rate or sodium and water excretion. Plasma renin activity and aldosterone remained unchanged. A Phase I study of 76 healthy volunteers suggested similar effects [64], and further investigations of cinaciguat are being planned.

SELECTIVE ADENOSINE RECEPTOR ANTAGONISTS (ROLOFYLLINE)

Selective adenosine receptor antagonists are not conventional vasodilators but mediate selective renal vasodilation. When elevated levels of sodium ions are detected in the distal tubule, the body attenuates excess salt and volume loss by decreasing the renal blood flow (and glomerular filtration rate). This compensatory mechanism, known as tubuloglomerular feedback (TGF), is also activated when AHF patients are given loop diuretics. TGF is mediated by adenosine binding to A_1 adenosine receptors on the afferent arterioles which lead to vasoconstriction of the arterioles and decrease in renal blood flow. This is obviously counterproductive in the management of AHF as progressively higher doses of loop diuretics will be required to overcome this mechanism and to successfully diurese patients. To break this cycle, selective A_1 adenosine receptor antagonists have been studied in the past few years.

Gottlieb et al. [65] showed that giving the adenosine A_1 receptor antagonist, BG9719, with furosemide may blunt the decrease in GFR from TGF in AHF. Rolofylline, an adenosine A_1 receptor antagonist, has been shown in studies with AHF patients to significantly increase both renal blood flow and glomerular filtration rate [66], increase diuresis and natriuresis with a concomitant preservation of renal function (Figure 6.8 A) [9, 67], and may induce improvement in dyspnea and have reno-protective effects that translate into trends in reduced rates of re-admission and death up to 2 months from treatment (Figure 6.8 B) [9]. The safety and efficacy of this drug continues to be studied in the Phase III PROTECT study, and if these results are replicated, will represent a significant advance in the care of patients.

Table 6.1 Effect of relaxin on primary treatment targets in the Pre-Relax-AHF study (adapted with permission from [10])

	Placebo (n=60)	Relaxin			
		10µg/kg/day (n=40)	30µg/kg/day (n=42)	100µg/kg/day (n=37)	250µg/kg/day (n=49)
Short term					
Proportion with moderately or markedly better dyspnoea at 6 h, 12 h, and 24 h (Likert)	14 (23%)	11 (28%); p=0.54	17 (40%); p=0.044	5 (14%); p=0.28	11 (22%); p=0.86
Dyspnoea AUC change from baseline to day 5 (VAS [mm*h])	1679 (2556)	2500 (2908); p=0.15	2567 (2898); p=0.11	2486 (2865); p=0.16	2155 (2338); p=0.31
Dyspnoea AUC change from baseline to day 14 (VAS [mm*h])	4621 (9003)	6366 (10078); p=0.37	8214 (8712); p=0.053	8227 (9707); p=0.064	6856 (7923); p=0.16
Worsening heart failure through day 5 (%)*	13 (21%)	8 (20%); p=0.75	5 (12%); p=0.29	5 (14%); p=0.40	5 (10%); p=0.15
Length of stay (days)	12.0 (7.3)	10.9 (8.5); p=0.36	10.2 (6.1); p=0.18	11.1 (6.6); p=0.75	10.6 (6.6); p=0.20
60 days					
Days alive out of hospital	44.2 (14.2)	47.0 (13.0); p=0.40	47.9 (10.1); p=0.16	48 (10.1); p=0.40	47.6 (12.0); p=0.048
KM cardiovascular death or readmission (HR, 95% CI)+	17.2%	10.1% (0.55, 0.17–1.77); p=0.32	2.6% (0.13, 0.02–1.03); p=0.053	8.4% (0.46, 0.13–1.66); p=0.23	6.2% (0.32, 0.09–1.17); p=0.085
KM all-cause death or readmission (HR, 95% CI)+	18.6%	12.5% (0.63, 0.22–1.81); p=0.39	7.6% (0.36, 0.10–1.29); p=0.12	10.9% (0.56, 0.18–1.76); p=0.32	8.3% (0.41, 0.13–1.28); p=0.12
180 days					
KM cardiovascular death (HR, 95% CI)++	14.3%	2.5% (0.19, 0.00–1.49); p=0.15	0.0% (0.00, 0.00–0.98); p=0.046	2.9% (0.23, 0.01–1.79); p=0.17	6.2% (0.56, 0.09–2.47); p=0.53
KM all-cause death (HR, 95% CI)+	15.8%	5.0% (0.34, 0.07–1.62); p=0.18	8.7% (0.54, 0.14–2.03); p=0.36	5.5% (0.41, 0.09–1.19); p=0.25	10.7% (0.08, 0.26–2.47); p=0.70

Data are number (%) or mean (SD), unless otherwise specified. AUC=area under the curve; CI=confidence interval; HR=hazard ratio; KM=Kaplan–Meier estimates of event rate at specified time; VAS=visual analogue scale.
*For Wilcoxon rank sum test of time to worsening heart failure up to day 5. Participants without Worsening heart failure were assigned a value of 6 days. +Fisher's exact test comparison of incidence densities. ++Analyses with safety population, which included one additional patient (n=38) in the 100 µg/kg per day group. Readmission to hospital included admission due to heart failure or renal failure.

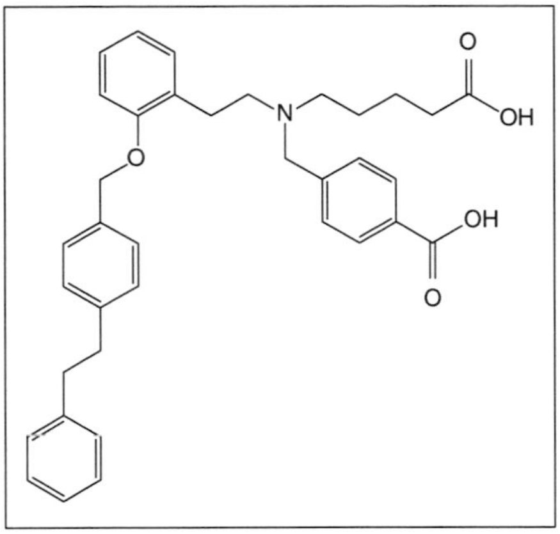

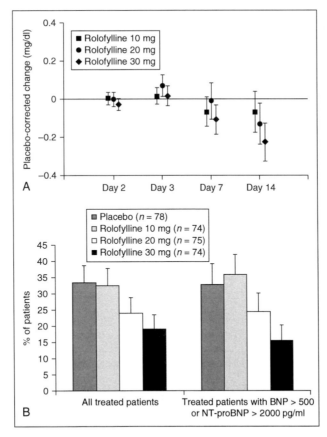

Figure 6.7 Cinaciguat (BAY 58-2667) (adapted with permission from [62]).

Figure 6.8 Results from the PROTECT Pilot study. (A) Placebo-corrected changes in serum creatinine from baseline (day 1) to days 2, 3, 7, and 14. $P=0.03$ for dose-related trend at 14 days. (Bars represent standard errors of the differences between active and placebo group mean changes.) (B) Proportion of patients dying of any cause or re-hospitalized for cardiovascular or renal causes during the 60-day follow-up period: bars represent standard errors of the proportions (adapted with permission from [9]).

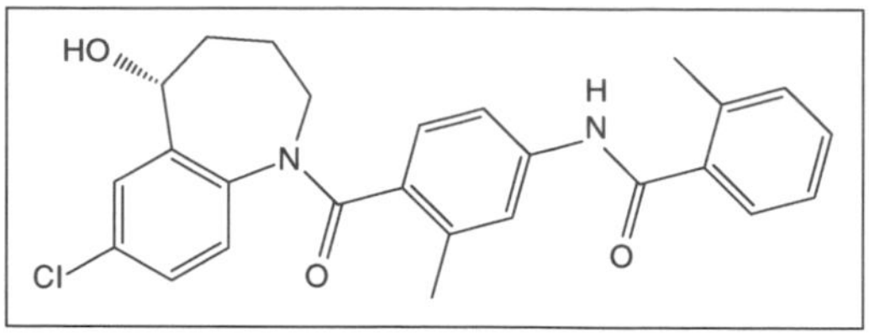

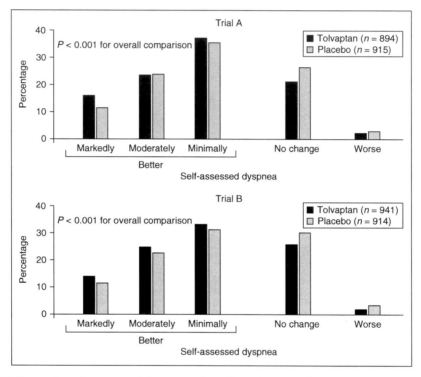

Figure 6.9 Structure of tolvaptan.

Figure 6.10 Change in patient-assessed dyspnea at day 1 for patients manifesting dyspnea at baseline (adapted with permission from [4]).

VASOPRESSIN ANTAGONISTS (TOLVAPTAN)

The vasopressin antagonists are also not typical vasodilators, but they have been shown to mediate diuresis in hypervolemia without significantly affecting natriuresis or potassium excretion. Arginine vasopressin (AVP, or vasopressin) is a neurohormone, produced in the hypothalamus, which controls both body water and blood pressure by regulating water excretion and vascular tone. AVP is normally released in response to increased plasma osmolality, hypovolemia or hypotension, and patients with AHF have increased concentrations of AVP [68]. AVP binds to V_2 receptors in the renal collecting duct which causes enhanced transcription and expression of aquaporin-2 proteins. These proteins then increase water absorption in the renal tubules. Elevated serum AVP can lead to hyponatremia, which in itself is a surrogate for poor prognosis in AHF as shown by the Outcomes of a Prospective Trial of Intravenous Milrinone for Exacerbations of Chronic Heart Failure (OPTIME-CHF) study [69]. Thus, in AHF patients, elevated AVP production possibly symbolizes a maladaptive response, similar to other neurohormones in the pathogenesis of HF.

Tolvaptan is a selective V_2 vasopressin antagonist which has been investigated in the last decade for the management of AHF (Figure 6.9). Tolvaptan has a higher binding affinity for V_2 receptors in the kidney than AVP and hence, competitively blocks AVP to prevent water reabsorption, increasing urine and free water clearance, improving hyponatremia, decreasing urine osmolality, while increasing renal blood flow and glomerular filtration rate by decreasing renovascular resistance. Multiple trials and subsequent post hoc analyses have substantiated the renal effects of tolvaptan. A relatively large pilot study randomized 319 patients hospitalized with HF to three doses of tolvaptan or placebo. This study demonstrated tolvaptan-related significant decreases in body weight, with no significant difference in worsening HF at 60 days after randomization. However, a post hoc, subgroup analysis revealed the intriguing finding that tolvaptan-treated patients had lower 60-day mortality compared to placebo. These findings provided the basis for the largest and most definitive study of tolvaptan, the Efficacy of Vasopressin Antagonism in Heart Failure Outcome Study with Tolvaptan (EVEREST) trial [70], a multicenter, international, randomized, double-blinded placebo-controlled trial which looked at the short- and long-term efficacy of the drug in patients hospitalized with HF. The study showed no difference in all cause mortality as compared to placebo, and secondary endpoints of cardiovascular mortality and worsening HF were also not different [71]. However, tolvaptan showed a small, but significant improvement in patient-assessed dyspnea on day 1 (Figure 6.10), total body weight, and day 7 edema [4]. The study also showed no harm in the long-term use of tolvaptan. In view of these findings, the role of tolvaptan in the treatment of patients with AHF remains unclear at this time.

CONCLUSION

Vasodilators remain important tools in the management of AHF, as emphasized in the current European Society of Cardiology heart failure guidelines. As demonstrated with data from studies on available conventional vasodilators, there may be beneficial effects in treating AHF. In addition, far from a death knell, there is a gradually increasing call to cautiously and appropriately increase the use of these agents. This call has the potential to change to an enthusiastic cheer, if any of the many exciting vasodilating drugs on the horizon fulfill their promise.

REFERENCES

1. Lloyd-Jones D, Adams R, Carnethon M et al. Heart disease and stroke statistics – 2009 update: a report from the American Heart Association Statistics Committee and Stroke Statistics Subcommittee. *Circulation* 2009; 119:480-486.
2. Teerlink JR. Overview of randomized clinical trials in acute heart failure syndromes. *Am J Cardiol* 2005; 96:59G-67G.
3. Cuffe MS, Califf RM, Adams KF Jr et al. Short-term intravenous milrinone for acute exacerbation of chronic heart failure: a randomized controlled trial. *JAMA* 2002; 287:1541-1547.
4. Gheorghiade M, Konstam MA, Burnett JC Jr et al. Short-term clinical effects of tolvaptan, an oral vasopressin antagonist, in patients hospitalized for heart failure: the EVEREST Clinical Status Trials. *JAMA* 2007; 297:1332-1343.
5. McMurray JJ, Teerlink JR, Cotter G et al. Effects of tezosentan on symptoms and clinical outcomes in patients with acute heart failure: the VERITAS randomized controlled trials. *JAMA* 2007; 298:2009-2019.

6. Teerlink JR, Malik FI, Clarke CP *et al.* The selective cardiac myosin activator, CK-1827452, increases left ventricular systolic function by increasing ejection time: results of a first-in-human study of a unique and novel mechanism. *J Card Fail* [Abstract] 2006; 12:763.

7. VMAC Investigators. Intravenous nesiritide vs nitroglycerin for treatment of decompensated congestive heart failure: a randomized controlled trial. *JAMA* 2002; 287:1531-1540.

8. Gheorghiade M, Blair JE, Filippatos GS *et al.* Hemodynamic, echocardiographic, and neurohormonal effects of istaroxime, a novel intravenous inotropic and lusitropic agent: a randomized controlled trial in patients hospitalized with heart failure. *J Am Coll Cardiol* 2008; 51:2276-2285.

9. Cotter G, Dittrich HC, Weatherley BD *et al.* The PROTECT pilot study: a randomized, placebo-controlled, dose-finding study of the adenosine A1 receptor antagonist rolofylline in patients with acute heart failure and renal impairment. *J Card Fail* 2008; 14:631-640.

10. Teerlink JR, Metra M, Felker GM *et al.* Relaxin for the treatment of patients with acute heart failure (Pre-RELAX-AHF): a multicentre, randomised, placebo-controlled, parallel-group, dose-finding phase IIb study. *Lancet* 2009; 373:1429-1439.

11. Gheorghiade M, Pang PS. Acute heart failure syndromes. *J Am Coll Cardiol* 2009; 53:557-573.

12. Cotter G, Moshkovitz Y, Kaluski E *et al.* The role of cardiac power and systemic vascular resistance in the pathophysiology and diagnosis of patients with acute congestive heart failure. *Eur J Heart Fail* 2003; 5:443-451.

13. Gheorghiade M, Zannad F, Sopko G *et al.* Acute heart failure syndromes: current state and framework for future research. *Circulation* 2005; 112:3958-3968.

14. Tsuyuki RT, McKelvie RS, Arnold JM *et al.* Acute precipitants of congestive heart failure exacerbations. *Arch Intern Med* 2001; 161:2337-2342.

15. Fonarow GC, Abraham WT, Albert NM *et al.* Factors identified as precipitating hospital admissions for heart failure and clinical outcomes: findings from OPTIMIZE-HF. *Arch Intern Med* 2008; 168:847-854.

16. Damman K, van Deursen VM, Navis G, Voors AA, van Veldhuisen DJ, Hillege HL. Increased central venous pressure is associated with impaired renal function and mortality in a broad spectrum of patients with cardiovascular disease. *J Am Coll Cardiol* 2009; 53:582-588.

17. Mullens W, Abrahams Z, Francis GS *et al.* Importance of venous congestion for worsening of renal function in advanced decompensated heart failure. *J Am Coll Cardiol* 2009; 53:589-596.

18. Dikshit K, Vyden JK, Forrester JS, Chatterjee K, Prakash R, Swan HJ. Renal and extrarenal hemodynamic effects of furosemide in congestive heart failure after acute myocardial infarction. *N Engl J Med* 1973; 288:1087-1090.

19. Metra M, Teerlink JR, Voors AA *et al.* Vasodilators in the treatment of acute heart failure: what we know, what we don't. *Heart Fail Rev* 2009; 14:299-307.

20. Dickstein K, Cohen-Solal A, Filippatos G *et al.* ESC Guidelines for the diagnosis and treatment of acute and chronic heart failure 2008: the Task Force for the Diagnosis and Treatment of Acute and Chronic Heart Failure 2008 of the European Society of Cardiology. Developed in collaboration with the Heart Failure Association of the ESC (HFA) and endorsed by the European Society of Intensive Care Medicine (ESICM). *Eur Heart J* 2008; 29:2388-2442.

21. Cotter G, Metzkor E, Kaluski E *et al.* Randomised trial of high-dose isosorbide dinitrate plus low-dose furosemide versus high-dose furosemide plus low-dose isosorbide dinitrate in severe pulmonary oedema. *Lancet* 1998; 351:389-393.

22. Sharon A, Shpirer I, Kaluski E *et al.* High-dose intravenous isosorbide-dinitrate is safer and better than Bi-PAP ventilation combined with conventional treatment for severe pulmonary edema. *J Am Coll Cardiol* 2000; 36:832-837.

23. Elkayam U, Akhter MW, Singh H, Khan S, Usman A. Comparison of effects on left ventricular filling pressure of intravenous nesiritide and high-dose nitroglycerin in patients with decompensated heart failure. *Am J Cardiol* 2004; 93:237-240.

24. Gori T, Parker JD. Nitrate-induced toxicity and preconditioning: a rationale for reconsidering the use of these drugs. *J Am Coll Cardiol* 2008; 52:251-254.

25. Nieminen MS, Brutsaert D, Dickstein K *et al.* EuroHeart Failure Survey II (EHFS II): a survey on hospitalized acute heart failure patients: description of population. *Eur Heart J* 2006; 27:2725-2736.

26. ADHERE Scientific Advisory Committee. Acute Decompensated Heart Failure National Registry (ADHERE®) Core Module Q1 2006 Final Cumulative National Benchmark Report: Scios, Inc., 2006.

27. Johnson W, Omland T, Hall C *et al.* Neurohormonal activation rapidly decreases after intravenous therapy with diuretics and vasodilators for class IV heart failure. *J Am Coll Cardiol* 2002; 39:1623-1629.

28. Mullens W, Abrahams Z, Francis GS *et al.* Sodium nitroprusside for advanced low-output heart failure. *J Am Coll Cardiol* 2008; 52:200-207.

29. Packer M, Meller J, Medina N, Gorlin R, Herman MV. Rebound hemodynamic events after the abrupt withdrawal of nitroprusside in patients with severe chronic heart failure. *N Engl J Med* 1979; 301:1193-1197.

30. Francis GS, Olivari MT, Goldsmith SR, Levine TB, Pierpont G, Cohn JN. The acute response of plasma norepinephrine, renin activity, and arginine vasopressin to short-term nitroprusside and nitroprusside withdrawal in patients with congestive heart failure. *Am Heart J* 1983; 106:1315-1320.

31. Mills RM, LeJemtel TH, Horton DP *et al.* Sustained hemodynamic effects of an infusion of nesiritide (human b-type natriuretic peptide) in heart failure: a randomized, double-blind, placebo-controlled clinical trial. Natrecor Study Group. *J Am Coll Cardiol* 1999; 34:155-162.

32. Colucci WS, Elkayam U, Horton DP *et al.* Intravenous nesiritide, a natriuretic peptide, in the treatment of decompensated congestive heart failure. Nesiritide Study Group. *N Engl J Med* 2000; 343:246-253.

33. Sackner-Bernstein JD, Kowalski M, Fox M, Aaronson K. Short-term risk of death after treatment with nesiritide for decompensated heart failure: a pooled analysis of randomized controlled trials. *JAMA* 2005; 293:1900-1905.

34. Sackner-Bernstein JD, Skopicki HA, Aaronson KD. Risk of worsening renal function with nesiritide in patients with acutely decompensated heart failure. *Circulation* 2005; 111:1487-1491.

35. Teerlink JR, Massie BM. Nesiritide and worsening of renal function: the emperor's new clothes? *Circulation* 2005; 111:1459-1461.

36. Aaronson KD, Sackner-Bernstein J. Risk of death associated with nesiritide in patients with acutely decompensated heart failure. *JAMA* 2006; 296:1465-1466.

37. Hernandez AF, O'Connor CM, Starling RC *et al.* Rationale and design of the Acute Study of Clinical Effectiveness of Nesiritide in Decompensated Heart Failure Trial (ASCEND-HF). *Am Heart J* 2009; 157:271-277.

38. Teerlink JR. The role of endothelin in the pathogenesis of heart failure. *Curr Cardiol Rep* 2002; 4:206-212.

39. Cernacek P, Stewart DJ. Immunoreactive endothelin in human plasma: marked elevations in patients in cardiogenic shock. *Biochem Biophys Res Commun* 1989; 161:562-567.

40. Cody RJ, Haas GJ, Binkley PF, Capers Q, Kelley R. Plasma endothelin correlates with the extent of pulmonary hypertension in patients with chronic congestive heart failure. *Circulation* 1992; 85:504-509.

41. Wei CM, Lerman A, Rodeheffer RJ *et al.* Endothelin in human congestive heart failure. *Circulation* 1994; 89:1580-1586.

42. Pacher R, Stanek B, Hulsmann M *et al.* Prognostic impact of big endothelin-1 plasma concentrations compared with invasive hemodynamic evaluation in severe heart failure. *J Am Coll Cardiol* 1996; 27:633-641.

43. Teerlink JR. Endothelins: pathophysiology and treatment implications in chronic heart failure. *Curr Heart Fail Rep* 2005; 2:191-197.

44. Schalcher C, Cotter G, Reisin L *et al.* The dual endothelin receptor antagonist tezosentan acutely improves hemodynamic parameters in patients with advanced heart failure. *Am Heart J* 2001; 142:340-349.

45. Torre-Amione G, Young JB, Durand J *et al.* Hemodynamic effects of tezosentan, an intravenous dual endothelin receptor antagonist, in patients with class III to IV congestive heart failure. *Circulation* 2001; 103:973-980.

46. Torre-Amione G, Durand JB, Nagueh S, Vooletich MT, Kobrin I, Pratt C. A pilot safety trial of prolonged (48 h) infusion of the dual endothelin-receptor antagonist tezosentan in patients with advanced heart failure. *Chest* 2001; 120:460-466.

47. Coletta AP, Cleland JG. Clinical trials update: highlights of the scientific sessions of the XXIII Congress of the European Society of Cardiology – WARIS II, ESCAMI, PAFAC, RITZ-1 and TIME. *Eur J Heart Fail* 2001; 3:747-750.

48. O'Connor CM, Gattis WA, Adams KF Jr *et al.* Tezosentan in patients with acute heart failure and acute coronary syndromes: results of the Randomized Intravenous TeZosentan Study (RITZ-4). *J Am Coll Cardiol* 2003; 41:1452-1457.

49. Torre-Amione G, Young JB, Colucci WS *et al.* Hemodynamic and clinical effects of tezosentan, an intravenous dual endothelin receptor antagonist, in patients hospitalized for acute decompensated heart failure. *J Am Coll Cardiol* 2003; 42:140-147.

50. Kaluski E, Kobrin I, Zimlichman R et al. RITZ-5: randomized intravenous TeZosentan (an endothelin-A/B antagonist) for the treatment of pulmonary edema: a prospective, multicenter, double-blind, placebo-controlled study. J Am Coll Cardiol 2003; 41:204-210.
51. Teerlink JR, McMurray JJ, Bourge RC et al. Tezosentan in patients with acute heart failure: design of the Value of Endothelin Receptor Inhibition with Tezosentan in Acute heart failure Study (VERITAS). Am Heart J 2005; 150:46-53.
52. Vesely DL. Urodilatin: a better natriuretic peptide? Curr Heart Fail Rep 2007; 4:147-152.
53. Drummer C, Kentsch M, Otter W, Heer M, Herten M, Gerzer R. Increased renal natriuretic peptide (urodilatin) excretion in heart failure patients. Eur J Med Res 1997; 2:347-354.
54. Elsner D, Muders F, Muntze A, Kromer EP, Forssmann WG, Riegger GA. Efficacy of prolonged infusion of urodilatin [ANP-(95-126)] in patients with congestive heart failure. Am Heart J 1995; 129:766-773.
55. Kentsch M, Ludwig D, Drummer C, Gerzer R, Muller-Esch G. Haemodynamic and renal effects of urodilatin bolus injections in patients with congestive heart failure. Eur J Clin Invest 1992; 22:662-669.
56. Mitrovic V, Luss H, Nitsche K et al. Effects of the renal natriuretic peptide urodilatin (ularitide) in patients with decompensated chronic heart failure: a double-blind, placebo-controlled, ascending-dose trial. Am Heart J 2005; 150:1239.
57. Mitrovic V, Seferovic PM, Simeunovic D et al. Haemodynamic and clinical effects of ularitide in decompensated heart failure. Eur Heart J 2006; 27:2823-2832.
58. Dickey DM, Burnett JC Jr, Potter LR. Novel bifunctional natriuretic peptides as potential therapeutics. J Biol Chem 2008; 283:35003-35009.
59. Lisy O, Huntley BK, McCormick DJ, Kurlansky PA, Burnett JC Jr. Design, synthesis, and actions of a novel chimeric natriuretic peptide: CD-NP. J Am Coll Cardiol 2008; 52:60-68.
60. Teichman SL, Unemori E, Dschietzig T et al. Relaxin, a pleiotropic vasodilator for the treatment of heart failure. Heart Fail Rev 2009; 14:321-329.
61. Dschietzig T, Teichman S, Unemori E et al. Intravenous recombinant human relaxin in compensated heart failure: a safety, tolerability, and pharmacodynamic trial. J Card Fail 2009; 15:182-190.
62. Evgenov OV, Pacher P, Schmidt PM, Hasko G, Schmidt HH, Stasch JP. NO-independent stimulators and activators of soluble guanylate cyclase: discovery and therapeutic potential. Nat Rev Drug Discov 2006; 5:755-768.
63. Boerrigter G, Costello-Boerrigter LC, Cataliotti A, Lapp H, Stasch JP, Burnett JC Jr. Targeting heme-oxidized soluble guanylate cyclase in experimental heart failure. Hypertension 2007; 49:1128-1133.
64. Frey R, Muck W, Unger S, Artmeier-Brandt U, Weimann G, Wensing G. Pharmacokinetics, pharmacodynamics, tolerability, and safety of the soluble guanylate cyclase activator cinaciguat (BAY 58-2667) in healthy male volunteers. J Clin Pharmacol 2008; 48:1400-1410.
65. Gottlieb SS, Brater DC, Thomas I et al. BG9719 (CVT-124), an A1 adenosine receptor antagonist, protects against the decline in renal function observed with diuretic therapy. Circulation 2002; 105:1348-1353.
66. Dittrich HC, Gupta DK, Hack TC, Dowling T, Callahan J, Thomson S. The effect of KW-3902, an adenosine A1 receptor antagonist, on renal function and renal plasma flow in ambulatory patients with heart failure and renal impairment. J Card Fail 2007; 13:609-617.
67. Givertz MM, Massie BM, Fields TK, Pearson LL, Dittrich HC. The effects of KW-3902, an adenosine A1-receptor antagonist, on diuresis and renal function in patients with acute decompensated heart failure and renal impairment or diuretic resistance. J Am Coll Cardiol 2007; 50:1551-1560.
68. Ho JE, Teerlink JR. Role of tolvaptan in acute decompensated heart failure. Expert Rev Cardiovasc Ther 2008; 6:601-608.
69. Klein L, O'Connor CM, Leimberger JD et al. Lower serum sodium is associated with increased short-term mortality in hospitalized patients with worsening heart failure: results from the Outcomes of a Prospective Trial of Intravenous Milrinone for Exacerbations of Chronic Heart Failure (OPTIME-CHF) study. Circulation 2005; 111:2454-2460.
70. Gheorghiade M, Orlandi C, Burnett JC et al. Rationale and design of the multicenter, randomized, double-blind, placebo-controlled study to evaluate the Efficacy of Vasopressin antagonism in Heart Failure: Outcome Study with Tolvaptan (EVEREST). J Card Fail 2005; 11:260-269.
71. Konstam MA, Gheorghiade M, Burnett JC Jr et al. Effects of oral tolvaptan in patients hospitalized for worsening heart failure: the EVEREST Outcome Trial. JAMA 2007; 297:1319-1331.

7

Fluid overload and cardiorenal syndrome in heart failure: two sides of the same coin?

L. Klein, J. B. O'Connell

INTRODUCTION

Over one million hospital admissions for decompensated heart failure (HF) occur yearly in the United States, with a similar number in Western Europe, accounting for two-thirds of the thirty billion dollars spent annually for this medical condition [1–4]. Data from multinational registries have shown that the majority of patients admitted with decompensated HF have signs and symptoms of fluid overload or congestion, rather than evidence of hypoperfusion or shock [5–8]. In most patients, the fluid accumulation and/or redistribution seem to be gradual processes that start several days to weeks before hospitalization, with a consequent increase in intracardiac filling pressures that translate into dyspnea on exertion, orthopnea and paroxysmal nocturnal dyspnea, leading eventually to hospital admissions [9, 10]. Congestion is often not adequately addressed during hospitalization, resulting in patients being discharged with improved symptoms yet persistently elevated filling pressures. This ultimately may lead to early re-admission when symptoms of congestion recur and contributes to increased short and long-term mortality [11–14]. Although pulmonary infections, myocardial ischemia, arrhythmias, and dietary and medication non-compliance are direct precipitants found in the majority of patients with decompensated HF [8], we submit that the underlying mechanism of fluid accumulation leading to clinical congestion and hospitalization is the result of the abnormal interaction between the cardiovascular system and kidney. This pathophysiological condition, in which combined cardiac and renal dysfunction amplifies progression of failure of the individual organs leading to increased morbidity and mortality, has been labeled cardiorenal syndrome [15]. Although precise criteria to define the cardiorenal syndrome are lacking, data from large epidemiological studies and clinical trials have shown that renal dysfunction in HF patients is associated with increased in-hospital [8, 16-18] and long-term mortality [17–20] and hospitalization rates [8, 16–18, 21]. Despite its poor prognosis, the pathophysiology has not been completely elucidated yet and treatment options are limited [22]. This review will highlight the current understanding of the pathophysiology of congestion and its precursor, the cardio renal syndrome, and describe current and future treatment strategies.

Liviu Klein, MD, MS, The Bluhm Cardiovascular Institute, The Feinberg School of Medicine, Northwestern Memorial Hospital, Chicago, IL, USA.

John B. O'Connell, MD, Executive Director, Heart Failure Program, St Joseph's Hospital, Atlanta, GA, USA.

PATHOPHYSIOLOGY OF CARDIORENAL SYNDROME LEADING TO CONGESTION

The water retention leading to volume overload in HF patients occurs due to an increase in total blood volume, primarily in the venous circulation. In normal subjects, an increase in total blood volume is associated with an increase in renal sodium and water excretion. However, in HF the integrity of the arterial circulation, not the blood volume, is the primary determinant of renal sodium and water handling [23]. The decrease in arterial pressure due to a decreased cardiac output results in the inhibition of high-pressure baroreceptor (located in the left ventricle, aortic arch and carotid sinus) discharge and subsequent activation of the sympathetic and renin-angiotensin-aldosterone systems (RAAS), vagal withdrawal, and non-osmotic vasopressin release [24]. In addition, the increase in stretch of the low-pressure atrial receptors results in secretion of atrial natriuretic peptide (ANP) and leads to an alteration in neural signaling to the hypothalamus and medulla with resultant increase in vasopressin synthesis and sympathetic discharge to the kidneys [25] (Figure 7.1).

Angiotensin II is a powerful vasoconstrictor of efferent glomerular arterioles, helping to maintain the glomerular perfusion pressure. It also acts directly on renal tubular epithelial cells, increasing proximal sodium reabsorption. By constricting the mesangial cells, angiotensin II decreases the effective area for filtration, further conserving sodium and water [26]. Angiotensin II also enhances the release of norepinephrine from renal nerve terminals and stimulates aldosterone production from the adrenal cortex [27]. Aldosterone promotes the retention of sodium in cortical collecting tubules and further activates the sympathetic system [28]. Altogether, these mechanisms are responsible for enhanced proximal sodium reabsorption and diminished sodium delivery to the collecting duct. The decreased sodium delivery to the collecting duct, coupled with a reduction in renal perfusion pressure results in further renin release.

Stimulation by direct renal sympathetic innervation and circulating catecholamines results in an increase in renal sodium reabsorption. This is achieved by alterations in local hemodynamics and direct tubular effects similar to those described for angiotensin II. By direct stimulation of renin production and the subsequent activation of angiotensin II, the sympathetic system further enhances sodium reabsorption [29].

The non-osmotic vasopressin release leads to activation of V2 receptors on the collecting duct which leads to aquaporin-2 water channel-mediated free water retention and contributes to development of hyponatremia [30, 31]. Vasopressin also increases urea permeability through activation of urea transporters, enabling urea to diffuse into the inner medullary interstitium and increasing its reabsorption and the serum blood urea nitrogen (BUN) concentration [32, 33]. In contrast, because creatinine is not reabsorbed but is in fact secreted by the kidney, BUN can rise in the absence of an increase in serum creatinine, causing the 'dissociation' between BUN and estimated glomerular filtration rate often seen in HF [34].

Adenosine and tubulo-glomerular feedback may also play a role in the pathophysiology of cardiorenal syndrome. Adenosine binds to receptors on the afferent arteriole and causes local vasoconstriction, thereby reducing renal blood flow. Stimulation of A1 adenosine receptors also increases sodium resorption in the proximal and distal tubules, leading to sodium and water retention [35]. An acute increase in the delivery of sodium in the distal tubule, seen with diuretic therapy, causes an increase in adenosine concentrations via tubulo-glomerular feedback at the macula densa and afferent arterioles, which subsequently reduces glomerular filtration rate [36].

Natriuretic peptides, including ANP and B-type natriuretic peptide (BNP), promote vasodilatation, as well as natriuresis and diuresis, thereby ameliorating the volume overload. By relaxing the mesangial cells, natriuretic peptides increase the effective area for filtration, an opposite effect to that of angiotensin II [37]. Natriuretic peptides also inhibit sodium reabsorption in collecting duct cells in the inner medulla [38]. At physiologic

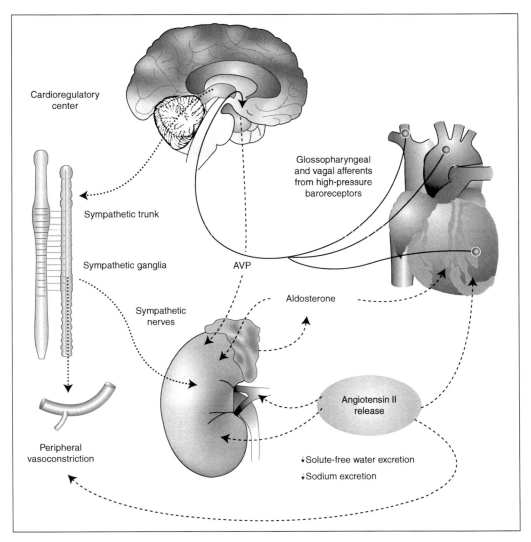

Figure 7.1 Neurohormonal activation in heart failure (adapted with permission from [23]). AVP = arginine vasopressin.

levels, these beneficial effects of natriuretic peptides are quickly overwhelmed by the continued neurohormonal activation that occurs in progressive HF. The exact mechanisms that mediate the attenuated response to natriuretic peptides remain poorly defined, but the decreased distal fluid delivery to the collecting duct (site of natriuretic peptide action) appears to be involved in natriuretic peptide resistance [39]. Moreover, a large part of the immunoreactive BNP in HF patients is made of pro-BNP that possesses significantly lower biological activity than the 32-amino acid hormone [40], leading to a discordance between the high circulating levels of immunoreactive BNP and hormone activity, suggesting that some patients may be in a state of natriuretic peptide deficiency.

In addition to neurohormonal influences, renal perfusion pressure is dependent on the trans-renal perfusion pressure (mean arterial pressure minus central venous pressure). Pulmonary hypertension, right ventricular dysfunction, and tricuspid regurgitation may

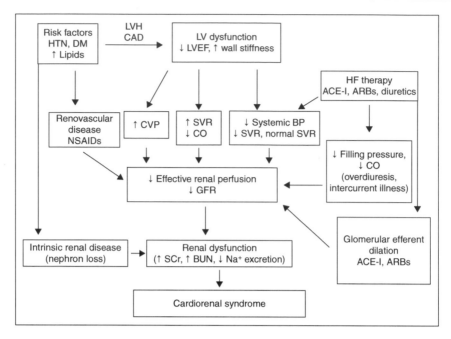

Figure 7.2 Pathophysiology of cardiorenal syndrome (adapted with permission from [41]).
ACE-I=angiotensin-converting-enzyme inhibitor; ARB=angiotensin receptor blocker; BP=blood pressure;
BUN=blood urea nitrogen; CAD=coronary artery disease; CO=cardiac output; CVP=central venous pressure;
DM=diabetes mellitus; GFR=glomerular filtration rate; HTN=hypertension; LV=left ventricular; LVEF=left
ventricular ejection fraction; LVH=left ventricle hypertrophy; NSAID=non-steroidal anti-inflammatory drug;
SCr=serum creatinine; SVR=systemic vascular resistance.

contribute to extremely high renal venous pressures and reduce renal perfusion pressure
dramatically [41] (Figure 7.2). In an elegant study, Firth *et al.* [42] evaluated the effect of
increasing venous pressure on glomerular filtration rate using an isolated rat kidney
preparation. Normal perfusion pressure was maintained while venous pressure was
increased in 6 mmHg steps. Increasing venous pressure above 14 mmHg produced significant reductions in glomerular filtration rate, sodium excretion, and fractional excretion of sodium, which resolved completely when venous pressure was restored to basal
levels [42]. This concept was validated in hospitalized HF patients, where central venous
pressure appeared to be the most important factor related to worsening renal function,
independent of cardiac output or pulmonary capillary wedge pressure [43]. In addition,
patients who were able to decrease their central venous pressure<8 mmHg, were less
likely to develop renal dysfunction during their hospital stay [43]. Increased renal venous
pressure in response to increased central venous pressure causes an increase in renal
interstitial pressure and in the hydrostatic pressure in Bowman's capsule [41]. As result,
angiotensin II concentration increases, leading to further sodium, water, and urea reabsorption in the proximal tubule [44]. Even the increase of intra-abdominal pressure by
external abdominal cuff compression in normal patients leads to a rise in renal vein pressure from 5 to 18 mmHg resulting in a 50% fall in urine output and 30% fall in glomerular
filtration rate [45, 46]. In hospitalized HF patients, an increase in intra-abdominal pressure is strongly correlated with poor renal function, while a reduction of intra-abdominal
pressure during hospital stay is strongly correlated with improvement in renal function
[47].

DIAGNOSIS AND MONITORING OPTIONS FOR CONGESTION

Increased filling pressures and volume overload are present for several days before hospital admission in the majority of patients with HF; however, congestion is often clinically silent in these patients [9, 10]. The ability to identify hemodynamic congestion before symptoms arise may help to avoid hospitalizations and reduce disease progression. Unfortunately, when compared to hemodynamic measurements, the signs and symptoms of HF demonstrate lower clinical accuracy. In a study by Mahdyoon *et al.* [48], only 32% of patients with pulmonary capillary wedge pressures >25 mmHg had moderate-to-severe pulmonary congestion detected by chest X-ray; moreover, 27% had no radiographic evidence of pulmonary congestion. Similarly, rales, edema, and elevated jugular venous pressure were absent in 41% of patients with pulmonary capillary wedge pressures >22 mmHg in another study [49]. Overall, the combination of clinical signs had only a 58% rate of sensitivity in detecting patients with elevated pulmonary capillary wedge pressure [49]. Increases in body weight are associated with hospitalization for HF and begin at least 1 week before admission [50]. Daily information about patients' body weight may identify a high-risk period during which interventions to avert decompensated HF that necessitates hospitalization may be beneficial [50].

Serum measurements of BNP or N-terminal pro-BNP (NT-proBNP) can be used as a surrogate marker of elevated pulmonary capillary wedge pressures [51, 52]. Although serum concentrations of BNP or NT-proBNP cannot be used to follow dynamic changes in congestion because their pattern of production and release is too slow to reliably mirror hemodynamic variations, having a baseline BNP concentration may help determine a patient's 'best' level and may be helpful in optimizing therapy [52].

Recently, two invasive methods to assess the development of pulmonary congestion have been introduced. Intrathoracic impedance measured by implantable cardiac defibrillators or cardiac resynchronization therapy devices has been inversely correlated with pulmonary capillary wedge pressure and fluid balance [10]. In the Medtronic Impedance Diagnostics in Heart Failure Patients Trial (MIDHeFT), intrathoracic impedance decreased before each admission by an average of 12% over an average of 18 days [10]. Impedance reduction began 15 days before the onset of worsening symptoms. Automated detection of impedance decreases had 77% sensitivity in detecting hospitalization for fluid overload. This method provides an early warning of congestion that may allow physicians to intervene by adding or titrating medications, possibly preventing the need for hospitalization [10].

A totally implantable continuous hemodynamic monitor has been developed for outpatient HF management. The Chronicle® device continuously measures and stores hemodynamic information that can be reviewed remotely [53]. Chronic studies comparing intracardiac pressure measurements recorded by the Chronicle® device with those obtained by a Swan-Ganz catheter have found the system to be safe, well tolerated, accurate, and stable over time [54]. Early experiences using the Chronicle® device information in clinical practice supported the use of intracardiac pressures to manage volume status [9]. Recently, the Chronicle® Offers Management to Patients with Advanced Signs and Symptoms of Heart Failure (COMPASS-HF) trial showed a non-significant 21% lower rate of all HF-related events in the Chronicle® arm compared with the control group. However, a retrospective analysis of the time to first HF hospitalization showed a 36% reduction in the relative risk of a HF-related hospitalization in the Chronicle® group [55]. The ongoing Reducing Events in Patients with Chronic Heart Failure (REDUCE-HF) study will assess the safety of the Chronicle® implantable cardiac defibrillator system and the effectiveness of a patient management strategy based on remote access to continuous intracardiac pressures in reducing HF-related events [56].

In addition, chronic hemodynamic monitoring of pulmonary artery and left atrial pressures by implanted devices is under clinical investigation [57, 58].

CURRENT TREATMENT STRATEGIES AND FUTURE DIRECTIONS

Since volume overload is central to the pathophysiology of most episodes of decompensated HF, relief of congestion is the primary goal in these patients. The oldest available therapy in this setting, diuretics, is dramatically effective. For the patient with normal blood pressure and intact renal function, diuretic therapy may be sufficient to relieve the acute symptoms of congestion. Continuous infusion of loop diuretics may provide greater diuresis and better safety profile compared with bolus injection. A meta-analysis of studies comparing continuous infusion versus bolus injection of loop diuretics in decompensated HF showed that urine output was greater in patients given continuous infusion, while electrolyte disturbances were similar between the two groups [59]. There were fewer adverse effects (tinnitus and hearing loss) after continuous infusion compared with bolus injection [59]. However, since the studies were small, mostly crossover trials and were relatively heterogeneous, evidence is insufficient to definitively recommend one method of administering loop diuretics, and further larger studies are needed. The addition of thiazide diuretics in combination with loop diuretics has been shown to improve efficacy and diuretic responsiveness in severe refractory HF, by preventing post-loop diuretic sodium retention [60, 61]. On the other hand, there are important limitations associated with the utility and tolerability of diuretic use. The greatest concerns include additional activation of the neurohormonal cascade, electrolyte depletion, worsening pre-renal azotemia despite ongoing extracellular fluid volume excess, arrhythmias, and renal injury. Use of parenteral loop diuretics such as furosemide has been shown to generate substantial activation of the RAAS that leads to further systemic vasoconstriction and fluid retention, which may further complicate the treatment of volume overload [62, 63]. In addition, parenteral furosemide administration in volume-overloaded patients has been demonstrated to acutely lower glomerular filtration rate despite increasing urine output, and to increase serum creatinine levels [63]. As even small increases in serum creatinine are associated with increased mortality, this risk of renal dysfunction should be carefully considered, and the patient receiving diuretic therapy should be followed very carefully for evidence of alterations in renal function [64–67]. Diuretic resistance is of particular concern in patients with advanced HF because of the need for escalating doses of diuretics to achieve the same or lesser levels of diuresis. The group with the highest risk appears to be the patients presenting with hyponatremia and hypervolemia who are poorly responsive to conventional doses of loop diuretics [68, 69]. Experimental studies also show that long-term sodium depletion caused by chronic loop diuretic use facilitates distal tubular hypertrophy and increases sodium reabsorption at the distal tubule. This can be overcome by the instituting a diuretic 'holiday' to allow the epithelial cells to recover [70].

Alternatives to diuretics or adjunctive approaches that allow for lower doses of diuretic therapy are currently being explored. These include non-pharmacologic strategies such as ultrafiltration, as well as alternative therapies that include positive inotropes, natriuretic peptides, vasopressin receptor antagonists, and adenosine receptor antagonists.

Ultrafiltration devices filter plasma water directly across a semipermeable membrane in response to a transmembrane pressure gradient. Extracellular fluid is thus removed while intravascular fluid volume is maintained, resulting in decreased ventricular filling pressures without significant changes in renal function [71]. Because both water and sodium are simultaneously moved across the membrane, the sodium concentration of the ultrafiltrate is similar to that of the overall blood plasma (isotonic fluid removal) in contrast to the diuretics, which remove only about a third of the plasma sodium (hypotonic fluid removal) [72]. Unlike diuretics, ultrafiltration has demonstrated the ability to mitigate RAAS activation and restore diuretic efficacy [73]. Recently, a peripherally inserted ultrafiltration device (Aquadex®) was approved by the Food and Drug Administration for therapy in HF. This device allows ultrafiltration to be performed at very low flows (40 ml/min) using only a peripheral intravenous catheter and a midline catheter in an antecubital vein, with < 40 ml of extracorporeal blood at any given time. After a series of small studies confirmed the safety of this technique [74], the Ultrafiltration Versus IV Diuretics for Patients Hospitalized for Acute Decompensated Heart Failure (UNLOAD) trial randomized 200 patients hospitalized for HF to peripheral ultrafiltration or standard intravenous diuretic therapy [75]. The primary endpoint of mean weight loss at 48 h was significantly better in patients receiving ultrafiltration compared with diuretic therapy and fewer patients receiving ultrafiltration required rescue therapy with vasoactive drugs [75]. Moreover, ultrafiltration was not associated with hypokalemia or adverse changes in serum creatinine and fewer patients in the ultrafiltration arm were readmitted for HF within 90 days of enrollment [75]. In clinical practice, caution must be exhibited to not overdiurese a patient, especially when ultrafiltration is used in combination with intravenous diuretics. In addition, the expense of treatment limits the potential use of ultrafiltration as a first-line strategy in all hospitalized patients with HF. Whether rescue therapy with ultrafiltration in patients with established cardiorenal syndrome will prove superior to standard care remains to be established.

Positive inotropic therapy is often used as an adjunct to diuretics in hospitalized HF patients because of the favorable hemodynamics and cardiac output achieved with this treatment. However, a randomized study in hospitalized patients found that not only did milrinone not improve symptoms or reduce hospitalization rates compared to placebo, but it increased the incidence of hypotension requiring intervention and atrial arrhythmias [76]. In addition, a recent retrospective analysis of the same study showed that milrinone did not improve outcomes, despite a minor improvement in renal function, contrary to the common belief that agents with positive inotropic effects may help patients with cardiorenal dysfunction [17]. Moreover, there was no difference in the proportion of patients who experienced worsening of their renal function during hospitalization between the placebo and milrinone groups [17]. Because of the important limitations and risks associated with inotropic therapy, it should be reserved for volume overload management only in patients with severe HF and low cardiac index.

Nesiritide (synthetic human BNP) is a potent vasodilator that has been shown to rapidly reduce filling pressures and improve dyspnea in hospitalized patients with HF [77, 78]. Studies, however, conflict on its effects on renal function, natriuresis, and diuresis. Wang et al. [79] examined the effects of a 24-h infusion of nesiritide versus placebo in 15 hospitalized patients with HF and volume overload. In this study, there were no differences in glomerular filtration rate, effective renal plasma flow, urine output, or sodium excretion for any time interval or for the entire 24-h period between the nesiritide and placebo [79]. A meta-analysis of randomized trials of nesiritide in hospitalized HF patients also suggested a possible adverse impact of nesiritide on renal function [80]. The B-Type Natriuretic Peptide in Cardiorenal Decompensation Syndrome (BNP-CARDS) trial randomized 75 consecutive hospitalized patients with HF and renal dysfunction to receive nesiritide or placebo for 48 h in addition to usual care [81]. There were no differences in changes in serum creatinine between the two groups. In addition, there were no differences in changes in weight, intravenous furosemide use, discontinuation of the infusion due to hypotension, or 30-day death/hospital re-admission [81]. A possible explanation for the disparate findings between this and other studies is the use of a bolus dose. It is plausible that any positive effects of nesiritide on glomerular filtration rate might be overcome by significant hypotension occurring with the bolus dose, possibly accounting for some of the worsened renal function seen in other retrospective analyses. The role of nesiritide as a renal-protective and diuresis-promoting therapy in HF remains promising but requires further study. The ASCEND-HF (Acute Study of Clinical Effectiveness of Nesiritide in Decompensated Heart Failure) is an ongoing large, multinational, randomized controlled trial that will evaluate the long-term clinical outcomes and benefit/risk profile of nesiritide in patients with acutely decompensated HF.

The Efficacy of Vasopressin Antagonism in Heart Failure Outcome Study With Tolvaptan (EVEREST) program evaluated short- and long-term effects of tolvaptan in patients admitted for decompensated HF [82, 83]. In the short-term trials, the primary endpoint (patient-assessed global clinical status and body weight reduction) was positive in favor of treatment with tolvaptan, driven by the reductions in body weight beyond that achieved with standard therapy alone and not by changes in global clinical status because the scores were almost identical between the groups [82]. The long-term follow-up trial was powered to assess all-cause mortality and cardiovascular death or HF hospitalization. Over a median of 10 months of follow-up, no effect was found compared with placebo on either endpoints despite effective short-term reductions in post-discharge body weight and improved serum sodium levels in hyponatremic patients. No excess adverse effects on renal function, heart rate, blood pressure, and serum potassium were reported [83]. Hence, the EVEREST data suggest that vasopressin antagonism in the hospitalized HF patients has potential benefit, including decreasing body weight by increasing urine output associated with improvement in dyspnea, without fostering abnormalities in electrolytes or renal function and normalizing serum sodium concentration in hyponatremic patients. The intravenous form of conivaptan as a several-day infusion also has undergone investigation for potential use in decompensated HF. A dose-ranging pilot study assessing the efficacy and safety of intravenous conivaptan in hospitalized HF patients found that conivaptan significantly increased urine output, was hemodynamically well tolerated, and had minimal excess adverse effects. No apparent significant change in respiratory symptoms or body weight was found [84]. Although vasopressin antagonists have the potential to promote free water excretion without compromising renal function, further studies are needed in order to evaluate their role in managing volume overload in HF patients.

Another promising new class of therapeutic agents is the A1 adenosine receptor antagonists. Several small studies have shown that different adenosine antagonists (BG9719, BG9928 and rolofylline) increase urine output, sodium excretion, and glomerular filtration rate in HF patients [85–87]. Addition to furosemide augmented urine output and restored the glomerular filtration rate to the level seen with the placebo infusion, suggesting a renoprotective effect against a furosemide-induced decline in glomerular filtration rate [88]. The Placebo-controlled Randomized study of rolofylline for patients hOspitalised with acute HF and volume Overload to assess Treatment Effect on Congestion and renal funcTion (PROTECT) in 304 hospitalized patients showed that rolofylline improved dyspnea, decreased the likelihood of worsening HF and improved renal function compared to placebo [89]. The ongoing Placebo-controlled Randomized Study of rolofylline for Patients Hospitalized with Worsening Renal Heart Failure Requiring Intravenous Therapy (REACH-UP) trial is aimed to evaluate the effect of rolofylline, in addition to standard therapy, on worsening HF, worsening renal function, and on mortality or re-admission for HF or worsening renal function [90]. The results of this larger study will determine whether A1 adenosine receptor antagonists will prevent worsening renal function and avoid diuretic resistance in patients with HF at risk for cardiorenal syndrome.

CONCLUSIONS

The management of volume overload in HF patients remains a clinical challenge owing to the lack of consistent data from randomized studies in this setting and the resulting lack of evidence-based treatment guidelines. The combined cardiac and renal dysfunction amplifies this issue and leads to cardiorenal syndrome. Patients hospitalized with HF are routinely discharged without achieving a clinically ideal volume state, but treatment goals are poorly defined and no clear criteria exist to direct clinicians in determining when the appropriate volume status has been reached. While diuretics remain necessary for reducing congestion, mounting evidence suggests that they may not be entirely benign and adjunctive strategies that permit lower doses of diuretic therapy, or alternative strategies that obviate the need for diuretic therapy represent important new directions for research.

REFERENCES

1. DeFrances CJ, Cullen KA, Kozak LJ. National Hospital Discharge Survey: 2005 annual summary with detailed diagnosis and procedure data. *Vital Health Stat 13* 2007; 165:1-209.
2. Nieminen MS, Böhm M, Cowie MR *et al.* ESC Committee for Practice Guideline. Executive summary of the guidelines on the diagnosis and treatment of acute heart failure: the Task Force on Acute Heart Failure of the European Society of Cardiology. *Eur Heart J* 2005; 26:384-416.
3. Rosamond W, Flegal K, Furie K *et al.* American Heart Association Statistics Committee and Stroke Statistics Subcommittee. Heart disease and stroke statistics – 2008 update: a report from the American Heart Association Statistics Committee and Stroke Statistics Subcommittee. *Circulation* 2008; 117:e25-e146.
4. Berry C, Murdoch DR, McMurray JJ. Economics of chronic heart failure. *Eur J Heart Fail* 2001; 3:283-291.
5. Cleland JG, Swedberg K, Follath F *et al.* Study Group on Diagnosis of the Working Group on Heart Failure of the European Society of Cardiology. The EuroHeart Failure survey programme – a survey on the quality of care among patients with heart failure in Europe. Part 1: patient characteristics and diagnosis. *Eur Heart J* 2003; 24:442-463.
6. Adams KF Jr, Fonarow GC, Emerman CL *et al.* ADHERE Scientific Advisory Committee and Investigators. Characteristics and outcomes of patients hospitalized for heart failure in the United States: rationale, design, and preliminary observations from the first 100,000 cases in the Acute Decompensated Heart Failure National Registry (ADHERE). *Am Heart J* 2005; 149:209-216.
7. Nieminen MS, Brutsaert D, Dickstein K *et al.* EuroHeart Survey Investigators. Heart Failure Association, European Society of Cardiology. EuroHeart Failure Survey II (EHFS II): a survey on hospitalized acute heart failure patients: description of population. *Eur Heart J* 2006; 27:2725-2736.
8. Fonarow GC, Abraham WT, Albert NM *et al.* OPTIMIZE-HF Investigators and Hospitals. Factors identified as precipitating hospital admissions for heart failure and clinical outcomes: findings from OPTIMIZE-HF. *Arch Intern Med* 2008; 168:847-854.
9. Adamson PB, Magalski A, Braunschweig F *et al.* Ongoing right ventricular hemodynamics in heart failure: clinical value of measurements derived from an implantable monitoring system. *J Am Coll Cardiol* 2003; 41:565-571.
10. Yu CM, Wang L, Chau E *et al.* Intrathoracic impedance monitoring in patients with heart failure: correlation with fluid status and feasibility of early warning preceding hospitalization. *Circulation* 2005; 112:841-848.
11. Gattis WA, O'Connor CM, Gallup DS *et al.* IMPACT-HF Investigators and Coordinators. Pre-discharge initiation of carvedilol in patients hospitalized for decompensated heart failure: results of the Initiation Management Pre-discharge: Process for Assessment of Carvedilol Therapy in Heart Failure (IMPACT-HF) trial. *J Am Coll Cardiol* 2004; 43:1534-1541.
12. Gheorghiade M, Gattis WA, O'Connor CM *et al.* for the Acute and Chronic Therapeutic Impact of a Vasopressin Antagonist in Congestive Heart Failure (ACTIV in CHF) Investigators. Effects of tolvaptan, a vasopressin antagonist, in patients hospitalized with worsening heart failure: a randomized controlled trial. *JAMA* 2004; 291:1963-1971.
13. Lucas C, Johnson W, Hamilton MA *et al.* Freedom from congestion predicts good survival despite previous class IV symptoms of heart failure. *Am Heart J* 2000; 140:840-847.
14. Drazner MH, Rame JE, Stevenson LW *et al.* Prognostic importance of elevated jugular venous pressure and a third heart sound in patients with heart failure. *N Engl J Med* 2001; 345:574-581.
15. National Heart, Lung, and Blood Institute: NHLBI Working Group – Cardio-Renal Connections in Heart Failure and Cardiovascular Disease – August 20, 2004. Available at http://www.nhlbi.nih.gov/meetings/workshops/cardiorenalhf-hd.htm. Accessed September 1, 2008.
16. Fonarow GC, Adams KF Jr, Abraham WT *et al.* Risk stratification for in-hospital mortality in acutely decompensated heart failure: classification and regression tree analysis. *JAMA* 2005; 293:572-580.
17. Klein L, Massie B, Leimberger J *et al.* Admission or changes in renal function during hospitalization for worsening heart failure predict post-discharge survival: results from the Outcomes of a Prospective Trial of Intravenous Milrinone for Exacerbations of Chronic Heart Failure (OPTIME-CHF). *Circ Heart Fail* 2008; 1:25-33.
18. Hillege HL, Nitsch D, Pfeffer MA *et al.* Renal function as a predictor of outcome in a broad spectrum of patients with heart failure. *Circulation* 2006; 113:671-678.

19. Dries DL, Exner DV, Domanski MJ et al. The prognostic implications of renal insufficiency in asymptomatic and symptomatic patients with left ventricular systolic dysfunction. *J Am Coll Cardiol* 2000; 35:681-689.

20. Lee DS, Austin PC, Rouleau JL et al. Predicting mortality among patients hospitalized for heart failure: derivation and validation of a clinical model. *JAMA* 2003; 290:2581-2587.

21. Krumholz HM, Chen YT, Wang Y et al. Predictors of readmission among elderly survivors of admission with heart failure. *Am Heart J* 2000; 139:72-77.

22. Kazory A, Ross EA. Contemporary trends in the pharmacological and extracorporeal management of heart failure: a nephrologic perspective. *Circulation* 2008; 117:975-983.

23. Schrier RW, Abraham WT. Hormones and hemodynamics in heart failure. *N Engl J Med* 1999; 341:577-585.

24. Schrier RW, Berl T. Non-osmolar factors affecting renal water excretion (first of two parts). *N Engl J Med* 1975; 292:81-88.

25. Schrier RW, Berl T. Non-osmolar factors affecting renal water excretion (second of two parts). *N Engl J Med* 1975; 292:141-145.

26. de Arriba G, Barrio V, Olivera A, Rodriguez-Puyol D, Lopez-Novoa JM. Atrial natriuretic peptide inhibits angiotensin II-induced contraction of isolated glomeruli and cultured glomerular mesangial cells of rats: the role of calcium. *J Lab Clin Med* 1988; 111:466-474.

27. Zimmerman BG. Adrenergic facilitation by angiotensin: does it serve a physiological function? *Clin Sci* 1981; 60:343-348.

28. Weber KT. Aldosterone and spironolactone in heart failure. *N Engl J Med* 1999; 341:753-755.

29. Packer M. Neurohormonal interactions and adaptations in congestive heart failure. *Circulation* 1988; 77:721-730.

30. Schrier RW, Berl T, Anderson RJ. Osmotic and non-osmotic control of vasopressin release. *Am J Physiol* 1979; 236:F321-F332.

31. Goldsmith SR, Francis GS, Cowley AW Jr, Levine TB, Cohn JN. Increased plasma arginine vasopressin levels in patients with congestive heart failure. *J Am Coll Cardiol* 1983; 1:1385-1390.

32. Goldsmith SR, Francis GS, Cowley AW Jr. Arginine vasopressin and the renal response to water loading in congestive heart failure. *Am J Cardiol* 1986; 58:295-299.

33. Schrier RW. Role of diminished renal function in cardiovascular mortality: marker or pathogenetic factor? *J Am Coll Cardiol* 2006; 47:1-8.

34. Schrier RW. Blood urea nitrogen and serum creatinine: not married in heart failure. *Circ Heart Fail* 2008; 1:2-5.

35. Dzau VJ. Renal and circulatory mechanisms in congestive heart failure. *Kidney Int* 1987; 31:1402-1415.

36. Elkayam U, Mehra A, Cohen G et al. Renal circulatory effects of adenosine in patients with chronic heart failure. *J Am Coll Cardiol* 1998; 32:211-215.

37. Stockand JD, Sansom SC. Regulation of filtration rate by glomerular mesangial cells in health and diabetic renal disease. *Am J Kidney Dis* 1997; 29:971-981.

38. Light DB, Schweibert EM, Karlson KH, Stanton BA. Atrial natriuretic peptide inhibits a cation channel in renal inner medullary collecting duct cells. *Science* 1989; 243:383-385.

39. Kalra PR, Anker SD, Coats AJS. Water and sodium regulation in chronic heart failure: the role of natriuretic peptides and vasopressin. *Cardiovasc Res* 2001; 51:495-509.

40. Liang F, O'Rear J, Schellenberger U et al. Evidence for functional heterogeneity of circulating B-type natriuretic peptide. *J Am Coll Cardiol* 2007; 49:1071-1078.

41. Fonarow GC, Heywood JT. The confounding issue of comorbid renal insufficiency. *Am J Med* 2006; 119:S17-S25.

42. Firth JD, Raine AE, Ledingham JG. Raised venous pressure: a direct cause of renal sodium retention in oedema? *Lancet* 1988; 331:1033-1035.

43. Mullens W, Abrahams Z, Francis GS et al. Importance of venous congestion for worsening of renal function in advanced decompensated heart failure. *J Am Coll Cardiol* 2009; 53:589-596.

44. Nohria A, Hasselblad V, Stebbins A et al. Cardiorenal interactions: insights from the ESCAPE trial. *J Am Coll Cardiol* 2008; 51:1268-1274.

45. Mullens W, Abrahams Z, Francis GS, Taylor DO, Starling RC, Tang WH. Prompt reduction in intra-abdominal pressure following large-volume mechanical fluid removal improves renal insufficiency in refractory decompensated heart failure. *J Card Fail* 2008; 14:508-514.

46. Mullens W, Abrahams Z, Skouri HN et al. Elevated intra-abdominal pressure in acute decompensated heart failure: a potential contributor to worsening renal function? *J Am Coll Cardiol* 2008; 51:300-306.

47. Damman K, Navis G, Smilde TDJ et al. Decreased cardiac output, venous congestion and the association with renal impairment in patients with cardiac dysfunction. *Eur J Heart Fail* 2007; 9:872-878.
48. Mahdyoon H, Klein R, Eyler W, Lakier JB, Chakko SC, Gheorghiade M. Radiographic pulmonary congestion in end-stage congestive heart failure. *Am J Cardiol* 1989; 63:625-627.
49. Chakko S, Woska D, Martinez H et al. Clinical, radiographic, and hemodynamic correlations in chronic congestive heart failure: conflicting results may lead to inappropriate care. *Am J Med* 1991; 90:353-359.
50. Chaudhry SI, Wang Y, Concato J, Gill TM, Krumholz HM. Patterns of weight change preceding hospitalization for heart failure. *Circulation* 2007; 116:1549-1554.
51. Logeart D, Thabut G, Jourdain P et al. Pre-discharge B-type natriuretic peptide assay for identifying patients at high risk of readmission after decompensated heart failure. *J Am Coll Cardiol* 2004; 43:635-641.
52. Wu AHB, Smith A, Wieczorek S et al. Biological variation for N-terminal pro- and B-type natriuretic peptides and implications for therapeutic monitoring of patients with congestive heart failure. *Am J Cardiol* 2003; 92:628-631.
53. Magalski A, Adamson P, Gadler F et al. Continuous ambulatory right heart pressure measurements with an implantable hemodynamic monitor: a multicenter, 12-month follow-up study of patients with chronic heart failure. *J Card Fail* 2002; 8:63-70.
54. Adamson PB, Kjellström B, Braunschweig F et al. Ambulatory hemodynamic monitoring from an implanted device: components of continuous 24-hour pressures that correlate to supine resting conditions and acute right heart catheterization. *Congest Heart Fail* 2006; 12:14-19.
55. Bourge RC, Abraham WT, Adamson PB et al. COMPASS-HF Study Group. Randomized controlled trial of an implantable continuous hemodynamic monitor in patients with advanced heart failure: the COMPASS-HF study. *J Am Coll Cardiol* 2008; 51:1073-1079.
56. Adamson PB, Conti JB, Smith AL et al. Reducing events in patients with chronic heart failure (REDUCE-HF) study design: continuous hemodynamic monitoring with an implantable defibrillator. *Clin Cardiol* 2007; 30:567-575.
57. Verdejo HE, Castro PF, Concepción R et al. Comparison of a radio frequency-based wireless pressure sensor to Swan-Ganz catheter and echocardiography for ambulatory assessment of pulmonary artery pressure in heart failure. *J Am Coll Cardiol* 2007; 50:2375-2382.
58. Rozenman Y, Schwartz RS, Shah H, Parikh KH. Wireless acoustic communication with a miniature pressure sensor in the pulmonary artery for disease surveillance and therapy of patients with congestive heart failure. *J Am Coll Cardiol* 2007; 49:784-789.
59. Salvador DR, Rey NR, Ramos GC, Punzalan FE. Continuous infusion versus bolus injection of loop diuretics in congestive heart failure. *Cochrane Database Syst Rev* 2005; 3:CD003178.
60. Dormans TP, Gerlag PG, Russel FG et al. Combination diuretic therapy in severe congestive heart failure. *Drugs* 1998; 55:165-172.
61. Dormans TP, Gerlag PG. Combination of high-dose furosemide and hydrochlorothiazide in the treatment of refractory congestive heart failure. *Eur Heart J* 1996; 17:1867-1874.
62. Ikram H, Chan W, Espiner EA, Nicholls MG. Haemodynamic and hormone responses to acute and chronic furosemide therapy in congestive heart failure. *Clin Sci* 1980; 59:443-449.
63. Francis GS, Siegel RM, Goldsmith SR, Olivari MT, Levine TB, Cohn JN. Acute vasoconstrictor response to intravenous furosemide in patients with chronic congestive heart failure: activation of the neurohumoral axis. *Ann Intern Med* 1985; 103:1-6.
64. Neuberg GW, Miller AB, O'Connor CM et al. for the PRAISE Investigators. Diuretic resistance predicts mortality in patients with advanced heart failure. *Am Heart J* 2002; 144:31-38.
65. Domanski M, Norman J, Pitt B, Haigney M, Hanlon S, Peyster E. Diuretic use, progressive heart failure, and death in patients in the Studies of Left Ventricular Dysfunction (SOLVD). *J Am Coll Cardiol* 2003; 42:705-708.
66. Hasselblad V, Gattis Stough W, Shah MR et al. Relation between dose of loop diuretics and outcomes in a heart failure population: results of the ESCAPE trial. *Eur J Heart Fail* 2007; 9:1064-1069.
67. Weinfeld MS, Chertow GM, Stevenson LW. Aggravated renal dysfunction during intensive therapy for advanced chronic heart failure. *Am Heart J* 1999; 138:285-290.
68. Ellison DH. Diuretic therapy and resistance in congestive heart failure. *Cardiology* 2001; 96:132-143.
69. Butler J, Forman DE, Abraham WT et al. Relationship between heart failure treatment and development of worsening renal function among hospitalized patients. *Am Heart J* 2004; 147:331-338.
70. Brater DC. Diuretic therapy. *N Engl J Med* 1998; 339:387-395.
71. Silverstein ME, Ford CA, Lysaght MJ et al. Treatment of severe fluid overload by ultrafiltration. *N Engl J Med* 1974; 291:747-751.

72. Agostoni PG, Marenzi GC, Pepi M *et al*. Isolated ultrafiltration in moderate congestive heart failure. *J Am Coll Cardiol* 1993; 21:424-431.

73. Forslund T, Riddervold F, Fauchald P *et al*. Hormonal changes in patients with severe chronic congestive heart failure treated by ultrafiltration. *Nephrol Dial Transplant* 1992; 7:306-310.

74. Bart BA, Boyle A, Bank AJ *et al*. Ultrafiltration versus usual care for hospitalized patients with heart failure: The Relief for Acutely Fluid-Overloaded Patients With Decompensated Congestive Heart Failure (RAPID-CHF) trial. *J Am Coll Cardiol* 2005; 46:2043-2046.

75. Costanzo MR, Guglin ME, Saltzberg MT *et al*. UNLOAD Trial Investigators. Ultrafiltration versus intravenous diuretics for patients hospitalized for acute decompensated heart failure. *J Am Coll Cardiol* 2007; 49:675-683.

76. Cuffe MS, Califf RM, Adams KF Jr *et al*. Outcomes of a Prospective Trial of Intravenous Milrinone for Exacerbations of Chronic Heart Failure (OPTIME-CHF) Investigators. Short-term intravenous milrinone for acute exacerbation of chronic heart failure: a randomized controlled trial. *JAMA* 2002; 287:1541-1547.

77. Colucci WS, Elkayam U, Horton DP *et al*. Intravenous nesiritide, a natriuretic peptide, in the treatment of decompensated congestive heart failure. Nesiritide Study Group. *N Engl J Med* 2000; 343:246-253.

78. Publication Committee for the VMAC (Vasodilatation in the Management of Acute CHF) Investigators. Intravenous nesiritide versus nitroglycerin for treatment of decompensated congestive heart failure: a randomized controlled trial. *JAMA* 2002; 287:1531-1540.

79. Wang DJ, Dowling TC, Meadows D *et al*. Nesiritide does not improve renal function in patients with chronic heart failure and worsening serum creatinine. *Circulation* 2004; 110:1620-1625.

80. Sackner-Bernstein JD, Skopicki HA, Aaronson KD. Risk of worsening renal function with nesiritide in patients with acutely decompensated heart failure. *Circulation* 2005; 111:1487-1491.

81. Witteles RM, Kao D, Christopherson D *et al*. Impact of nesiritide on renal function in patients with acute decompensated heart failure and pre-existing renal dysfunction a randomized, double-blind, placebo-controlled clinical trial. *J Am Coll Cardiol* 2007; 50:1835-1840.

82. Konstam MA, Gheorghiade M, Burnett JC Jr *et al*. Efficacy of Vasopressin Antagonism in Heart Failure Outcome Study With Tolvaptan (EVEREST) Investigators. Effects of oral tolvaptan in patients hospitalized for worsening heart failure: the EVEREST Outcome Trial. *JAMA* 2007; 297:1319-1331.

83. Gheorghiade M, Konstam MA, Burnett JC Jr *et al*. Efficacy of Vasopressin Antagonism in Heart Failure Outcome Study With Tolvaptan (EVEREST) Investigators. Short-term clinical effects of tolvaptan, an oral vasopressin antagonist, in patients hospitalized for heart failure: the EVEREST Clinical Status Trials. *JAMA* 2007; 297:1332-1343.

84. Udelson JE, Smith WB, Hendrix GH *et al*. Acute hemodynamic effects of conivaptan, a dual V(1A) and V(2) vasopressin receptor antagonist, in patients with advanced heart failure. *Circulation* 2001; 104:2417-2423.

85. Gottlieb SS, Brater DC, Thomas I *et al*. BG9719 (CVT-124), an A1 adenosine receptor antagonist, protects against the decline in renal function observed with diuretic therapy. *Circulation* 2002; 105:1348-1353.

86. Givertz MM, Massie BM, Fields TK, Pearson LL, Dittrich HC. CKI-201 and CKI-202 Investigators. The effects of KW-3902, an adenosine A1-receptor antagonist, on diuresis and renal function in patients with acute decompensated heart failure and renal impairment or diuretic resistance. *J Am Coll Cardiol* 2007; 50:1551-1560.

87. Dittrich HC, Gupta DK, Hack TC *et al*. The effect of KW-3902, an adenosine A1 receptor antagonist, on renal function and renal plasma flow in ambulatory patients with heart failure and renal impairment. *J Card Fail* 2007; 13:609-617.

88. Greenberg B, Thomas I, Banish D *et al*. Effects of multiple oral doses of an A1 adenosine antagonist, BG9928, in patients with heart failure: results of a placebo-controlled, dose-escalation study. *J Am Coll Cardiol* 2007; 50:600-606.

89. Cleland JG, Coletta AP, Yassin A *et al*. Clinical trials update from the American College of Cardiology 2008: CARISMA, TRENDS, meta-analysis of Cox-2 studies, HAT, ON-TARGET, HYVET, ACCOMPLISH, MOMENTUM, PROTECT, HORIZON-HF and REVERSE. *Eur J Heart Fail* 2008; 10:614-620.

90. Chaparro S, Dittrich HC, Tang WHW. Rolofylline (KW-3902): a new adenosine A1-receptor antagonist for acute congestive heart failure. *Future Cardiol* 2008; 4:117-123.

8

Should we use endomyocardial biopsy more often in heart failure diagnosis?

K. L. Baughman

INTRODUCTION

The fundamental value of inspecting heart muscle tissue in patients with heart muscle disorders is intuitive. In the same way coronary angiography leads to a better understanding of the diagnosis and treatment of coronary disease, and cardiac catheterization to the understanding and treatment of valvular heart disease, examination of heart tissue should guide the understanding of cardiac muscle disease. Enthusiasm of the cardiovascular community for endomyocardial biopsy has varied in the 50 years since its introduction, but waned considerably after the release of the Myocarditis Treatment Trial [1] which demonstrated disparities in the histopathologic diagnosis of myocarditis and failure of immunosuppressive therapy to favorably alter the course of this illness [1]. Over the course of the last several years, the tools utilized to evaluate heart muscle tissue have expanded dramatically. At the time of the Myocarditis Treatment Trial standard investigation included hematoxylin and eosin histologic staining, electron microscopy and a limited number of special stains for immunopathologic assessment. We now have the ability to use histologic markers for cellular components, and have expanded our molecular and cellular tests to include polymerase chain reaction enhancement of viral pathogens, and sophisticated genetic analysis.

Clinicians recognize that not all cardiomyopathies are idiopathic in origin and that not all non-ischemic cardiomyopathies are 'viral'. Determining the etiology of cardiomyopathy is important for prognosis and potential treatment. As demonstrated by Felker [2], in patients with similar degrees of heart dysfunction, the outcome varied dramatically based on the established diagnosis after complete evaluation, including heart biopsy (Figure 8.1).

NON-BIOPSY ANALYSIS

The diagnosis of the etiology of the heart muscle disorder often does not require heart biopsy. The diagnosis can be made with a careful history, physical examination, blood work, echocardiogram, cardiac catheterization, or coronary angiogram [3]. Historical clues to the diagnosis include a significant past history of hypertension, usually with systolic pressures in excess of 200 mm of mercury, poor blood pressure control, or hypertensive crises. Patients with ischemic heart disease should have a documented history of a myocardial infarction, have undergone bypass or stent placement or have had a catheterization demonstrating the narrowing of the coronary artery of greater than 50% (Box 1). Individuals with recognized

The late **Kenneth Lee Baughman**, MD, Formerly Professor of Medicine, Harvard Medical School, Director, Advanced Heart Disease Section, Brigham & Women's Hospital, Boston, MA, USA.

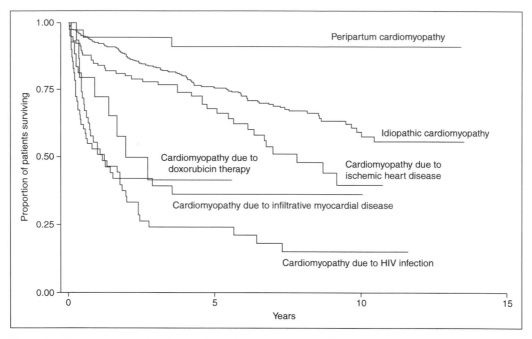

Figure 8.1 In a large series of patients submitted to endomyocardial biopsy to evaluate new onset heart dysfunction, Felker demonstrated a significant difference in long-term outcome based on the final diagnosis [2].

Box 1 Diagnostic tests to be done before biopsy

All	*Select populations*
History	Coronary angiogram
Examination	Cardiac catheterization
EKG	MRI
CXR	Special blood/urine studies
Echocardiogram	
TSH	
ANA	
ANA = antinuclear antibody; CXR = chest X-ray; EKG = electrocardiogram; MRI = magnetic resonance imaging; TSH = thyroid stimulating hormone.	

congenital heart diseases which predispose to left or right ventricular dysfunction as they age, need little further analysis. Patients with first degree relatives having an established dilated or hypertrophic cardiomyopathy, should generally not be considered for biopsy. Women who are within the last month of pregnancy or within 5 months of delivery, presenting with a new onset of cardiac dysfunction with no other apparent etiology have peripartum cardiomyopathy, which rarely should be evaluated with biopsy. Finally, a careful history of exposure to cardiotoxins including chemotherapy (adriamycin and cytoxan), alcohol (greater than eight ounce of ethanol per day for 6 months), or illicit drugs such as cocaine, usually need no further evaluation.

Table 8.1 Histologic diagnosis by heart biopsy

	Fulminant	*Acute*	*Chronic active*	*Chronic persistent*
Onset	Distinct	Indistinct	Indistinct	Indistinct
LV function	Severe dysfunction	Moderate dysfunction	Moderate dysfunction	No dysfunction
Biopsy	Multiple foci	Active or borderline	Active or borderline	Active or borderline
Clinical history	Recovery or death	Incomplete DCM	Restrictive CM	Normal LV function
Histologic outcome	Complete resolution	Complete resolution	Giant cells-fibrosis	Ongoing

CM = cardiomyopathy; DCM = dilated cardiomyopathy; LV = left ventricular.

Physical examination may strongly indicate a valvular abnormally or a significant AV communication. Similarly, there may be physical examination changes to suggest metabolic disorders (thyroid disease, hemochromatosis). Non-invasive imaging, particularly echocardiography, may demonstrate a primary valvular disorder, multi-segment dysfunction compatible with ischemic heart disease, or show non-myocardial etiologies of heart failure (HF) such as pericardial diffusion or constriction.

All patients presenting with new onset left ventricular compromise should have a careful history as outlined above, complete physical examination, an electrocardiogram, chest X-ray, echocardiogram, and blood work for antinuclear antibodies and thyroid stimulating hormone. The latter blood tests are performed to ensure that subtle connective tissue or thyroid abnormalities are not present. Patients with suspected disorders based on the above analysis, should undergo specific testing. Those displaying signs of growth hormone excess should have growth hormone measured. Individuals who's findings are compatible with pheochromocytoma should have appropriate measurement of free catechols and urinary vanillyl mandelic acid (VMA). Human immunodeficiency virus (HIV) should be analyzed in those hosts with concerning risk factors. Coronary angiography should be performed in men over 45 years of age and women over 50 years of age with appropriate risk factors (hypertension, diabetes, smoking, high cholesterol, family history). If there is a suggestion of a primary valvular abnormality or a constrictive restrictive processes, cardiac catheterization is most beneficial.

DIAGNOSIS BY ENDOMYOCARDIAL BIOPSY

Heart biopsy can establish the histopathologic diagnosis of a number of disorders (Table 8.1) including vascular, restrictive, malignancy, and inflammatory states.

The risks of endomyocardial biopsy are dependent on the operator and experience with the technique. Most series that have reported the risk of endomyocardial biopsy have not prospectively and diligently evaluated the risks of the procedure, including complications associated with venous or arterial access [4, 5]. In a prospective series of 546 cardiomyopathy patients submitted to diagnostic endomyocardial biopsy, Deckers reported 2.7% complication rate with vascular access in the 3.3% risk during the biopsy itself [6]. Most of the risks (arrhythmia and conduction abnormalities) resolved without therapy. Nonetheless, death can occur and was recorded in 0.5% of those biopsied. Death results from myocardial perforation with pericardial tamponade in patients with a very narrow margin for hemodynamic

Box 2

Endomyocardial biopsy may be of benefit even when no specific histological diagnosis is established.

Box 3

Definitions of class and levels of evidence.
Class
I – Evidence or general agreement of benefit
II – Conflicting evidence or divergence of opinion
IIa – weight of evidence favors
IIb – usefulness less well established
III – Evidence or general agreement not useful
Level of evidence
A – Multiple randomized clinical trials
B – Limited randomized trials, non-randomized trials or registry
C – Expert consensus

compromise and the potential to clot a portion of their acute blood loss in the pericardial space preventing full removal percutaneously. The risk may be increased in those with bleeding disorders or on anticoagulants and those with increased right ventricular systolic or diastolic pressure. The risk of biopsy is therefore dependent on the skill of the operator and the status of the patients and their ability to undergo diagnostic procedures.

Endomyocardial biopsy is of benefit, even if no definitive histopathologic diagnosis is demonstrated (Box 2) [7–10]. Patients with idiopathic cardiomyopathy display evidence of hypertrophy, interstitial fibrosis, and nuclear enlargement. Quantitating these changes allows the clinician an understanding of the duration of illness and the potential for clinical improvement with treatment (Box 3). Similarly, the finding of replacement fibrosis (large areas of myocyte loss with fibrotic infiltration), pigment laden macrophages, and macrophage removal of dead myocytes may confirm the diagnosis of ischemic cardiomyopathy in patients who are too ill to undergo standard cardiac catheterization, or have compromised renal function preventing dye exposure.

BIOPSY GUIDELINES

Guidelines have recently been released evaluating the role of endomyocardial biopsy in the management of cardiovascular disease [11]. These guidelines help the clinician determine what patient populations should be submitted to heart biopsy (Table 8.2). These recommendations are based primarily upon expert consensus as there are a limited number of prospective randomized trials of biopsy proven disorders. Nonetheless, two clinical presentations have warranted recommendations for which there is general agreement that the procedure is beneficial, useful, and effective. These include new onset HF of less than 2 weeks duration associated with normal sized or dilated left ventricle and hemodynamic compromise or the new onset of HF of 2 weeks to 3 months duration associated with a dilated left ventricle and new ventricular arrhythmias, second and third degree heart block, or failure to respond to usual care within 1 to 2 weeks. Each of these has specific histopathologic entities associated with them.

Table 8.2 The Role of Endomyocardial Biopsy in 14 Clinical Scenarios

Scenario number	Clinical scenario	Class of recommendation (I, IIa, IIb, III)	Level of evidence (A, B, C)
1	New-onset heart failure of <2 *weeks'* duration associated with a normal-sized or dilated left ventricle and hemodynamic compromise	I	B
2	New-onset heart failure of 2 *weeks'* to 3 months' duration associated with a dilated left ventricle and new ventricular arrhythmias, second- or third-degree heart block, or failure to respond to usual care within 1 to 2 weeks	I	B
3	Heart failure of >3 *months'* duration associated with a dilated left ventricle and new ventricular arrhythmias, second- or third-degree heart block, or failure to respond to usual care within 1 to 2 weeks	IIa	C
4	Heart failure associated with a DCM of any duration associated with suspected allergic reaction and/or eosinophilia	IIa	C
5	Heart failure associated with suspected anthracycline cardiomyopathy	IIa	C
6	Heart failure associated with unexplained restrictive cardiomyopathy	IIa	C
7	Suspected cardiac tumors	IIa	C
8	Unexplained cardiomyopathy in children	IIa	C
9	New-onset heart failure of 2 *weeks'* to 3 *months'* duration associated with a dilated left ventricle, without new ventricular arrhythmias or second- or third-degree heart block, that responds to usual care within 1 to 2 weeks	IIb	B
10	Heart failure of >3 *months'* duration associated with a dilated left ventricle, without new ventricular arrhythmias or second- or third-degree heart block, that responds to usual care within 1 to 2 weeks	IIb	C
11	Heart failure associated with unexplained HCM	IIb	C
12	Suspected ARVD/C	IIb	C
13	Unexplained ventricular arrhythmias	IIb	C
14	Unexplained atrial fibrillation	III	C

(With permission from [11]).

Patients with unexplained new onset HF of less than 2 weeks duration associated with normal sized or dilated left ventricles with hemodynamic compromise define fulminant myocarditis [12–15]. This is often due to an immediate post-viral infection or autoimmune response. Patients in this category often require pressor or mechanical support. The ventricle is usually thickened, presumable due to myocardial edema, and may not be dilated but is always hypofunctional. Heart biopsies from this group show characteristic Dallas criteria confirmed myocarditis (Box 4). Immunosuppressive therapy is not beneficial to this group and they either die or have recovered virtually completely within 2 weeks. The prognosis for this group is excellent, even after long-term follow up [12].

Box 4

Histologic 'Dallas' Criteria
Inflamatory infiltrate
- lymphocytic
- focal/diffuse
Myocyte destruction
- necrosis
- damage
Borderline myocarditis
Sparse inflamatory infiltrate
No light microscopic myocyte destruction
(Reference [53])

Box 5

Biopsy should be performed in patients when the differential diagnosis includes:
- Fulminant myocarditis
- Giant cell myocarditis.

Box 6

Biopsy should be strongly considered when the differential diagnosis includes:
Sarcoidosis
Allergen or eosinophil related
Antracycline exposure
Restrictive cardiomyopathy
Cardiac tumors
Unexplained cardiomyopathy in children

Patients with this hemodynamic and clinical presentation may also display necrotizing eosinophilic myocarditis or giant cell myocarditis [16]. These disorders have a very poor prognosis. Necrotizing eosinophilic myocarditis displays not only eosinophilic myocardial infiltrates associated with an inflammatory response, but severe myocyte necrosis [17, 18]. Giant cell myocarditis is usually more subtle in presentation but may display a fulminant pattern. Giant cell myocarditis is associated with an inflammatory infiltrate, giant cells, myocyte necrosis, scar tissue, and a poor prognosis. Both of these disorders may respond to immunosuppressive therapy [16–19] (Box 5).

Patients with unexplained new onset HF of 2 weeks to 3 months duration associated with a dilated left ventricle and new ventricular arrhythmias or heart block which fails to respond to therapy within 1 to 2 weeks of treatment should also be biopsied. Patients who fail to respond to treatment, or show a progressive course, within 3 months of their presentation should be considered to have giant cell myocarditis [16, 20]. This disorder has a very poor prognosis with an overall survival of under 6 months. Giant cell myocarditis is often associated with pre-existent autoimmune diseases or drug sensitivity. Patients present with aggressive HF, progressive ventricular arrhythmias, or heart block. Immunosuppressive therapy has been demonstrated in non-randomized observations to improve the prognosis compared to those without the treatment, from three to 12 months

[16]. There are some data to suggest that aggressive immunosuppressive therapy may be of some benefit; however, no prospective randomized trials have been reported to confirm this.

Therefore, patients in these two categories should undergo endomyocardial biopsy, even if this means transferring the patient to a center where biopsies are performed.

Six additional scenarios have been classified as conditions for which there is conflicting evidence and/or divergence of opinion about the usefulness or efficacy of treatment but for which the weight of evidence is in favor of usefulness or efficacy. These conditions are briefly outlined below (Box 6).

Endomyocardial biopsy is thought to be reasonable in the clinical setting of unexplained HF of greater than 3 months duration associated with a dilated left ventricle and ventricular arrhythmias, heart block, or failure to respond to usual care within 1 to 2 weeks. Patients in this clinical presentation should be evaluated for cardiac sarcoidosis [21–24]. Heart biopsy shows inflammation associated with non-cacseating granuloma and fibrosis. Unfortunately, the sensitivity of heart biopsy for sarcoidosis, even in those who have clinically suspected disease, is only 20 to 30% because of the spotty nature of the involvement [22]. Cardiac sarcoidosis may be present without other systemic manifestations of the inflammatory disease and the frequency of cardiac involvement is much higher (25%) than those with clinical manifestations (5%) [22]. Cardiac sarcoidosis is an indication for corticoid steroid therapy, although this recommendation is based on non-prospective non-randomized treatment studies [25–27]. There is a high frequency of ventricular arrhythmias and sudden cardiac death and knowledge of cardiac sarcoidosis may inform the insertion of an implantable cardioverter defibrillator (ICD) [22, 27–30].

Endomyocardial biopsy is 'reasonable' in patients with HF and dilated cardiomyopathy of any duration associated with an allergic reaction with or without eosinophilia. Two other myocardial disorders associated with the eosinophils may be diagnosed by endomyocardial biopsy. Hypersensitivity myocarditis is the association of an eosinophilic myocardial infiltrate (with limited myocyte necrosis) and often subtle deterioration in ventricular performance [31]. This is often seen in patients with established heart disease who are initiated on medication or remedy which is an allergen. Clinical deterioration may include worsening HF, ventricular arrhythmias, or sudden death. This may be seen in 2.4 to 7.0% explanted hearts at transplant or autopsy [32]. Recognition of this disorder may allow withdrawal of the responsible agent and treatment with corticosteroids.

Eosinophilic myocarditis is an eosinophilic infiltrate associated with myocardial dysfunction in individuals with a known eosinophilic disorder. The infiltrate may be associated with worsening heart function or endocardial fibrosis. This condition often improves as the eosinophilic disorder is appropriately treated and eosinophil count decreases.

Anthracycline exposure is also noted as a reasonable indication for heart biopsy. The presentation of cardiac dysfunction may follow administration of anthracyclines by many years [33, 34]. In addition, other chemotherapeutic agents, including cytoxan and herceptin, may expose or exacerbate pre-existent subclinical cardiovascular disease related to anthracycline toxicity. Electron microscopic assessment of endomyocardial biopsy specimens allows determination of the degree of adriamycin exposure experienced by the myocyte [35, 36]. This may be helpful to evaluate anthracyclines as the cause of cardiotoxicity in a patient presenting with cardiac dysfunction and prior exposure to this agent or at risk of cardiac damage by additional anthracycline or cardiotoxic chemotherapeutic agent administration [37, 38].

Patients presenting with restrictive cardiomyopathy will have a diagnosis established by endomyocardial biopsy (Table 8.3) [39–42]. Most frequently, patients present with an infiltrative abnormality. Of these diagnoses, amyloidosis is the most frequent. Endomyocardial biopsy allows confirmation of the diagnosis, which significantly influences general and specific management. Tissue analysis techniques also allow determination the nature of the amyloid (primary, myeloma related, senile, inherited or secondary). These categories often

Table 8.3 Presentation of patients with restrictive cardiomyopathy

Non-infiltrative	Infiltrative	Storage
Idiopathic	Amyloid	Hemochromatosis
Familial	Sarcoid	Fabry's
Hypertrophic	Gaucher's	Glycogen
Scleroderma	Hurler's	
Diabetic	Fatty	

Box 7

Biopsy should be considered when the following diagnoses are considered:
▣ Myocarditis
▣ Autoimmune cardiomyopathy
▣ Hypertrophic cardiomyopathy
▣ ◆ Fabry
  ◆ Pompe
▣ Arrhythmogenic right ventricular dysplasia

trigger further assessment and, on occasion, qualify patients for aggressive solid organ and bone marrow transplantation [43–45]. Patients with storage disease, particular Fabre's and glycogen storage disease, may present with similar echocardiograhpic findings. Endomyocardial biopsy allows clinicians to differentiate myocardial from endocardial disorders. Most importantly, in patients presenting with constrictive or restrictive findings, a normal endomyocardial biopsy provides significant evidence that the hemodynamic compromise is due to pericardial as opposed to myocardial disease.

Cardiac tumors are yet another indication for endomyocardial biopsy. Tumors appearing within the heart are usually metastatic in nature [46]. Therefore, in most instances, the diagnosis can be established by other means. If endomyocardial biopsy is considered, one must ensure the diagnosis cannot be established using International Carotid Stenting Study (ICSS) invasive techniques, and that the ability to obtain diagnostic tissue is high with limited risk. These techniques are usually performed under transesophageal or transthoracic echocardiographic guidance [47, 48].

Heart biopsy is also thought to be 'reasonable' in unexplained cardiomyopathy found in children [49]. Children have a higher incidence of myocarditis accounting for their new onset heart dysfunction than adults [50, 51]. Biopsy may allow not only confirmation of the histologic diagnosis but, when combined with the polymerase chain reaction, also identify the causative agent.

Five additional scenarios have garnered a less robust recommendation. In this category, the authors identified conflicting evidence, but noted that the usefulness or efficacy is less well established and the recommendation is almost entirely dependent on consensus opinion (Box 7).

Heart biopsy may be considered with unexplained HF of 2 weeks to 3 months duration associated with the dilated left ventricle without evidence of arrhythmia or heart block. Similarly, heart biopsy may be considered in the setting of unexplained HF of greater than 3 months duration without arrhythmia or heart block.

These recommendations reflect our current uncertainty in diagnosing histologic myocarditis or other indicators of autoimmune damage in patients with new onset cardiomyopathy [1]. The Myocarditis Treatment Trial demonstrated that, as defined by the Dallas criteria (see Box 4), patients with new onset HF and myocarditis were not improved by treatment with immunosuppressive therapy [1, 52]. Similarly, Parrillo demonstrated in patients

Box 8

Limitations of Dallas criteria:
Sampling error
Inter-observer variability in diagnosis
Lack of correlation with PCR demonstrated viral infection
Lack of correlation with treatment results
(Reference [55])
PCR = polymerase chain reaction.

with established cardiomyopathy, even with interstitial inflammation, that corticosteroids provided no benefit in heart function [53] in the long term. McNamara utilized intravenous immunoglobulin for non-ischemic cardiomyopathy and demonstrated no difference in outcome relative to those who received placebo and standard management [54]. The studies by Mason and McNamara were remarkable for the significant spontaneous improvement in the 'control' group's ejection fraction.

The Dallas criteria may not be appropriate to make the diagnosis of myocarditis given the sampling error, focal nature of disease, inter-observer variability in tissue diagnosis, failure of diagnosis to influence response to therapy, and lack of the diagnosis to correlate with polymerase chain reaction-proven myocarditis [55–58] (Box 8).

Two recent trials, utilizing different markers of immune up regulation, have demonstrated improvement with immunosuppressive therapy. Patients with immune up regulation, characterized by human leukocyte antigen (HLA) staining displayed an improvement in functional capacity and ejection fraction with immunosuppressive therapy [59, 60]. Frustaci evaluated 112 patients with myocarditis, demonstrated that 41 had progressive HF. All patients were treated with prednisone and azathrioprine and the 20 who responded with an improvement in ejection fraction, had anti-heart antibodies but no evidence of viral persistence [61]. Therefore, there may be criteria which would allow us to determine, in the more chronic dilated cardiomyopathy category, based on viral persistence and autoimmune up regulation, which patients may respond to immunosuppressive therapy.

Heart biopsy is considered in patients with apparent hypertrophic cardiomyopathy. Inherited hypertrophic cardiomyopathy rarely deserves endomyocardial biopsy. The same echocardiographic and clinical pattern, however, may be seen in patients with amyloidosis, or infiltrative diseases including Fabrey's and Pompe's. These disorders can usually be diagnosed by other techniques.

Heart biopsy may be considered in patients suspected to have arrhythmogenic right ventricular dysplasia (ARVD) [62, 63]. The value of endomyocardial biopsy in patients with presumed ARVD is currently being explored in an international prospective trial. A diagnosis of ARVD can usually be established by non-invasive techniques including echocardiography, computed tomography (CT), or cardiac magnetic resonance imaging [64]. Biopsy may demonstrate myocyte replacement by fibrofatty tissue and inflammation [65, 66]. The most diagnostic sites for endomyocardial biopsy are those which are highest risk for myocardial perforation, including the apex and the right ventricular outflow track. Therefore, the risk: benefit ratio must be considered in evaluating patients with this suspected disorder.

Endomyocardial biopsy may be considered in an unexplained ventricular arrhythmias, but currently has no role in the setting of unexplained atrial fibrillation (Box 9) [67–69]. Patients with life threatening arrhythmias, without apparent structural heart disease, occasionally have histologic abnormalities demonstrated by endomyocardial biopsy [70–72]. Rarely have these findings been associated with treatment options which alter outcome.

Box 9

Biopsy has little role in ventricular arrhythmia of unknown etiology
No apparent role in atrial fibrillation.

Box 10

Heart biopsy in research:
- Molecular diagnosis
- Genetic diagnosis
- Cell therapy

Nonetheless, Vignola [67] and Frustaci [73] have reported the finding of significant myocardial inflammation in patients with unexplained ventricular arrhythmias or sudden cardiac arrest and no other apparent cardiac disorders. Vignole demonstrated a diminished ability to provoke arrhythmias in five of six patients treated with immunosuppressive therapy [67]. There are no randomized prospective trials that demonstrate improved outcome with patients in this category.

Endomyocardial biopsy should be considered in individuals with unexplained ventricular arrhythmias where knowledge of the presence of organic heart disease of any type (myocardial inflammation, fibrosis or hypertrophy) would influence the placement of an ICD.

HEART BIOPSIES AS A RESEARCH TOOL

Heart biopsy allows the sampling of heart tissue. Our ability to analyze this material has increase dramatically in the last decade. The polymerase chain reaction now allows us to determine whether or not a viral pathogen is present in the myocardium. Similarly, we have been able to assess the genetic makeup of dysfunctional tissue or alteration in protein expression [74–78]. Samples are also being utilized for cell therapy and potential cardiac replacement [79] (Box 10).

SUMMARY

The guidance provided by the writing committee has helped establish standards for the performance of endomyocardial biopsy. To this point, heart biopsies have been performed primarily in centers that have experience with the procedure based on assessment and treatment of patients with heart transplantation. These centers will similarly likely be the early adapters of advanced histologic, molecular, and cellular techniques to analyze cardiac tissue. It is anticipated that this enhanced diagnostic yield will result in better understanding of the cause of heart muscle disorders and inform its treatment. In the interim, it is clear that certain clinical scenarios of heart dysfunction mandate heart biopsy analysis, while others are considered appropriate. While the diagnosis of the etiology of heart muscle dysfunction can be made by history, examination, echocardiography, catheterization, or coronary angiography, there remains a broad spectrum of patients who are without a diagnosis at the completion of this analysis. In the past, even using current endomyocardial biopsy techniques, 50% of those submitted to biopsy have no etiology found [2]. That number is expected to diminish rapidly with the enhanced diagnostic and therapeutic approaches outlined above. Currently, we are not using endomyocardial biopsy often enough in the diagnosis of HF, but this will inevitably change.

REFERENCES

1. Mason JW, O'Connell JB, Hershkowitz A *et al*. A clinical trial of immunosuppressive therapy for myocarditis. The Myocarditis Treatment Trial Investigators. *N Engl J Med* 1995; 333:269-275.
2. Felker GM, Thompson RE, Hare JM *et al*. Underlying causes and long-term survival in patients with initially unexplained cardiomyopathy. *New Engl J Med* 2000; 342:1077-1084.
3. Felker GM, Hu W, Hare JM *et al*. The spectrum of dilated cardiomyopathy. The Johns Hopkins experience with 1,278 patients. *Medicine* (Baltimore) 1999;78: 270-283.
4. Fowles RE, Mason, JW. Endomyocardial biopsy. *Ann Intern Med* 1982; 97:885-894.
5. Sekiguchi M, Take M. World survey of catheter biopsy of the heart. In: Sekiguchi M, eds. *Cardiomyopathy: Clinical, Pathological and Theoretical Aspects*. Baltimore: University Park Press, 1980, pp 217-225.
6. Deckers JW, Hare JM, Baughman KL. Complications of transvenous right ventricular endomyocardial biopsy in adult patients with cardiomyopathy: a seven-year study of 546 consecutive diagnostic procedures in a tertiary referral center. *J Am Coll Cardiol* 1992; 19:43-47.
7. Veinot JP, Ghadially FN, Walley VM. Light microscopy and ultrastructure of the blood vessel and heart. In: Silver MD, eds. *Cardiovascular Pathology*. Philadelphia: Churchill Livingstone, 2001, pp 30-53.
8. Virmani R, Burke A, Farb A, Atkinson J *Cardiovascular Pathology*. Philadelphia: WB Saunders, 2001.
9. Cunningham KS, Veinot JP, Butany J. An approach to endomyocardial biopsy interpretation. *J Clin Pathol* 2006; 59:121-129.
10. Veinot JP. Diagnostic endomyocardial biopsy pathology: general biopsy considerations, and its use for myocarditis and cardiomyopathy: a review. *Can J Cardiol* 2002; 18:55-65.
11. Cooper LT, Baughman KL, Feldman AM *et al*. The role of endomyocardial biopsy in the management of cardiovascular disease. *Circulation* 2007; 116:2216-2233.
12. McCarthy RE 3rd, Boehmer JP, Hruban RH *et al*. Long-term outcome of fulminant myocarditis as compared with acute (nonfulminant) myocarditis. *N Engl J Med* 2000; 342:690-695.
13. Amabile N, Fraisse A, Bouvenot J *et al*. Outcome of acute fulminant myocarditis in children. *Heart* 2006; 92:1269-1273.
14. Felker GM, Boehmer JP, Hruban RH *et al*. Echocardiographic findings in fulminant and acute myocarditis. *J Am Coll Cardiol* 2000; 36:227-232.
15. Dec GW Jr, Palacios IF, Fallon JT *et al*. Active myocarditis in the spectrum of acute dilated cardiomyopathies: clinical features, histologic correlates, and clinical outcome. *N Engl J Med* 1985; 31: 885-890.
16. Cooper LT Jr, Berry GJ, Shabetai R. Idiopathic giant cell myocarditis: natural history and treatment. Multicenter Giant Cell Myocarditis Study Group Investigators. *N Engl J Med* 1997; 336:1860-1866.
17. Herzog CA, Snover DC, Stanley NA. Acute necrotizing eosinophilic myocarditis. *Br Heart J* 19847; 52: 343-348.
18. deMello DE, Liapis H, Jureidini S *et al*. Cardiac localization of eosinophilic-granule major basic protein in acute necrotizing myocarditis. *N Engl J Med* 1990; 323:1542-1545.
19. Daniels PR, Berry GJ, Tazelaar HD, Cooper LT Jr. Giant cell myocarditis as a manifestation of drug hypersensitivity. *Cardiovasc Pathol* 2000; 9:287-291.
20. Shields RC, Tazelaar HD, Berry GJ, Cooper LT Jr. The role of right ventricular endomyocardial biopsy for idiopathic giant cell myocarditis. *J Card Fail* 2002; 8:74-78.
21. Okura Y, Dec GW, Hare JM *et al*. A multicenter registry comparison of cardiac sarcoidosis and idiopathic giant-cell myocarditis. *Circulation* 2000; 102:II-788.
22. Silverman KJ, Hutchins GM, Bulkley BH. Cardiac sarcoid: a clinicopathologic study of 84 unselected patients with systemic sarcoidosis. *Circulation* 1978; 58:1204-1211.
23. Sekiguchi M, Yazaki Y, Isobe M, Hiroe M. Cardiac sarcoidosis: diagnostic, prognostic, and therapeutic considerations. *Cardiovasc Drug Ther* 1996; 10:495-510.
24. Uemura A, Morimoto S, Hiramitsu *et al*. Histologic diagnostic rate of cardiac sarcoidosis: evaluation of endomyocardial biopsies. *Am Heart J* 1999; 138:299-302.
25. Cooper L, Okura Y, Hare J *et al*. Survival in biopsy-proven cardiac sarcoidosis is similar to survival in lymphocytic myocarditis and dilated cardiomyopathy. In: Kimchi A, ed. *Heart Disease: New Trends in Research, Diagnosis, and Treatment: Proceedings of the 2nd International Congress on Heart Disease*. Pianoro (Bologna) Italy: Medimond Medical Publications, 2001, pp 491-496.
26. Ardehali H, Howard DL, Hariri A *et al*. A positive endomyocardial biopsy result for sarcoid is associated with poor prognosis in patients with initially unexplained cardiomyopathy. *Am Heart J* 2005; 150:459-463.

27. Takada K, Ina Y, Yamamoto M *et al*. Prognosis after pacemaker implantation in cardiac sarcoidosis in Japan: clinical evaluation of corticosteroid therapy. *Sarcoidosis* 1994; 11:113-117.
28. Bellhassen B, Pines A, Laniado S. Failure of corticosteroids to prevent induction of ventricular tachycardia in sarcoidosis. *Chest* 1989; 95:918-920.
29. Bajaj AK, Kopelman HA, Echt DS. Cardiac sarcoidosis with sudden death: treatment with the automatic implantable cardioverter defibrillator. *Am Heart J* 1988; 116:557-560.
30. Winters SL, Cohen M, Greenberg S *et al*. Sustained ventricular tachycardia associated with sarcoidosis: assessment of the underlying cardiac anatomy and the prospective utility of programmed ventricular stimulation, drug therapy, and an implantable antitachycardia device. *J Am Coll Cardiol* 1991; 18:937-943.
31. Taliercio CP, Olney BA, Lie JT. Myocarditis related to drug hypersensitivity. *Mayo Clin Proc* 1985; 60: 463-468.
32. Spear GS. Eosinophilic explant carditis with eosinophilia: hypersensitivity to dobutamine infusion. *J Heart Lung Transplant* 1995; 14:755-760.
33. Meinardi MT, van der Graaf WT, van Veldhuisen DJ *et al*. Detection of anthracycline-induced cardiotoxicity. *Cancer Treatment Recovery* 1999; 25:237-247.
34. Bristow MR. Lopez MB, Mason JW *et al*. Efficacy and cost of cardiac monitoring in patients receiving doxorubicin. *Cancer* 1982; 50:32-41.
35. Mackay B, Ewer MS, Carrasco CH, Benjamin RS. Assessment of anthracycline cardiomyopathy by endomyocardial biopsy. *Ultrastruct Pathol* 1994; 18:203-211.
36. Torti, FM, Bristow MM, Lum BL *et al*. Cardiotoxicity of epirubicin and doxorubicin: assessment by endomyocardial biopsy. *Cancer Res* 1986; 46:3722-3727.
37. Billingham ME, Mason JW, Bristow MR, Daniles JR. Anthracycline cardiomyopathy monitored by morphologic changes. *Cancer Treat Rep* 1975; 62:865-872.
38. Torti Fm, Bristow MR, Howes AE *et al*. Reduced cardiotoxicitiy of doxorubicin delivered on a weekly schedule: assessment by endomyocardial biopsy. *Ann Inter Med* 1983; 99:745-749.
39. Kushwaha SS, Fallon JT, Fuster V. Restrictive cardiomyopathy. *N Engl J Med* 1997; 336:267-276.
40. Asher CR, Klein AL. Diastolic heart failure: restrictive casrdiomyopathy, constrictive pericarditis, and cardiac tamponade: clinical and echocardiographic evaluation. *Cardiol Rev* 2002; 10:218-229.
41. Yazdani K, Maraj S, Amanullah AM. Differentiating constrictive pericarditis from restrictive cardiomyopathy. *Rev Cardiovasc Med* 2005; 6:61-71.
42. Olson, LJ, Edwards ED, McCall, JT *et al*. Cardiac iron deposition in idiopathic hemochromatosis: histologic and analytic assessment of 14 hearts from autopsy. *J Am Coll Cardiol* 1987; 10:1239-1243.
43. Falk RH. Diagnosis and management of the cardiac amyloidosis. *Circulation* 2005; 112:2047-2060.
44. Rahman JE, Helou EF, Gelzer-Bell R *et al*. Noninvasive diagnosis of biopsy-proven cardiac amyloidosis. *J Am Coll Cardiol* 2004; 43:410-415.
45. Pellikka PA, Holmes DR Jr, Edwards WD *et al*. Endomyocardial biopsy in 30 patients with primary amyloidosis and suspected cardiac involvement. *Arch Intern Med* 1988; 148:662-666.
46. Flipse TR, Tazelaar HD, Holmes DR Jr. Diagnosis of malignant cardiac disease by endomyocardial biopsy. *Mayo Clin Proc* 1990; 65:1415-1422.
47. Scott PJ, Ettles DF, Rees MR, Williams GJ. The use of combined transesophageal echocardiography and fluoroscopy in the biopsy of a right atrial mass. *Br J Radiol* 1990; 63:222-224.
48. Burling F, Devlin G, Heald S. Primary cardiac lymphoma diagnosed with transesophageal echocardiography-guided endomyocardial biopsy. *Circulation* 2000; 101:179-181.
49. Towbin J. Cardiomyopathy and heart transplantation in children. *Curr Opin Cardiol* 2002; 17:274-279.
50. Bowles NE, Ni J, Kearney DL *et al*. Detection of viruses in myocardial tissues by polymerase chain reaction: evidence of adenovirus as a common cause of myocarditis in children and adults. *J Am Coll Cardiol* 2003; 42:466-472.
51. Martin AB, Webber S, Fricker FJ *et al*. Acute myocarditis: rapid diagnosis by PCR in children. *Circulation* 1994; 90:330-339.
52. Aretz HT, Billingham MR, Edwards WD *et al*. Myocarditis: a histopathologic definition and classification. *Am J Cardiovasc Pathol* 1987; 1:3-14.
53. Parrillo JE. Inflammatory cardiomyopathy (myocarditis): which patients should be treated with anti-inflammatory therapy? *Circulation* 2001; 104:4-6.
54. McNamara DM, Holubkov R, Starling RC *et al*. Controlled trial of intravenous immune globulin in recent-onset dilated cardiomyopathy. *Circulation* 2001; 103:2254-2259.
55. Baughman KL. Diagnosis of myocarditis: death of Dallas criteria. *Circulation* 2006; 113:593-595.

56. Bowles NE, Ni J, Kearney DL *et al*. Detection of viruses in myocardial tissues by polymerase chain reaction: evidence of adenovirus as a common cause of myocarditis in children and adults. *J Am Coll Cardiol* 2003; 42:466-472.

57. Kuhl U, Pauschinger M, Noutsias M *et al*. High prevalence of viral genomes and multiple viral infections in the myocardium of adults with 'idiopathic' left ventricular dysfunction. *Circulation* 2005; 111:887-893.

58. Tschope C, Bock CT, Kasner M *et al*. High prevalence of cardiac parvovirus B19 genome in endomyocardial biopsies from patients with suspected myocarditis or idiopathic left ventricular dysfunction. *Z Kardiol* 2004; 93:300-309.

59. Wojnicz R, Nowalany-Kozielska E, Wojciechowska C *et al*. Randomized, placebo-controlled study for immunosuppressive treatment of inflammatory dilated cardiomyopathy: two-year follow-up results. *Circulation* 2001; 104:39-45.

60. Herskowitz A, Ahmed-Ansari A, Neumann DA *et al*. Induction of major histocompatability complex antigens within the myocardium of patients with active myocarditis: a nonhistologic marker of myocarditis. *J Am Coll Cardiol* 1990; 15:624-632.

61. Frustaci A, Chimenti C, Calabrese F *et al*. Immunosuppressive therapy for active lymphocytic myocardtis: virological and immunologic profile of responders versus nonresponders. *Circulation* 2003; 6:857-863.

62. Kies P, Bootsma M, Bax J *et al*. Arrthymogenic right ventricular dysplasia/cardiomyopathy: screening, diagnosis, and treatment. *Heart Rhythm* 2006; 3:225-234.

63. Hulot JS, Jouven X, Empana JP *et al*. Natural history and risk stratification of arrhythmogenic right ventricular dysplasia/cardiomyopathy. *Circulation* 2004; 110:1879-1884.

64. Tandri H, Castillo E, Ferrari VA *et al*. Magnetic resonance imaging of arrhythmogenic right ventricular dysplasia: sensitivity, specificity, and observer variability of fat detection versus functional analysis of the right ventricle. *J Am Coll Cardiol* 2006; 48:2277-2284.

65. Basso C, Thiene G. Adipositas cordis, fatty infiltration of the right ventricle, and arrhythmogenic right ventricular cardiomyopathy: just a matter of fat? *Cardiovasc Pathol* 2005; 14:37-41.

66. Basso C, Ronco F, Abudureheman A, Thiene G. In vitro validation of endomyocardial biopsy for the in vivo diagnosis or arrhythmogenic right ventricular cardiomyopathy. *Eur Heart J* 2006; 27:960.

67. Vignola PA, Aonuma K, Swaye PS *et al*. Lymphocytic myocarditis presenting as unexplained ventricular arrhythmias: diagnosis with endomyocardial biopsy and respond to immunosuppression. *J Am Coll Cardiol* 1984; 4:812-819.

68. Yonesaka S, Takahashi T, Tomimoto K *et al*. Clinical and histopatholgical studies in children with supraventricular tachycardia. *Jpn Circ J* 1996; 60:560-566.

69. Teragaki M, Toda I, Sakamoto K *et al*. Endomyocardial biopsy findings in patient with atrioventricualr block in the absence of apparent heart disease. *Heart Vessels* 1999; 14:170-176.

70. Hosenpud JD, McAnulty JH, Niles NR. Unexpected myocardial disease in patient with life threatening arrhythmias. *Br Heart J* 1986; 56:55-61.

71. Oakes DF, Manolis AS, Estes NA 3rd. Limiited clinical utility of endomyocardial biopsy in patients presenting with ventricular tachycardia without apparent structural heart disease. *Clin Cardiol* 1992; 15:24-28.

72. Sugrue DD, Holmes DR Jr., Gersh BJ *et al*. Cardiac histologic findings in patients with life-threatening ventricular arrhythmias of unknown origin. *J Am Coll Cardiol* 1984; 4:952-957.

73. Frustaci A, Bellocci F, Olsen EG. Results of biventricular endomyocardial biopsy in survivors of cardiac arrest with apparently normal hearts. *Am J Cardiol* 1994; 74:890-895.

74. Feldman AM, Ray PE, Silan CM *et al*. Selective gene expression in failing human heart: quantification of steady-state levels of messenger RNA in endomyocardial biopsies using the polymerase chain reaction. *Circulation* 1991; 83:1866-1872.

75. Ladenson PA, Sherman, SI, Baughma KL *et al*. Reversible alterations in myocardial gene expression in a young man with dilated cardiomyopathy and hypothyroidism. *Proc Natl Acad Sci USA* 1992; 89:5251-5255.

76. Bristow MR, Minobe WA, Raynolds MV *et al*. Reduced beta 1 receptor messenger RNA abundance in the failing human heart. *J Clin Invest* 1993; 92:2737-2745.

77. Lowes BD, Zolty R, Minobe WA *et al*. Serial gene expression profiling in the intact human heart. *J Heart Lung Transplant* 2006; 25:579-588.

78. Cook SA, Rosenzweig A. DNA microarrays: implications for cardiovascular medicine. *Circ Res* 2002; 91:559-564.

79. Smith RR, Barile L, Cho HC *et al*. Regenerative potential of cardiosphere-derived cells expanded from percutaneous endomyocardial biopsy specimens. *Circulation* 2007; 115:896-908.

9

Prescribing exercise training for patients with heart failure

S. D. Russell

INTRODUCTION

The understanding of the therapy of heart failure (HF) has changed dramatically over the years. Until the publication of trials showing efficacy in the late 1990s, beta blockers were considered to be contraindicated in HF because of their negative inotropic effects. Similarly, exercise was strongly discouraged because of its presumed detrimental effects on the heart. McDonald *et al.* [1] described their experience with prolonged bed rest and found that 40% of the patients had a normalization of heart size. Others felt that bed rest increased renal blood flow which therefore improved urine output and enhanced pharmacological diuresis [2].

During the 1980s many studies demonstrated the safety of exercise and cardiac rehabilitation in post-myocardial infarction patients [3] and that experience was quickly transferred over to HF patients. Since then, many studies have evaluated the safety and efficacy of exercise testing and exercise training programs in patients with HF [4–18]. As will be reviewed, improvements in functional capacity and quality of life (QoL) were demonstrated with a variety of different exercise regimens. Based on that data, a large clinical trial evaluating the effects of exercise training in HF patients was performed and recently presented. The objective of this chapter is to review the physiologic abnormalities that are present in HF patients and the effects of those abnormalities on exercise, review the effects of exercise on functional capacity, quality of life, and morbidity and mortality, and finally to discuss how to prescribe exercise regimens for people with HF.

CARDIAC PHYSIOLOGY DURING EXERCISE IN HF

HF can be caused by a number of different conditions; however, the end result is progressive impairment of functional capacity and progressive symptoms of exertional dyspnea and fatigue. These symptoms all result from a reduction in cardiac output and the subsequent adaptations that the body makes to respond to that lack of blood delivery. There are a number of factors that contribute to the limitations to exercise in patients with HF. These include decreased cardiac output, decreased skeletal muscle blood flow, early anaerobic energy metabolism, increased pulmonary capillary wedge pressure, and excessive pulmonary dead space and ventilation [19]. Although the exact contribution of heart versus the periphery to the exercise limitation is unclear, it is quite clear that both have limitations that probably contribute.

Stuart D. Russell, MD, FACC, Associate Professor of Medicine, Chief, Heart Failure and Transplantation, Division of Cardiology, Johns Hopkins School of Medicine, Baltimore, MD, USA.

Some of the seminal work examining the central hemodynamic response to exercise was performed at Duke University in the late 1980s and early 1990s. Higginbotham, Sullivan, and Cobb performed a number of exercise tests with invasive monitoring while measuring both oxygen consumption and ejection fraction in both normal patients and those with HF [19–21]. They found that HF patients have an increased resting heart rate, but a reduction in heart rate at peak exercise [20]. Similarly, stroke volume was reduced at both rest and peak exercise and therefore the cardiac output was reduced. Of interest, the central arterio-venous oxygen difference was increased at rest and at peak exercise was similar to the A-V oxygen difference in normal controls. However, it is not clear that these central cardiac changes are solely responsible for the exercise limitations of these patients. Various interventions such as inotropes or vasodilators that improve cardiac output and leg blood flow do not improve exercise tolerance [22–24].

Due to these findings, many investigators have examined the peripheral muscle response to exercise and found significant abnormalities. Leg blood flow is reduced due to low cardiac output, but also increased leg vascular resistance and abnormal arteriolar constriction [20, 21, 25]. There are also many intrinsic skeletal muscle changes that limit exercise. These include reduced skeletal muscle capillary density, change in skeletal muscle fiber type with a shift from oxidative type I fiber to glycolytic type II muscle fiber, a reduction in oxidative enzymes in the Kreb's cycle, a decrease in mitochondrial size and number, an increase in inflammatory markers, and a reduction in muscle mass and strength [25]. One could certainly hypothesize that some of these adaptations that occur could be improved by exercise training.

EFFECTS OF EXERCISE TRAINING IN HF PATIENTS

Numerous studies have evaluated the physiological, psychological, and morbidity and mortality effects of exercise training in HF patients [4–18]. Most of these have been small, single center studies looking at a variety of mechanistic changes with exercise. More recently, the results of a large, 2300 patient trial was presented at the 2008 American Heart Association meeting [26, 27]. These studies have examined a number of different endpoints including functional capacity, quality of life, adverse events, and morbidity and mortality.

FUNCTIONAL CAPACITY

The major results of the randomized trials are outlined in Table 9.1. A number of small studies have examined the effects of exercise training on changes in functional capacity [4–17]. With the exception of one small trial of 22 patients showing no benefit [13], all of the studies demonstrated a significant increase in oxygen consumption and/or exercise time. Most trials show an early improvement in oxygen consumption within 2 to 3 months that is sustained throughout the duration of exercise training. The 6 min walk test has not been as well studied and has shown less consistent results. In the two largest training trials by Belardinelli and McKelvie, despite a significant improvement in peak oxygen consumption in the training groups both the training and control groups had an increase in the 6 min walk distance and there was no significant difference between them [14, 16]. Based on these results, patients can be told to anticipate an improvement in their ability to perform maximal activities.

QUALITY OF LIFE

Similar to the improvements in functional capacity, most of the studies that have examined quality of life using a variety of different methodologies have shown improvements [4–6, 12–14]. Comparing the two large studies, McKelvie et al. [16] found a non-statistically significant trend towards improvement using the Minnesota Living with Heart Failure ques-

Table 9.1 Results of randomized, controlled trials of exercise training

	Number trained	Change in exercise time	Change in peak VO$_2$	Change in QoL	Adverse events	Morbidity and mortality
Coats [4]	11	Increase	2.4 ml/kg/min	Improve	None	
Coats [5]	17	Increase	2.4 ml/kg/min	Improve		
Koch [6]	12	Increase		Improve	None	
Belardinelli [7]	36		15%		None	No difference
Hambrecht [8]	12		31%		None	
Kiilavuori [9]	8		15%			
Keteyian [10]	21	Increase	231 ml/min		None	
Kiilavuori [11]	12	Increase	2.4 ml/kg/min			
Keteyian [12]	26	Increase	2.3 ml/kg/min	Improve		
Willenheimer [13]	22		No change	Improve	None	
Belardinelli [14]	50		2.9 ml/kg/min	Improve	None	Improved
Hambrecht [15]	36	Increase	4.8 ml/kg/min		None	
McKelvie [16]	90		104 ml/min	No	None	No difference
Nilsson [17]	40	Increase		Improve		
HF-ACTION [26, 27]	1159	Increase	0.6 ml/kg/min	Improve		No difference

tionnaire. This contrasts with the Belardinelli study which showed an improvement in quality of life using the same test that appeared to parallel the improvement in peak oxygen consumption [14]. In general, it is safe to tell patients that they can usually expect to feel better with an exercise training regimen than without.

MORBIDITY AND MORTALITY

Until the presentation of the recent Heart Failure and A Controlled Trial Investigating Outcomes of Exercise TraiNing (HF-ACTION) trial which will be presented below, only two of the exercise training studies included the endpoints of morbidity and mortality [14, 16]. Belardinelli *et al.* [14] randomized 110 patients to exercise training or usual care. The training group exercised three times a week at 60% of peak oxygen consumption for 8 weeks and then twice a week for a year. Ninety-four of the 110 patients completed the training regimen. Exercise training was associated with a reduction in mortality (9 in exercise arm versus 20 in usual care) and HF hospitalizations (5 vs.14). This contrasts with the findings of McKelvie *et al.* [16]. In their study of 181 patients, the exercise training group exercised three times a week for 30 min at 60–70% of their heart rate response. Despite demonstrating an increase in oxygen consumption in the exercise group, there were no significant differences in mortality, HF hospitalizations, or the composite of mortality and worsening HF.

The contrasting long-term data on outcomes for exercise training in HF set the stage for the HF-ACTION trial. This trial was designed as a 3000 patient multicenter, randomized trial of exercise training initially using supervised exercise training sessions followed by home based exercise. To facilitate home exercise, all patients in the exercise arm were given either a treadmill or exercycle.

HF-ACTION TRIAL

The results of the HF-ACTION trial were first presented at the 2008 meeting of the American Heart Association [26, 27]. This was a 2331 patient randomized trial of aerobic exercise training versus usual care. Enrollment criteria included an ejection fraction less than 35%, New York Heart Association functional class II–IV HF symptoms, and the ability to participate in an exercise program. The patients were randomized in a 1:1 manner and stratified by enrolling center and by the etiology of their HF. Patients in the exercise training arm underwent 36 supervised exercise training sessions. Patients were asked to return every 3 months to reinforce the exercise regimen. The amount of exercise performed was monitored by both patient diary and a heart rate monitor to evaluate adherence. In both arms of the trial, all patients had optimization of their medical care in a standardized fashion. Additionally, all patients received HF education about diet and routine phone calls to assess how they were doing. The primary endpoint of the trial was all-cause mortality and all-cause hospitalization over a 2 year period. Additionally, secondary endpoints such as quality of life measurements (Kansas City Cardiomyopathy Questionnaire, Beck Depression Inventory, and the Multidimensional Scale of Perceived Social Support) and functional capacity measurements (6 min walk distance, peak oxygen consumption) were measured.

The exercise training protocol involved aerobic exercise only using a combination of treadmill and cycle based activities. The target heart rate range initially was 60% of the patient's heart rate reserve which over time could be increased to 70%. The goal was for the patients to have a total exercise time of 30 min with a 10 min warm up and cool down period. Once independent, the patients were encouraged to increase their activity to 40 min. Upper body exercises (arm ergometer, dual-action cycle, and rowing machines) and strength training were not permitted.

There was a statistically significant improvement in exercise capacity at both 3 months and 1 year with exercise training compared to the usual care group. Both 6 min walk distance (5 – usual care – vs. 20 meters – training, $P < 0.0001$) and peak oxygen consumption (0.2 vs. 0.6 ml/kg/min, $P < 0.0001$) increased at 3 months. At 1 year, the difference in 6 min walk distance (12 vs. 13 meters) disappeared but the change in peak oxygen consumption (0.1 vs. 0.7 ml/kg/min, $P < 0.0001$) was still significant. Of interest, this improvement in peak oxygen consumption was less than what was seen in prior exercise training trials [4, 5, 7–12, 14–16] and is also less than the effect seen with biventricular pacing in HF patients [28].

In addition to a lack of clinically significant improvement in exercise capacity, there also was no difference in the primary outcome of all-cause mortality and hospitalization between the two groups (hazard ratio [HR] 0.93; 95% confidence interval [CI]; 0.84–1.02). The authors did perform a prespecified secondary analysis adjusting patients for major prognostic factors including HF etiology, exercise capacity, ejection fraction, history of atrial fibrillation/ flutter, and incidence of depression and found a reduction in the endpoint after that adjustment. Finally, the authors also showed an improvement in quality of life with exercise [27]. Further details of this trial will hopefully be published in the near future.

One can make several conclusions based on the results of this study. First, exercise is safe and results in significant improvements in exercise capacity, albeit less than in smaller single center trials. One could hypothesize that the training effect was less because the centers did not have the same specialized effort that was performed in the smaller trials. It is still unclear if mortality would be reduced with a larger training effect. Second, perhaps the type of exercise performed and the duration of exercise is important. Others have shown that other types of exercise training result in further improvements in exercise capacity which might reflect on outcomes in a more positive fashion. Third, even with no improvement in clinical outcomes, for patients that have a chronic disease like HF the improvements in quality of life are reason enough to exercise. Finally, there are many substudies and further analyses that need to be performed in this trial. Hopefully, an evaluation of the effects of

Table 9.2 Potential benefits of exercise in congestive heart failure

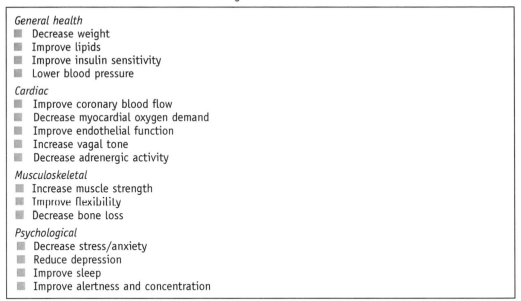

General health
- Decrease weight
- Improve lipids
- Improve insulin sensitivity
- Lower blood pressure

Cardiac
- Improve coronary blood flow
- Decrease myocardial oxygen demand
- Improve endothelial function
- Increase vagal tone
- Decrease adrenergic activity

Musculoskeletal
- Increase muscle strength
- Improve flexibility
- Decrease bone loss

Psychological
- Decrease stress/anxiety
- Reduce depression
- Improve sleep
- Improve alertness and concentration

exercise duration, the frequency of exercise, the amount of training effect, differences in functional class and exercise, and others will be performed to help further understand both the mechanism of benefit and the group of patients who do benefit from exercise training.

HOW TO PRESCRIBE EXERCISE TRAINING

As listed in Table 9.2, there are many benefits to exercise training. For one person, exercise may be prescribed to promote a healthier lifestyle and to help reduce chronic risk factors such as hypertension and diabetes through weight loss. For another, the goal may be to improve physical fitness, muscle strength, and endurance. The prescription for these two people would be quite different and the first part of an exercise prescription should be adapted to the needs and goals of the individual person. For most patients with HF, the goal should be both to adapt a healthier lifestyle focused on weight reduction and blood pressure control as well as to improve fitness and endurance. This improvement in endurance will increase their ability to perform daily activities and improve their quality of life. Additionally, one must ensure that exercise is safe for the patient.

Prior to initiating an exercise program, all patients should have a comprehensive evaluation of both their HF therapy and their current physical state. Patients that are volume overloaded should be diuresed to euvolemia prior to initiating an exercise routine. For patients with an ischemic etiology of HF or those without a prior assessment of their coronary artery status, an evaluation to rule out active ischemia should be performed. This test is also helpful for setting up the exercise prescription.

One should also strongly consider performing metabolic gas exchange during the exercise test. In addition to evaluating exercise induced ischemia many studies have shown that both peak oxygen consumption and the slope of ventilation to carbon dioxide production are helping for evaluating prognosis [29–37]. One can also rule out pulmonary limitations to exercise and develop a baseline to measure potential functional capacity improvements using this test.

Table 9.3 Borg Rate of Perceived Exertion (RPE) scale [38]

Scale	Symptom
6	
7	Very, very light
8	
9	Very light
10	
11	Fairly light
12	
13	Somewhat hard
14	
15	Hard
16	
17	Very hard
18	
19	Very, very hard
20	

Based on the safety of exercise shown in the HF-ACTION trial, one should use a similar intensity of exercise when making an exercise prescription. Patients were started at 60% of their heart rate reserve and then increased to 70% over time.

CALCULATION OF HEART RATE RESERVE

Heart rate reserve = Maximum heart rate – resting heart rate
Training heart rate = Heart rate reserve x desired intensity (e.g. 60%)

Once the training heart rate is established, allow a 10 beat per minute range around that target heart rate (if training heart rate is 110, set a goal heart rate range of 105–115 beats per minute). One additional benefit of a metabolic exercise test is that the ventilatory threshold can be measured. Ideally, one would want the exercise training range to be just below the heart rate at ventilatory threshold.

Because of the chronotropic incompetence and use of beta blockers in patients with HF, many patients will have a very small heart rate reserve and therefore their target heart rate will not be much above their resting heart rate. One can also set the exercise training target of to a value of 11–14 on the Borg Rate of Perceived Exertion scale as shown in Table 9.3 [38]. This rate is usually below the ventilatory threshold and corresponds with a level of exertion that will provide a training effect.

In addition to prescribing a heart rate range, one must also prescribe the type, duration, and frequency of exercise. For most patients, aerobic exercise on either a treadmill or exercycle is preferred. The duration of exercise should be based on the patient's current fitness level. An advanced NYHA functional class III patient might start at 10 min a day. An NYHA functional class I patient may be able to start at 30 min a session. All patients should work up to 30–40 min of exercise per session including warm-up and warm down. The frequency of exercise should start at three times a week (at a minimum) and build up to 5–6 days a week. Table 9.4 outlines an example of a possible training regimen.

Although exercise at a cardiac rehabilitation facility would be ideal for patients with HF, the reality is that, in America, it is rarely covered by insurance and many patients can not

Table 9.4 Sample training regimen, based on the HF-ACTION exercise training program [18]

Stage	Week	Exercise frequency (per week)	Exercise intensity (%HRR)	Exercise duration (min)
Initial	1–2	3	60	15–30
Improvement	3–6	3–5	70	30–35
Maintenance	13+	5	70	40

HRR = heart rate reserve; min = minute.

Table 9.5 Tips for maintaining an exercise regimen

- Set short- and long-term goals
- Give rewards for achieving goals
- Remind yourself of the reasons to exercise
- Exercise with others
- Make exercise more entertaining (bring music, different location)

afford to participate in cardiac rehabilitation. This does not mean that they can't exercise however. Patients can still be given an exercise prescription and told to exercise outdoors or at their local shopping mall or large, warehouse type store. Also, some patients may not want to check their heart rate. Set their exercise prescription at a walk rate where they can just carry on a conversation without long pauses because of breathlessness or to a rate of perceived exertion. However, even if patients can't afford cardiac rehab they should still have an evaluation for ischemia prior to initiating this program.

There is little data about resistance training in HF patients and more research should be performed [39, 41]. If performed, patients should use low resistance, high repetition methods and avoid any body building type activities.

Once the exercise intensity, duration, and frequency are established, there are some practical matters that the patient must be counseled about. First, a slow warm-up from rest is important. This has been shown to reduce the risk of musculoskeletal injury and possibly reduce the risk of ischemia and arrhythmias [42]. This should last between 5 and 10 min and consist of stretching exercise followed by a slow build up in aerobic activity to the prescribed level. Similarly, after exercise, patients should undergo a cool-down period of lower exercise intensity followed again by stretching exercises prior to stopping the exercise period. This as well should be done over a 10 min period. At first, patients may have a 10 min warm-up, 5 min exercise period, and a 10 min cool down period. Overtime, they should slowly build up their exercise period to a goal of 40 min per session as outlined in Table 9.4.

Finally, although patients may be quite motivated to exercise at first, over time the frequency, intensity, and duration of exercise may start to be reduced. One benefit of a cardiac rehab center is that the personnel at the center can help with motivation. Short of that, giving patients some motivational hints as outlined in Table 9.5 may help them to keep exercising. Additionally, similar to asking about weighing themselves, taking their meds, and HF symptoms, questions about exercise should be considered part of the routine visit with your HF patients.

Table 9.6 Contraindications to exercise training (adapted with permission [39])

Absolute
- Progressive worsening of exercise tolerance or dyspnea at rest or on exertion over previous 3 to 5 days
- Significant ischemia at low levels of exercise
- Acute systemic illness
- Uncontrolled diabetes
- Recent embolism
- Thrombophlebitis
- Active pericarditis or myocarditis
- Moderate to severe aortic stenosis
- Regurgitant valvular heart disease requiring surgery
- Myocardial infarction within the previous month
- New onset atrial fibrillation

Relative
- 4 pound increase in weight over 1 to 3 days
- Continuous or intermittent inotropic therapy
- Decrease in systolic blood pressure with exercise
- New York Heart Association functional class IV symptoms
- Rest or exertion induced arrhythmias
- Supine resting heart rate > 100 beats per minute

SAFETY

The safety of exercise training in patients with HF was reported in most of the exercise training trials [4, 6–8, 10, 13–16, 40]. None of the trials reported any complications of either exercise testing or training. This emphasizes the importance of a baseline exercise test to evaluate for ischemia. All of these trials performed such a test and did not enroll patients with active ischemia. Remember that many patients were excluded from these trials if they had comorbidites that increased the risk of exercise. Common contraindications to exercise training are outlined in Table 9.6.

There are a few practical points that should be mentioned about safety during exercise. Exercise outdoors during extremes of temperature or humidity should be cautioned against. Exposure to the cold is associated with cutaneous vasoconstriction which will increase peripheral vascular resistance and blood pressure. This puts an added stress on the HF heart and in theory could exacerbate symptoms. Similarly, exercise in the heat or humidity also puts a stress on the heart with increased myocardial oxygen demand and systemic vasodilation. The increased distribution of blood to the extremities for cooling may limit leg blood flow and decrease exercise tolerance. One other caution is that it is important to maintain hydration during exercise in the heat. HF patients may have trouble replacing the proper amounts of fluid and should be careful with their volume replacement.

CONCLUSION

Although the HF-ACTION trial showed no mortality benefit, importantly it also demonstrated that exercise is both safe and improves quality of life in HF patients. With the wealth of data showing improvements in quality of life and functional capacity, exercise training should be added to the therapeutic regimen of all HF patients. Further studies should be performed to evaluate the effects of resistance training, but it is quite clear that aerobic exercise is safe for patients without ischemia and easy to prescribe.

REFERENCES

1. McDonald CD, Burch GE, Walsh JJ. Prolonged bed rest in the treatment of idiopathic cardiomyopathy. *Am J Med* 1972; 52:41-50.
2. Working Group on Cardiac Rehabilitation and Exercise Physiology and Working Group on Heart Failure of the European Society of Cardiology. Recommendations for exercise training in chronic heart failure patients. *Eur Heart J* 2001; 22:125-135.
3. Oldridge NB, Guyatt GH, Rimm AA. Cardiac rehabilitation after myocardial infarction. Combined experience of randomized clinical trials. *JAMA* 1988; 260:945-950.
4. Coats AJS, Adamopoulos S, Meyer TE, Conway J, Sleight P. Effects of physical training in chronic heart failure. *Lancet* 1990; 335:63-66.
5. Coats AJS, Adamopoulos S, Radaelli A *et al.* Controlled trial of physical training in chronic heart failure. Exercise performance, hemodynamics, ventilation, and autonomic function. *Circulation* 1992; 85:2119-2131.
6. Koch M, Douard H, Broustet JP. The benefit of graded physical exercise in chronic heart failure. *Chest* 1992; 101:231S-235S.
7. Belardinelli R, Georgiou D, Cianci G, Berman N, Ginzton L, Purcaro A. Exercise training improves left ventricular diastolic filling in patients with dilated cardiomyopathy. Clinical and prognostic implications. *Circulation* 1995; 91:2775-2784.
8. Hambrecht R, Niebauer J, Fiehn E *et al.* Physical training in patients with stable chronic heart failure: effects on cardiorespiratory fitness and ultrastructural abnormalities of leg muscles. *J Am Coll Cardiol* 1995; 25:1239-1249.
9. Kiilavuori K, Toivonen L, Naveri H, Leinonen H. Reversal of autonomic derangements by physical training in chronic heart failure assessed by heart rate variability. *Eur Heart J* 1995; 16:490-495.
10. Keteyian SJ, Levine AB, Brawner CA *et al.* Exercise training in patients with heart failure. A randomized, controlled trial. *Ann Intern Med* 1996; 124:1051-1057.
11. Kiilavuori K, Sovijarvi A, Naveri H, Ikonen T, Leinonen H. Effect of physical training on exercise capacity and gas exchange in patients with chronic heart failure. *Chest* 1996; 111:985-991.
12. Keteyian SJ, Brawner CA, Schairer JR *et al.* Effects of exercise training on chronotropic incompetence in patients with heart failure. *Am Heart J* 1999; 138:233-240.
13. Willenheimer R, Erhardt L, Cline C, Rydberg E, Israelsson B. Exercise training in heart failure improves quality of life and exercise capacity. *Eur Heart J* 1998; 19:774-781.
14. Belardinelli R, Georgiou D, Cianci G, Purcaro A. Randomized, controlled trial of long-term moderate exercise training in chronic heart failure. Effects on functional capacity, quality of life, and clinical outcome. *Circulation* 1999; 99:1173-1182.
15. Hambrecht R, Gielen S, Linke A *et al.* Effects of exercise training on left ventricular function and peripheral resistance in patients with chronic heart failure. *JAMA* 2000; 283:3095-3101.
16. McKelvie RS, Teo KK, Roberts R *et al.* Effects of exercise training in patients with heart failure: The Exercise Rehabilitation Trial (EXERT). *Am Heart J* 2002; 144:23-30.
17. Nilsson BB, Westheim A, Risberg MA. Long-term effects of a group-based high-intensity aerobic interval-training program in patients with chronic heart failure. *Am J Cardiol* 2008; 102:1220-1224.
18. Whellan DJ, O'Connor CM, Lee KL *et al.* On behalf of the HF-ACTION trial investigators. Heart Failure and A Controlled Trial Investigating Outcomes of Exercise TrainNing (HF-ACTION): design and rationale. *Am Heart J* 2007; 153:201-211.
19. Sullivan MJ, Cobb FR. Central hemodynamic response to exercise in patients with chronic heart failure. *Chest* 1992; 101:340S-346S.
20. Sullivan MJ, Knight JD, Higginbotham MB, Cobb FR. Relation between central and peripheral hemodynamics during exercise in patients with chronic heart failure: muscle blood flow is reduced with maintenance of arterial perfusion pressure. *Circulation* 1989; 80:769-781.
21. Sullivan MJ, Cobb FR. Dynamic regulation of leg vasomotor tone in patients with chronic heart failure. *J Appl Physiol* 1991; 71:1070-1075.
22. Maskin CS, Forman R, Sonnenblick EH, Frishman WH, LeJemtel TH. Failure of dobutamine to increase exercise capacity despite hemodynamic improvement in severe chronic heart failure. *Am J Cardiol* 1983; 51:177-182.
23. Wilson JR, Martin JL, Ferraro N, Weber KT. Effect of hydralazine on perfusion and metabolism in the leg during upright bicycle exercise in patients with heart failure. *Circulation* 1983; 68:425-432.

24. Wilson JR, Martin JL, Ferraro N. Impaired skeletal muscle nutritive flow during exercise in patients with congestive heart failure: role of cardiac pump dysfunction as determined by the effect of dobutamine. *Am J Cardiol* 1984; 53:1308-1315.

25. Duscha BD, Schulze PC, Robbins JL, Forman DE. Implications of chronic heart failure on peripheral vasculature and skeletal muscle before and after exercise training. *Heart Fail Rev* 2008; 13:21-37.

26. O'Connor CM, Whellan DJ, Lee KL et al; HF-ACTION Investigators. Efficacy and safety of exercise training in patients with chronic heart failure: HF-ACTION randomized controlled trial. *JAMA* 2009; 301:1439-1450.

27. Flynn KE, Piña IL, Whellan DJ et al; HF-ACTION Investigators. Effects of exercise training on health status in patients with chronic heart failure: HF-ACTION randomized controlled trial. *JAMA* 2009; 301:1451-1459.

28. Young JB, Abraham WT, Smith AL et al. Multicenter InSync ICD Randomized Clinical Evaluation (MIRACLE ICD) Trial Investigators. Combined cardiac resynchronization and implantable cardioversion defibrillation in advanced chronic heart failure: the MIRACLE ICD Trial. *JAMA* 2003; 289:2685-2694.

29. Mancini DM, Eisen H, Kussmaul W, Mull R, Edmunds LH, Wilson JR. Value of peak exercise oxygen consumption for optimal timing of cardiac transplantation in ambulatory patients with heart failure. *Circulation* 1991; 83:778-786.

30. Peterson LR, Schechtman KB, Ewald GA et al. Timing of cardiac transplantation in patients with heart failure receiving b-adrenergic blockers. *J Heart Lung Transplant* 2003; 22:1141-1148.

31. Chua TP, Ponikowski P, Harrington D et al. Clinical correlates and prognostic significance of the ventilatory response to exercise in chronic heart failure. *J Am Coll Cardiol* 1997; 29:1585-1590.

32. Robbins M, Francis G, Pashkow RJ et al. Ventilatory and heart rate responses to exercise. Better predictors of heart failure mortality than peak oxygen consumption. *Circulation* 1999; 100:2411-2417.

33. Francis DP, Shamim W, Davies LC et al. Cardiopulmonary exercise testing for prognosis in chronic heart failure: continuous and independent prognostic value from Ve/VCO$_2$ slope and peak VO$_2$. *Eur Heart J* 2000; 21:154-161.

34. Kleber FX, Vietzke G, Wernecke KD et al. Impairment of ventilatory efficiency in heart failure. Prognostic impact. *Circulation* 2000; 101:2803-2809.

35. Gitt AK, Wasserman K, Kilkowski C et al. Exercise anaerobic threshold and ventilatory efficiency identify heart failure patients for high risk of early death. *Circulation* 2002; 106:3079-3084.

36. Arena R, Humphrey R. Comparison of ventilatory expired gas parameters used to predict hospitalization in patients with heart failure. *Am Heart J* 2002; 143:427-432.

37. Arena R, Myers J, Aslam SS, Varughese EB, Peberdy MA. Peak VO$_2$ and Ve/VCO$_2$ slope in patients with heart failure: a prognostic comparison. *Am Heart J* 2004; 147:354-360.

38. Borg G. Perceived exertion as an indicator of somatic stress. *Scand J Rehabil Med* 1970; 2-3:92-98.

39. Working Group on Cardiac Rehabilitation and Exercise Physiology and Working Group on Heart Failure of the European Society of Cardiology. Recommendations for exercise training in chronic heart failure patients. *Eur Heart J* 2001; 22:125-135.

40. Keteyian SJ, Isaac D, Thadani U et al; HF-ACTION Investigators. Safety of symptom-limited cardiopulmonary exercise testing in patients with chronic heart failure due to severe left ventricular systolic dysfunction. *Am Heart J* 2009; 158(4 Suppl):S72-S77.

41. Myers J. Principles of exercise prescription for patients with chronic heart failure. *Heart Fail Rev* 2008; 13:61-68.

42. Balady GJ, Berra KA, Golding LA et al. General principles of exercise prescription. In: Franklin BA, ed. ACSM's Guidelines for Exercise Testing and Prescription, 6th edition. Philadelphia: Lippincott Williams and Wilkins, 2000, pp 137-164.

10

How does metabolic syndrome lead to heart failure?

M. T. Reddy, H. O. Ventura

INTRODUCTION

Metabolic syndrome is a constellation of factors that predispose an individual to increased cardiovascular mortality and morbidity. It is also known as the insulin resistance syndrome or syndrome X.

While recognized as early as the 1920s [1], it was not until the 1980s [2] that researchers developed a deeper understanding of the role a combination of risk factors such as insulin resistance, dyslipidemia and hypertension (HTN) played in the pathogenesis of cardiovascular disease. Metabolic syndrome was not officially defined until 1999 when the World Health Organization (WHO) published the first guidelines on this disease process [3]. Since then several different definitions have been proposed by various organizations around the world including the European Group for study of Insulin Resistance (EGIR) [4], the Adult Treatment Panel (ATP) III definition (in 2002 [5] and updated in 2005 [6]) and the International Diabetes Federation (IDF) definition in 2004 [7]. While all the definitions are similar and include common components of glucose intolerance, obesity, HTN and dyslipidema they differ in their clinical cut-offs for the above measures and have different inclusion criteria.

DEFINITION

In the US, per the ATP III guidelines published by the National Cholesterol Education Program (NCEP) a patient with three or more of the five risk factors in Table 10.1 meets criteria for metabolic syndrome. One advantage of this definition of metabolic syndrome is that the parameters used are easily and routinely measured clinically and can therefore ostensibly be widely introduced in clinical practice.

The WHO guidelines focus on insulin resistance as noted below. A patient with insulin resistance plus two other conditions as noted in Table 10.2 meets criteria for metabolic syndrome. One disadvantage of this classification is that it involves measurements that are not routinely carried out in clinical practice and that may preclude its widespread introduction in clinical practice. Nevertheless, as the first official definition of metabolic syndrome it was an important step forward in the understanding of metabolic syndrome.

The multitude of definitions for metabolic syndrome has led to some confusion in clinical practice. Based on the actual definition the prevalence of this disease varies somewhat [8, 9].

Madhavi T. Reddy, MD, Fellow in Cardiology, University of Illinois, Chicago, IL, USA.

Hector O. Ventura, MD, FACC, FACP, FASH, Section Head, Cardiomyopathy and Heart Transplantation, John Ochsner Heart and Vascular Institute, Ochsner Health System, New Orleans, LA, USA.

Table 10.1 ATP III clinical identification of the metabolic syndrome

1. Abdominal obesity, given as waist circumference	
Men	>102 cm (40 in)
Women	>88 cm (35 in)
2. Triglycerides	>150 mg/dl
3. HDL cholesterol	
Men	>40 mg/dl
Women	>50 mg/dl
4. Blood pressure	>130/85 mmHg
5. Fasting glucose	>110 mg/dl

Table 10.2 WHO criteria for metabolic syndrome

1. Insulin resistance, identified by one of the following:
   - Type 2 diabetes;
   - Impaired fasting glucose;
   - Impaired glucose tolerance; or
   - For those with normal fasting glucose levels (<110 mg/dl), glucose uptake below the lowest quartile for background population under investigation under hyperinsulinemic, euglycemic conditions

Plus any two of the following:
2. Antihypertensive medication and/or high blood pressure (>140 mmHg systolic or >90 mmHg diastolic)
3. Plasma triglycerides >150 mg/dl (>1.7 mmol/l)
4. HDL cholesterol >35 mg/dl (>0.9 mmol/l) in men or >39 mg/dl (1.0 mmol/l) in women
5. BMI >30 kg/m^2 and/or waist:hip ratio >0.9 in men, >0.85 in women
6. Urinary albumin excretion rate >20 g/min or albumin:creatinine ratio >30 mg/g

Despite the confusion on the definition of this syndrome, several epidemiologic studies have shown that metabolic syndrome confers a two-fold risk for coronary heart disease (CHD) [10–15]. However, the degree of association beyond routine risk factors is still a topic of much debate [16–20]. Metabolic syndrome is also associated with other diseases for example, type 2 diabetes and polycystic ovarian disease. The relationship between metabolic syndrome and heart failure (HF) has been less well studied and remains to be elucidated.

DOES METABOLIC SYNDROME LEAD TO HF?

The question of whether metabolic syndrome is an independent risk factor for HF is an important one but to date there have been few studies to investigate this. Whether the concurrence of these specific factors puts any given individual at a risk beyond what is expected based on the known associations of each risk factor with HF is also unknown. In the next few paragraphs we will summarize the trials that have investigated the relationship between metabolic syndrome and HF.

The Uppsala Longitudinal Study of Adult Men (ULSAM) trial is a well-conducted cohort study of 2314 Swedish middle-aged men, in which researchers showed that metabolic syndrome is a significant predictor of HF [21]. All 50 year old men in Uppsala County during the years 1970–1974 were invited to enroll in the ULSAM cohort. 82 % (2322 men) enrolled in the study and were followed till age 70. Eight men were excluded because of presence of CHD or valvular disease at baseline. During median follow-up of 20.1 years, 100 patients were diagnosed with definite HF based on hospital discharge codes and external review of patient charts by two separate researchers. After adjusting for other known risk factors for HF (including interim myocardial infarction, hypertension, diabetes mellitus, left ventricular hypertrophy [LVH], smoking and body mass index [BMI]) the presence of metabolic syndrome at baseline conferred a hazard ratio (HR) of 1.80 (confidence interval [CI] 1.11–2.91) for the subsequent development of HF in middle-aged men. Interestingly, apart from myocardial infarction and HTN, metabolic syndrome was a stronger predictor of subsequent HF than diabetes, LVH, tobacco use and BMI alone. This study was the first one to show that metabolic syndrome is a strong independent predictor of subsequent HF in a cohort of middle-aged Swedish men without CHD or valvular disease. In addition, given the strength of the association, metabolic syndrome may provide a valuable tool in the prediction of HF in the patient without traditional HF risk factors. A limitation of this study was that it was restricted to middle-aged men of Swedish background. In addition, the study authors used BMI instead of waist circumference as one of the markers of metabolic syndrome which may not be a valid substitution given the importance of abdominal obesity in the pathogenesis of metabolic syndrome.

Disparate findings were reported in a recently published study based on the Multi-Ethnic Study of Atherosclerosis (MESA) cohort [22]. MESA is a community based cohort study of 6814 men and women of Caucasian (38%), African (28%), Hispanic (22%) and Chinese (12%) background. Patients were recruited between 2002 and 2006 from six different states in the United States and followed for a median of 4 years. Unlike the Swedish cohort, MESA included participants of both genders (3601 or 53% women) and a wider age range (45 to 84 years). Seventy-nine out of 6814 MESA patients developed HF during follow-up. The metabolic syndrome was observed in 2362 participants (34.7%) at baseline. In unadjusted models, participants who met ATP III criteria for the metabolic syndrome at baseline were at higher risk of developing HF (HR 2.04 ; CI 1.31–3.17). However, once adjusted for conventional risk factors for HF (including age, gender, hypertension, diabetes, LVH, obesity, serum total cholesterol, and current cigarette smoking, baseline left ventricular [LV] function) as well as interim myocardial infarction this relationship was no longer significant with a HR of 1.60 (CI 0.89–2.87). These results show that although the metabolic syndrome is strongly associated with incident congestive heart failure (CHF), this association is largely explained by its specific risk factor components.

How do we explain the differences in these two studies? First, follow-up time in the MESA study was only 4 years when compared to the follow-up time of 20 years in the Uppsala cohort. Therefore, a longer follow-up time might have increased statistical power in the MESA trial in the detection of a significant association between metabolic syndrome and HF. Secondly, gender and racial differences in the association between metabolic syndrome may have diluted the effect seen in the MESA trial. Given the conflicting results of these trials, further research is necessary to elucidate the causal relationship if any between metabolic syndrome and HF.

PATHOPHYSIOLOGY

The pathophysiology linking metabolic syndrome and HF is multifactorial and appears to be mediated by insulin resistance, obesity and inflammatory activation.

INSULIN RESISTANCE

Metabolic syndrome as a disease of insulin resistance was first articulated by Reaven in 1988. In his ground-breaking lecture, Reaven postulated that insulin resistance and resulting hyperglycemia caused a compensatory hyperinsulinemia which turn increased glucose uptake and decreased glucose production. Although the hyperinsulinemia was an appropriate compensatory mechanism it lead to myriad adverse side-effects such as HTN [23], ventricular remodeling [23], activation of the sympathetic nervous system [24], increased oxidative stress [25] and immune activation [26], all of which contribute to HF [27–29] as shown below.

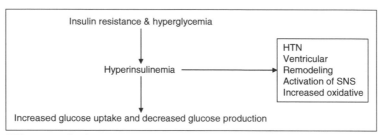

SNS = sympathetic nervous system.

Insulin resistance was recently shown to be an independent risk factor for mortality in patients with stable chronic HF [30]. 105 male patients with stable HF secondary to ischemic (63%) or non-ischemic (37%) etiology were prospectively followed for a mean follow-up period of 44 months. Insulin sensitivity (IS) was assessed from glucose and insulin dynamic profiles during an intravenous glucose tolerance test. Patients with IS below the median value had worse survival than patients with IS above the median value (relative risk [RR] 0.38; 95% CI 0.21–0.67). IS remained an independent predictor for survival after adjustment of confounding variables (RR 0.56; 95% CI 0.35–0.89).

OBESITY

Obesity is a growing pandemic worldwide [31, 32]. Obesity predisposes to the development of several conventional risk factors for HF. The risk of developing diabetes, hypertension, or dyslipidemia starts to increase from a BMI of as low as $21\,kg/m^2$ [33, 34]. Diabetes, HTN and dyslipidemia have all been shown to predispose to HF.

In addition, obesity likely leads to ventricular hypertrophy independent of development of other risk factors. For example, LV dilation and hypertrophy may result from chronic volume overload as a consequence of an elevated cardiac output even in normotensive individuals. In a substudy of 3922 adults enrolled in the Framingham Heart Study [35], body mass index strongly correlated with LV mass. After adjusting for age and blood pressure, body mass index remained a strong independent predictor of LV mass, LV wall thickness, and LV internal dimension. This observation was substantiated by findings in adolescents and young adults enrolled in the Strong Heart Study (SHS) and the Bogalusa Heart Study. In the SHS substudy [36], a total of 460 unselected American Indian adolescent participants age 14–20 years were enrolled. LV hypertrophy was more common in obese (33.5%) than in overweight (12.4%) and normal weight (3.5%) participants. The stroke volume was 79.5 ml in obese participants and increased compared with both overweight (76.5 ml) and normal weight participants (73.1 ml) indicating increased cardiac workload. These findings were corroborated in other ethnicities in the Bogalusa Heart Study where a strong association between LV mass in childhood and young adults across BMI quartiles in both whites and blacks was demonstrated [37].

INFLAMMATORY ACTIVATION

Inflammation has been associated with both metabolic syndrome and HF and inflammatory activation may be an important mediator of HF in the patient with metabolic syndrome.

Several studies have shown that elevated inflammatory markers are associated with HF [38, 39]. For example in the ULSAM cohort, a community-based prospective study of 2314 middle-aged men free from HF, myocardial infarction, and valvular disease at baseline, erythrocyte sedimentation rate (ESR) was analyzed in multivariable models together with established risk factors for HF (hypertension, diabetes, electrocardiographic LVH, smoking, obesity, and serum cholesterol) and hematocrit. ESR was an independent predictor of HF (HR 1.46 for highest quartile vs. the lowest, 95% CI 1.04–2.06) [38].

Similarly, in a substudy of 732 Framingham study subjects (mean age 78 years, 67% women) free of prior MI and HF, 56 subjects (35 women) developed HF during mean follow-up of 5.2 years. After adjustment for established risk factors, including the occurrence of myocardial infarction on follow-up, subjects with elevated levels of three biomarkers (serum IL-6 and tumour necrosis factor (TNF)-α > median values, C-reative protein [CRP] > or = 5 mg/dl) had a markedly increased risk of HF (HR 4.07 [95% CI 1.34–12.37], $P = 0.01$) compared with the other subjects [39].

Most recently, in the MESA trial, markers of systemic inflammation were significant predictors of HF [22]. Among these markers, IL-6 was the strongest predictor in the unadjusted models (HR of 1.84 for each SD increase in log serum IL-6). A serum CRP > 5 mg/dl was also significantly associated with an increase in the risk of HF (HR 1.87; 95% CI 1.16–3.00) [22].

Inflammation may therefore be an important component of the relationship between metabolic syndrome and HF. Several studies have evaluated the relationship of CRP with metabolic syndrome and HF. In the West of Scotland Coronary Prevention Study (WOSCOPS), a primary prevention trial that demonstrated the effectiveness of pravastatin in preventing coronary morbidity and mortality, 6595 moderately hypercholesterolemic men with no history of myocardial infarction were randomly assigned to pravastatin (40 mg daily) or placebo and followed for an average of 4.9 years. The corresponding HRs for men in the low-CRP/no metabolic syndrome ($n = 3017$), high-CRP/no metabolic syndrome ($n = 862$), low-CRP/yes metabolic syndrome ($n = 1166$), and high-CRP/yes metabolic syndrome ($n = 612$) groups were 1.0 (referent), 1.6 (95% CI 1.3–2.1), 1.6 (95% CI 1.2–2.1), and 2.75 (95% CI 2.1–3.6), respectively, for CHD events [40].

A similar relationship was seen in the Women's Health Study (WHS) substudy [41], a trial of aspirin and vitamin E in primary prevention. In brief, American women aged 45 years and over with no prior history of cardiovascular disease or cancer were enrolled between November 1992 and July 1995. Analysis was limited to the 14719 WHS participants not using hormone replacement therapy (HRT) and free of diabetes at study entry. The age-adjusted relative risks of future cardiovascular events for women in the low-CRP/no metabolic syndrome, high-CRP/no metabolic syndrome, low-CRP/yes metabolic syndrome, and high-CRP/yes metabolic syndrome groups were 1.0 (referent), 1.5 (95% CI 1.0–2.2), 2.3 (95% CI 1.6–3.3), and 4.0 (95% CI 3.0–5.4), respectively [41]. In both trials, CRP added important and independent prognostic information in terms of future cardiovascular risk.

TREATMENT

While sufficient evidence does not exist to prove that metabolic syndrome causes HF some proponents nevertheless advocate recognition and treatment of this syndrome. Currently, treatment of metabolic syndrome consists of treatment of its components and does not involve a specialized approach to the syndrome or its underlying pathology as a whole [42, 43]. Because excess visceral adiposity is a key feature of metabolic syndrome, therapeutic approaches that focus on reducing visceral adipose tissue could have a major impact on the clustering abnormalities of this disease.

The NCEP-ATP III guidelines [42] specify weight loss as the primary recommended treatment for metabolic syndrome. A realistic goal for overweight/obese persons is to reduce body weight by 7% to 10% over a period of 6 to 12 months. Weight reduction should be combined with a daily minimum of 30 min of moderate-intensity physical activity. Other possible targets include treatment of insulin resistance (with metformin or thiazolidinediones), high low-density lipoprotein (LDL) (especially in the presence of other cardiovascular risk factors) and HTN (according to JNC 7 recommendations). However, the NCEP-ATP III guidelines do not recommend any specific class of agents as there are few trials looking into precise agents for the treatment of metabolic syndrome.

One such trial was derived from the Antihypertensive and Lipid-Lowering Treatment to Prevent Heart Attack (ALLHAT) cohort [44]. The choice of initial antihypertensive regimen in the patient with metabolic syndrome and HTN is unclear. Angiotensin-converting-enzyme inhibitors (ACE-I) and/or angiotensin receptor blockers (ARBs) were favored as an initial choice because of their favorable profile in patients with diabetes.

ALLHAT is a multicenter randomized clinical trial designed to determine whether the occurrence of fatal CHD or non-fatal myocardial infarction (MI) is lower in high-risk hypertensive patients whose antihypertensive treatment began with a calcium channel blocker (CCB) (amlodipine) or an ACE inhibitor (lisinopril) compared with a thiazide-like diuretic (chlorthalidone). Researchers performed a post hoc analysis to evaluate differences in risk of metabolic, cardiovascular disease (CHD), and renal outcomes in non-diabetic participants with or without metabolic syndrome, according to their initial antihypertensive medication assignment. 8013 patients with metabolic syndrome and 9502 patients without metabolic syndrome were followed for a mean duration of 4.9 years (maximum 8.1 years). In participants with metabolic syndrome, there were no significant differences in the primary endpoint (non-fatal MI or CHD death) for either amlodipine vs. chlorthalidone (RR 0.96 [95% CI 0.79–1.16]) or lisinopril vs. chlorthalidone (1.05 [CI 0.88–1.27]). Those with the metabolic syndrome assigned to lisinopril compared with chlorthalidone were significantly more likely to experience HF (1.31 [CI 1.04–1.64]). However, in those with metabolic syndrome, fasting glucose levels were 3 to 7 mg/dl lower in the amlodipine and lisinopril groups than in the chlorthalidone group. This suggests that diuretics are the preferred initial treatment for HTN in older individuals with the metabolic syndrome compared with ACE inhibitors and CCBs, despite the higher incidence of new diabetes for the chlorthalidone group [44].

CONCLUSION

An estimated 47 million US residents and around a quarter of the world's adult population have metabolic syndrome [8, 9]. With rising rates of obesity worldwide, the prevalence of metabolic syndrome is projected to increase proportionally. Patients with metabolic syndrome are more likely to have a heart attack or stroke or develop diabetes compared with people without the syndrome. Metabolic syndrome may also contribute to the growing public health burden of HF. It is vital that a universal definition and treatment strategy be established for metabolic syndrome. Further research is also urgently needed on its underlying pathophysiology and relationship with HF.

REFERENCES

1. Kylin E. Studien uber das Hypertonie-Hyperglyka 'mie-Hyperurika' miesyndrom. *Zentralbl Inn Med* 1923; 44:105–127.
2. Reaven GM. Banting lecture 1988: role of insulin resistance in human disease. *Diabetes* 1988; 37:1595–1607.
3. World Health Organization. Definition, diagnosis and classification of diabetes mellitus and its complications: report of a WHO Consultation. Part 1: diagnosis and classification of diabetes mellitus. Geneva, Switzerland: World Health Organization; 1999. Available at: http://whqlibdoc.who.int/hq/1999/WHO_NCD_NCS_99.2.pdf. Accessed 29 April 2008.
4. Balkau B, Charles MA. Comment on the provisional report from the WHO consultation. *Diabet Med* 1999; 16:442-443.

5. Third report of the National Cholesterol Education Program (NCEP) expert panel on detection, evaluation, and treatment of high blood cholesterol in adults (Adult Treatment Panel III). Final report. *Circulation* 2002; 106:3143–3421.
6. Grundy SM, Brewer HB, Cleeman JI *et al*. Definition of metabolic syndrome. Report of the National Heart, Lung, and Blood Institute/American Heart Association Conference on Scientific Issues Related to Definition. *Circulation* 2004; 109;433-438.
7. The IDF consensus worldwide definition of the metabolic syndrome. Available at: http://www.idf.org/home/index.cfm?node=1429. Accessed 2 May 2008.
8. Ford ES, Giles WH, Dietz WH. Prevalence of the metabolic syndrome among US adults: findings from the Third National Health and Nutrition Examination Survey. *JAMA* 2002; 287:356–359.
9. Dunstan DW, Zimmet PZ, Welborn TA *et al*. The rising prevalence of diabetes and impaired glucose tolerance. The Australian Diabetes, Obesity and Lifestyle Study. *Diabetes Care 2002*; 25:829-834.
10. Lakka HM, Laaksonen DE, Lakka TA *et al*. The metabolic syndrome and total and cardiovascular disease mortality in middle-aged men. *JAMA* 2002; 288:2709–2716.
11. Nigam A, Bourassa MG, Fortier A *et al*. The metabolic syndrome and its components and the long-term risk of death in patients with coronary heart disease. *Am Heart J* 2006; 151:514-521.
12. Malik S, Wong ND, Franklin SS *et al*. Impact of the metabolic syndrome on mortality from coronary heart disease, cardiovascular disease, and all causes in United States adults. *Circulation* 2004; 110:1245-1250.
13. Hunt KJ, Resendez RG, Williams K *et al*. National cholesterol education program versus World Health Organization metabolic syndrome in relation to all-cause and cardiovascular mortality in the San Antonio Heart Study. *Circulation* 2004; 110:1251-1257.
14. Yusuf S, Hawken S, Ounpuu S *et al*. Effect of potentially modifiable risk factors associated with myocardial infarction in 52 countries (the INTERHEART study): case-control study. *Lancet* 2004; 364:937-952.
15. Despre's JP, Poirier P, Bergeron J *et al*. From individual risk factors and the metabolic syndrome to global cardiometabolic risk. *Eur Heart J* 2008(suppl B):B24-B33.
16. Wannamethee SG, Shaper AG, Lennon L *et al*. Metabolic syndrome vs Framingham risk score for prediction of coronary heart disease, stroke, and type 2 diabetes mellitus. *Arch Intern Med* 2005; 165:2644-2650.
17. Stern MP, Williams K, Gonzalez-Villalpando C *et al*. Does the metabolic syndrome improve identification of individuals at risk of type 2 diabetes and/or cardiovascular disease? *Diabetes Care* 2004; 27:2676-2681.
18. McNeill AM, Rosamond WD, Girman CJ *et al*. The metabolic syndrome and 11-year risk of incident cardiovascular disease in the Atherosclerosis Risk in Communities study. *Diabetes Care* 2005; 28:385-390.
19. Wang J, Ruotsalainen S, Moilanen L *et al*. The metabolic syndrome predicts cardiovascular mortality: a 13-year follow-up study in elderly non-diabetic Finns. *Eur Heart J* 2007; 28:857–864.
20. Cull CA, Jensen CC, Retnakaran R *et al*. Impact of the Metabolic Syndrome on Macrovascular and Microvascular Outcomes in Type 2 Diabetes Mellitus United Kingdom Prospective Diabetes Study 78. *Circulation* 2007; 116:2119-2126.
21. Ingelsson E, Arnlov J, Lind L *et al*. Metabolic syndrome and risk for heart failure in middle-aged men. *Heart* 2006; 92:1409-1413.
22. Bahrami H, Bluemke DA, Kronmal R *et al*. Novel metabolic risk factors for incident heart failure and their relationship with obesity. The MESA (Multi-Ethnic Study of Atherosclerosis) Study. *J Am Coll Cardiol* 2008; 51:1775-1783.
23. Holmang A, Yoshida N, Jennische E *et al*. The effects of hyperinsulinemia on myocardial mass, blood pressure regulation and central haemodynamics in rats. *Eur J Clin Invest* 1996; 26:973-978.
24. Anderson EA, Hoffman RP, Balon TW *et al*. Hyperinsulinemia produces both sympathetic neural activation and vasodilation in normal humans. *J Clin Invest* 1991; 87:2246-2252.
25. Doehner W, Anker SD, Coats AJ. Defects in insulin action in chronic heart failure. *Diabetes Obes Metab* 2000; 2:203–212.
26. Anker SD, von Haehling S. Inflammatory mediators in chronic heart failure: an overview. *Heart* 2004; 90:464–470.
27. Swan JW, Anker SD, Walton C *et al*. Insulin resistance in chronic heart failure: relation to severity and etiology of heart failure. *J Am Coll Cardiol* 1997; 30:527–532.

28. Paolisso G, De Riu S, Marrazzo G, Verza M, Varricchio M, D'Onofrio F. Insulin resistance and hyperinsulinemia in patients with chronic congestive heart failure. *Metabolism* 1991; 40:972–977.

29. Swan JW, Walton C, Godsland IF, Clark AL, Coats AJS, Oliver MF. Insulin resistance in chronic heart failure. *Eur Heart J* 1994; 15:1528–1532.

30. Doehner W, Rauchhaus M, Ponikowski P *et al.* Impaired insulin sensitivity as an independent risk factor for mortality in patients with stable chronic heart failure. *J Am Coll Cardiol* 2005; 46:1019–1026.

31. World Health Organization. Obesity: preventing and managing the global epidemic. WHO Technical Report Series number 894. Geneva: WHO, 2000.

32. Flegal KM, Carroll MD, Ogden CL *et al.* Prevalence and trends in obesity among US adults, 1999–2000. *JAMA* 2002; 288:1723–1727.

33. Haslam DW, James WP. Obesity. *Lancet* 2005; 366:1197–1209.

34. Yusuf S, Hawken S, Ounpuu S *et al.* Obesity and the risk of myocardial infarction in 27,000 participants from 52 countries: a case-control study. *Lancet* 2005; 366:1640–1649.

35. Lauer MS, Anderson KM, Kannel WB, Levy D. The impact of obesity on left ventricular mass and geometry. The Framingham Heart Study. *JAMA* 1991; 266:231–236.

36. Chinali M, de Simone G, Roman MJ *et al.* Impact of obesity on cardiac geometry and function in a population of adolescents: the Strong Heart Study. *J Am Coll Cardiol* 2006; 47:2267–2273.

37. Li X, Li S, Ulusoy E, Chen W, Srinivasan SR, Berenson GS. Childhood adiposity as a predictor of cardiac mass in adulthood: the Bogalusa Heart Study. *Circulation* 2004; 110:3488–3492.

38. Ingelsson E, Arnlov J, Sundstrom J *et al.* Inflammation, as measured by the erythrocyte sedimentation rate, is an independent predictor for the development of heart failure. *J Am Coll Cardiol* 2005; 45:1802–1806.

39. Vasan RS, Sullivan LM, Roubenoff R *et al.* Inflammatory markers and risk of heart failure in elderly subjects without prior myocardial infarction; the Framingham Heart Study. *Circulation* 2003; 107:1486–1491.

40. Sattar N, Gaw A, Scherbakova O *et al.* Metabolic syndrome with and without C-reactive protein as a predictor of coronary heart disease and diabetes in the West of Scotland Coronary Prevention Study. *Circulation* 2003; 108:414-419.

41. Ridker PM, Buring JE, Cook NR *et al.* C-reactive protein, the metabolic syndrome and risk of incident cardiovascular events; an 8-year follow-up of 14719 initially healthy American women. *Circulation* 2003; 107:391-397.

42. Grundy SM, Hansen B, Smith SS *et al.* Clinical management of metabolic syndrome. Report of the American Heart Association/National Heart, Lung, and Blood Institute/American Diabetes Association Conference on Scientific Issues Related to Management. *Circulation* 2004; 109:551-556.

43. Orchard TJ, Temprosa M, Goldberg R *et al.* The effect of metformin and intensive lifestyle intervention on the metabolic syndrome: the Diabetes Prevention Program randomized trial. *Ann Intern Med* 2005; 142:611–619.

44. Black H, Davis B, Barzilay J *et al.* Metabolic and clinical outcomes in nondiabetic individuals with the metabolic syndrome assigned to chlorthalidone, amlodipine, or lisinopril as initial treatment for hypertension. A report from the Antihypertensive and Lipid-Lowering Treatment to Prevent Heart Attack Trial (ALLHAT). *Diabetes Care* 2008; 31:353-360.

11

Obesity and heart failure: too much of a bad thing is good?

C. J. Lavie, R. V. Milani, H. O. Ventura

INTRODUCTION

Obesity is a chronic medical problem that is increasing in epidemic proportions in most of the world and especially in westernized society [1–3]. In the United States (US), nearly 70% of the adult population are classified as either overweight or obese, compared with less than 25% 40 years ago [4, 5]. The distribution of obese in the US has also shifted in a skewed fashion such that the proportion of morbid obesity has increased even more so than over-weightness and obesity [3]. In fact, recent evidence indicates that obesity is associated with more morbidity than smoking, alcoholism and poverty combined, and if current trends continue, obesity may soon overtake cigarette abuse as the leading cause of preventable death in the US [6–8]. The World Health Organization estimates that more than one billion people are overweight globally, and this organization predicts that this number will increase to nearly 1.5 billion by 2015 [9]. If the obesity epidemic continues in the US, and we fail to stop current trends, it has been predicted that we may soon witness an abrupt end or even a reversal of the steady climb in life expectancy [9, 10].

There are numerous adverse affects of obesity on general and, particularly, cardiovascular (CV) health [8]. Clearly, obesity has numerous pathological affects on arterial pressure as well as CV structure and systolic and diastolic left ventricular (LV) function, thus contributing substantially to its role in hypertension (HTN), coronary heart disease (CHD), atrial fibrillation (AF), as well as systolic and non-systolic heart failure (HF) [3, 8, 11–14].

In this chapter, we review the affects of obesity on pathophysiology, hemodynamics, LV structure and function, as well as the epidemiology of HF. However, despite the fact that obesity is a powerful risk factor for premature HF, substantial evidence is also reviewed demonstrating that in clinical cohorts with HF, overweight and obese patients with HF tend to have a more favorable short- and long-term prognosis than leaner patients with HF. Considering this, we also discuss the implications of whether obesity should be treated with purposeful weight reduction strategies.

Carl J. Lavie, MD, FACC, FACP, FCCP, Medical Director, Cardiac Rehabilitation and Prevention, Director, Stress Testing Laboratory, John Ochsner Heart and Vascular Institute, Ochsner Health System, New Orleans, LA, USA.

Richard V. Milani, MD, FACC, FAHA, Vice-Chairman, Department of Cardiology, John Ochsner Heart and Vascular Institute, Ochsner Health System, New Orleans, LA, USA.

Hector O. Ventura, MD, FACC, FACP, FASH, Section Head, Cardiomyopathy and Heart Transplantation, John Ochsner Heart and Vascular Institute, Ochsner Health System, New Orleans, LA, USA.

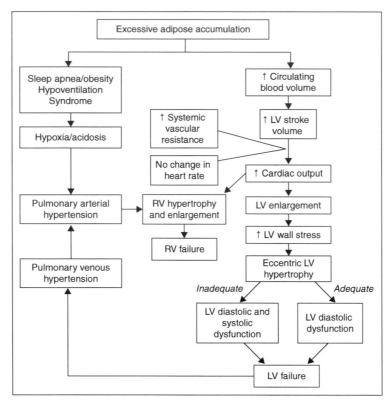

Figure 11.1 Pathophysiology of obesity and cardiomyopathy (with permission from [21]).

EFFECTS OF OBESITY ON PATHOPHYSIOLOGY, HEMODYNAMICS, LV STRUCTURE AND FUNCTION

The fat cell itself plays a substantial role in the pathogenesis of obesity as well as its complications [1, 15]. The adipocytes in obese subjects generate increased levels of the hormone leptin, which controls food intake and energy metabolism, and may be especially related with CV diseases [15, 16]. Exactly how leptin plays a role in the development of CV disease and HF is not completely understood but is likely multifactorial. Leptin may be involved with impaired baroreceptor control of vagal and neural outflow, and elevated levels of leptin are associated with increased sympathetic activation seen in obesity [16-18]. Alterations in sympathovagal balance may be an important cause of increased CV events and mortality [19]. Additionally, leptin has been suggested as playing a significant role in HTN, impairment in cardiac contractility, LV apoptosis, and reperfusion injury [16, 20].

Obesity may also have numerous adverse affects on hemodynamics as well as LV structure and function (Figure 11.1) [21]. Obesity increases total blood volume, which leads to increases in cardiac output and cardiac workload [21–24]. At any given level of blood pressure, obese patients have lower total peripheral resistance but a higher cardiac output. Most of this higher cardiac output is due to an increased blood volume and subsequent stroke volume, but other mechanisms play a role especially in early obesity including heightened sympathetic activation, heart rate and contractility [1, 25]. The Frank Starling curve is shifted to the left due to increases in filling pressure and volume, thus increasing total cardiac workload.

The increases in LV filling pressure and volume in overweight and obese patients often lead to substantial LV dilatation [8, 11, 21, 22, 26, 27]. Although obesity is a major cause of elevated arterial pressure and the development of HTN, even independent of arterial pressure, obesity increases the risk of all types of LV structural abnormalities, including concentric remodeling as well as eccentric and concentric LV hypertrophy [1, 28]. In addition to increasing the development of LV structural abnormalities, the increase in circulating blood volume as well as substantial LV diastolic abnormalities predispose the obese patient to the development of left atrial enlargement and increased risk of AF [28–31].

Particularly when combined with HTN and the above mentioned structural abnormalities, obesity has many adverse effects on LV function, especially diastolic abnormalities [1, 21, 32, 33]. However, early in obesity, subtle systolic abnormalities may be present [34] preload dependent indices of systolic function, such as ejection fraction or velocity of circumferential fiber shortening, remain preserved possibly due to increased LV blood volume and LV filling. However, preload independent indices, such as end-systolic stress/end-systolic volume index, demonstrates reduced LV contractility [34]. Clearly, as obesity progresses, there are significant adverse affects on both systolic and diastolic ventricular function [21, 35, 36].

Additionally, obesity leads to more frequent and complex ventricular arrhythmias, especially when combined with HTN and eccentric LVH [25, 27]. Moreover, due to prolongation in the Q-T interval, increased prevalence of late potentials, and abnormalities in the autonomic nervous system, obesity may increase the risk of sudden cardiac death [2, 16–19, 37–39].

EPIDEMIOLOGY OF OBESITY IN HF

Since obesity has adverse effects on LV structure and function, it is not surprising that it may increase the risk of HF [11, 13]. In a study of 5881 Framingham Heart Study participants, Kenchaiah et al. [40] demonstrated that during a 14-year follow-up period, for every 1 kg/m^2 increment in body mass index (BMI), the risk of HF increased by 5% in men and 7% in women. In fact, they noted a graded increase in the risk of HF across all categories of BMI (Figure 11.2) [40], suggesting a causal relationship between excess body weight and the development of HF. In a study by Alpert et al. [41] of 74 morbidly obese patients, nearly one-third had clinical evidence of HF, and the probability of HF increased dramatically with increased duration of morbid obesity (Figure 11.3) [41]. In fact, at 20 and 25 years of obesity duration, the probability of HF was 66% and 93%, respectively.

IMPACT OF OBESITY ON CLINICAL ASSESSMENT

Obesity may have significant impact on the history, physical examination, and diagnostic tests related with HF. Since obesity is often accompanied by considerable deconditioning, the symptoms in obese patients may appear out of proportion to the severity of clinical HF [42, 43]. In other words, this could cause the obese HF patient to present earlier with less advanced disease. On physical examination, marked obesity may make it considerably more difficult to visualize the neck veins, to hear extra cardiac sounds, and to fully evaluate for cardiopulmonary disease. Additionally, the large chest wall and abdominal mass may make it difficult to evaluate for pleural effusions and ascites. Although the evaluation of peripheral edema may likewise be more difficult with marked obesity, these patients often have considerable venous disease, due to increased intravascular volume as well as high-volume lymphatic overload as well as reduced physical activity, often leading to venous insufficiency and more peripheral edema independent of HF [1, 44].

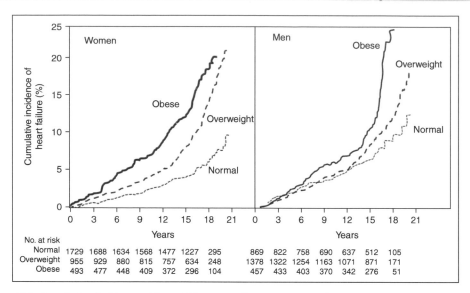

Figure 11.2 Cumulative incidence of heart failure according to category of BMI at the baseline examination. Obese indicates BMI of 30.0 kg/m²; overweight, BMI of 25.0 to 29.9 kg/m²; normal, BMI of 18.5 to 24.9 kg/m² (with permission from [40]).

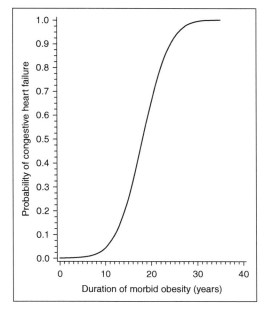

Figure 11.3 Sigma curve showing the probability of heart failure as a function of duration of morbid obesity (with permission from [41]).

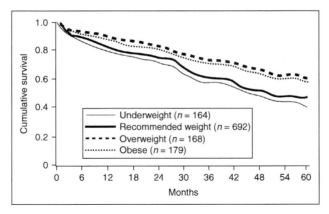

Figure 11.4 Risk-adjusted survival curves for the four BMI categories at 5 years in a study of 1203 individuals with moderate to severe heart failure. Survival was significantly better in the overweight and obese categories (with permission from [46]).

In addition, studies have suggested a close relationship between the natriuretic peptide system and adiposity, including in HF, and Mehra *et al.* [45] have demonstrated reduced levels of natriuretic peptide in obese patients with HF. This line of evidence lends further credence to the explanation that obese patients with HF may present earlier from a symptomatic standpoint. On the other hand, since natriuretic peptide levels are often used by clinicians to aid in the diagnosis of clinical HF, lower circulating levels in obesity may make the diagnosis more difficult, particularly in overweight/obese patients with relatively mild degrees of HF. Likewise on X-ray films of the chest, the lungs often appear less expanded and the cardiac size relatively enlarged, also potentially affecting the diagnosis of HF in obesity. Finally, and perhaps most importantly, many clinicians rely heavily on Doppler echocardiographic data in the diagnosis of HF, and many obese patients have technically difficult transthoracic echocardiographic studies, although advances in technology are currently allowing the transthoracic echocardiogram to be interpreted even in most cases of extreme obesity.

IMPACT OF OBESITY ON PROGNOSIS—THE 'OBESITY PARADOX'

Although obesity has adverse affects on LV structure and function and increases the prevalence of HF, numerous studies have now noted a powerful 'obesity paradox' in which overweight and obese patients with HF appear to have a better clinical prognosis in both short- and long-term studies compared with their leaner counterparts with similar HF [3, 13]. One of the earliest studies to demonstrate the relationship between obesity and HF mortality was published by Horwich and colleagues (Figure 11.4) [46]. In fact, in a relatively small study of 209 patients with chronic systolic HF being evaluated for heart transplantation (HT), we demonstrated that both higher BMI and higher percent body fat were independent predictors of better event-free survival (Figure 11.5) [47]. In our study, for every 1% increase in percent body fat, we observed a >13% reduction in major clinical events (cardiac death or urgent HT). Moreover, preliminary data in a much larger cohort of nearly 1000 patients with chronic systolic HF from our institution also demonstrated that higher percent body fat was one of the strongest independent predictors of better total survival [48].

This 'obesity paradox' has been examined in a recent meta-analysis by Oreopoulos *et al.* [49] of nine observation HF studies ($n = 28\,209$) with an average follow-up of just under 3 years. This analysis demonstrated that compared to HF patients without elevated BMI, overweight and obese HF patients had significant 19% and 40% reductions, respectively in CV mortality, with 16% and 33% reductions, respectively in all-cause mortality. Fonarow *et al.* [50] evaluated 108 927 decompensated HF patients in a large registry and found that higher BMI was associated with lower mortality (for every $1/kg/min^2$ increase in BMI, mortality was reduced by 10%).

The reasons for this puzzling paradox are difficult to elucidate. As mentioned earlier, obese patients may present with symptoms earlier with less advanced disease due to their deconditioning, restrictive lung disease (which may itself induce symptoms out of proportion to HF), as well as the lower levels of circulating atrial natriuretic peptides [42, 43, 45]. Also, since HF is a catabolic state and wasting disorder, obese patients with HF may have more metabolic reserve which may provide protection [51–54]. Additionally, none of these studies accounted for non-purposeful weight loss. Cytokines and neuroendocrine profiles of obese may also be protective [49]. Adipose tissue itself produces soluble tumor necrosis factor alpha (TNF-α) receptors, and this could play a protective role in obese patients with HF by at least partially neutralizing the adverse biological effects of TNF-α [55]. Obese with HF may have altered responses of the sympathetic nervous system and renin angiotensin aldosterone systems [56, 57]. Obese may have higher circulating levels of lipoproteins that may bind and detoxify lipopolysaccharides that play a role in stimulating release of inflammatory cytokines, which may also protect the obese HF patient [51, 58, 59]. Finally, since obesity raises levels of arterial pressure, obese HF patients often have more HTN and may tolerate more and higher doses of various cardioprotective medications [49].

IMPACT OF OBESITY IN CARDIOPULMONARY STRESS TESTING (CPX)

CPX has emerged as a leading modality to assess prognosis in HF [60, 61]. A detailed discussion of the use of CPX and clinical HF is beyond the scope of this chapter. However, from a simple practical standpoint, many clinicians rely heavily on peak oxygen consumption (VO_2) to determine functional capacity and to predict prognosis in HF. Initially, Mancini *et al.* [62] recommended peak VO_2 of 14 ml/kg/min as a cutoff for risk stratification and as a discriminator for those being considered for HT. Clearly patients with peak $VO_2 > 18$ ml/kg/ min have a very good prognosis, whereas those with values <10 ml/kg/min have a poor prognosis [63]. However, in between these extremes, CPX may not be as valuable. Importantly, CPX may lose prognostic power in certain subgroups with high percentage of body fat, such as women and obese, since typically peak VO_2 is corrected for total as opposed to lean body mass, despite the fact that adipose tissue does not utilize much oxygen or receive substantial perfusion. We have demonstrated that correcting peak VO_2 for lean as opposed to total body mass, using a cutoff of 19 ml/kg/min (lean) performed considerably better than uncorrected peak VO_2 (Figure 11.6), [64] which may be particularly applicable to obesity (Table 11.1) [64, 65]. Likewise, we also demonstrated that peak O_2 pulse, which represents peak VO_2/peak heart rate, also predicted prognosis better than uncorrected indices (Figure 11.7) [66].

SHOULD OBESITY BE TREATED?

Some long-term studies have suggested that weight loss in overweight and obesity is associated with increased mortality, leading to suggestions that purposeful weight loss may not be beneficial and may even be detrimental in patients with CV diseases, including HF [46, 67–70]. In contrast, however, studies assessing mortality based on body fat and lean mass rather than BMI or total weight also have suggested that subjects losing body fat rather than lean mass have a lower mortality [69, 71].

Clearly in CHD and HTN, small studies have suggested considerable benefits of purposeful weight loss, including lower clinical events [72]. Only minimal data is available on

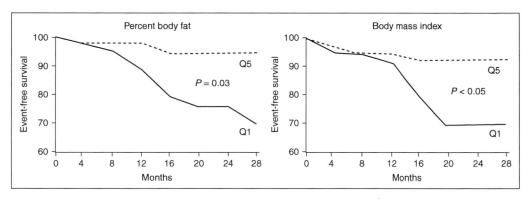

Figure 11.5 Kaplan–Meier major event-free survival curves (freedom from cardiovascular death or urgent transplantation) in patients in quintiles (Q) 1 and 5 for percent body fat (left panel) and BMI (right panel) (with permission from [47]).

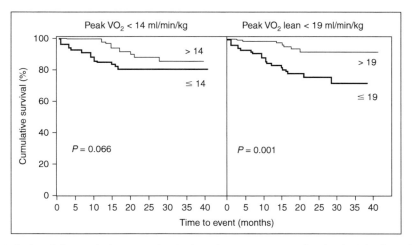

Figure 11.6 Kaplan–Meier survival curves using both peak oxygen consumption (peak VO_2) of 14 ml/kg/min and peak oxygen consumption adjusted to lean body mass (peak VO_2 lean) of 19 ml/kg/min as cutoffs, showing a stronger prognostic value to the fat-adjusted peak VO_2 by log-rank testing (adapted with permission from [64]).

Table 11.1 Impact of obesity on cardiopulmonary stress test results and prognosis (adapted with permission from [64, 65])

Parameter	Obese (n = 76)	Lean (n = 43)	P-value	Obese (n = 76)	Non-obese (n = 133)	P-value
Age, years	51±12	57±14	<0.02	51±12	56±12	<0.01
BMI, kg/m²	34.6±4.3	22.7±1.8	<0.0001	34.6±4.3	25.8±2.7	<0.0001
Peak VO_2, ml/kg/min	14.5+4.9	17.7±7.4	<0.01	14.5±4.9	17.0±6.3	<0.01
Anaerobic threshold, ml/kg/min	11.8±3.6	14.2±5.0	=0.02	11.8±3.6	13.4±4.2	=0.02
Peak VO_2 (lean), ml/kg/min	20.9±6.5	22.2±9.0	=0.36	20.9±6.5	22.1±7.8	=0.28
Major events, %	10.5%	21%	=0.11	10.5%	15%	=0.35

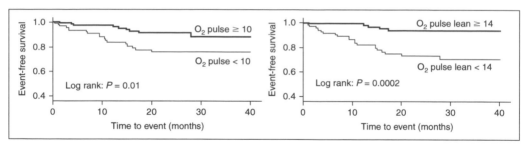

Figure 11.7 Kaplan–Meier survival curves using both peak oxygen pulse (O_2 pulse) 10 ml/beat and peak oxygen pulse lean (O_2 pulse lean) 14 ml/beat as cutoffs for predicting event-free survival (adapted with permission from [66]).

weight loss in obesity HF. In a small study of only 14 morbidly obese patients who achieved marked weight loss (> 30% of body weight) after gastroplasty, functional class improved in twelve patients by an average of at least one functional class; weight loss was also associated with marked improvements in LV chamber size, LV end-systolic wall stress, as well as systolic and diastolic LV function [41]. More marked weight reduction with bariatric surgical procedures have also been associated with short- and long-term improvements in CV morbidity and mortality, although short-term affects on blood pressure do not seem to be maintained long-term [73–75]. Realizing that the jury is still out regarding purposeful weight loss and its impact on morbidity and mortality in HF, including the risk and benefits of bariatric surgery in this group of patients, the 'weight' of evidence currently supports purposeful weight loss, particularly with strategies that do not produce reductions in lean body mass, in patients with marked obesity and HF, despite its 'obesity paradox' [76, 77].

CONCLUSIONS

This chapter reviews the complex relationship between obesity and HF. Despite adverse affects on hemodynamics and LV structure and function and being a powerful risk factor for HF, overweightness and obesity seems to favorably influence HF prognosis. Further studies are needed to better elucidate the mechanisms of this puzzling 'obesity paradox' as well as to confirm the impact of purposeful weight reduction on HF treatment and prognosis.

REFERENCES

1. Poirier P, Giles TD, Bray GA et al. Obesity and cardiovascular disease: pathophysiology, evaluation, and effect of weight loss: an update of the 1997 American Heart Association Scientific Statement on obesity and heart disease from the obesity committee of the Council on Nutrition, Physical Activity, and Metabolism. Circulation 2006; 113:898-918.
2. Klein S, Burke LE, Bray GA et al. Clinical implications of obesity with specific focus on cardiovascular disease: a statement for professionals from the American Heart Association Council on Nutrition, Physical Activity, and Metabolism: endorsed by the American College of Cardiology Foundation. Circulation 2004; 110:2952-2967.
3. Artham SM, Lavie CJ, Milani RV, Ventura HO. The obesity paradox: impact of obesity on the prevalence and prognosis of cardiovascular diseases. Postgrad Med 2008; 120:34-41.
4. Flegal JN, Carroll MD, Ogden CL, Johnson CL. Prevalence and trends in obesity among US adults, 1999-2000. JAMA 2002; 288:1723-1727.

5. Manson JE, Bassuk SS. Obesity in the United States: a fresh look at its high toll. *JAMA* 2003; 289:229-230.

6. Allison DB, Fontaine KR, Manson JE, Stevens J, VanItallie TB. Annual deaths attributable to obesity in the United States. *JAMA* 1999; 282:1530-1538.

7. Sturm R, Well KB. Does obesity contribute as much to morbidity as poverty or smoking? *Public Health* 2001; 115:229-235.

8. Lavie CJ, Milani RV. Obesity and cardiovascular disease: the hippocrates paradox? *J Am Coll Cardiol* 2003; 42:677-679.

9. World Health Organization. Definition, diagnosis, and classification of diabetes mellitus and its complications: report of a WHO consultation. Geneva: *WHO*, 1999.

10. Ford ES, Capewell S. Coronary heart disease mortality among young adults in the US from 1980 through 2002: concealed leveling of mortality rates. *J Am Coll Cardiol* 2007; 50:2128-2132.

11. Lavie CJ, Milani RV, Mehra MH, Ventura HO, Messerli FH. Obesity, weight reduction and survival in heart failure. *J Am Coll Cardiol* 2002; 39:1563.

12. Lavie CJ, Messerli FH. Cardiovascular adaptation to obesity and hypertension. *Chest* 1986; 90:275-279.

13. Artham SM, Lavie CJ, Patel HM, Ventura HO. Impact of obesity on the risk of heart failure and its prognosis. *J Cardiometab Syndr* 2008; 3:155-161.

14. Miller MT, Lavie CJ. Impact of obesity on the pathogenesis and prognosis of coronary heart disease. *J Cardiometab Syndr* 2008; 3:162-167.

15. Martin SS, Qasim A, Reilly MP. Leptin resistance. *J Am Coll Cardiol* 2008; 52:1201-1210.

16. Lavie CJ, Milani RV, Ventura HO. Untangling the heavy cardiovascular burden of obesity. *Nat Clin Pract Cardiovasc Med* 2008; 5:428-429.

17. Esler M, Straznicky N, Eikelis N, Masuo K, Lambert G, Lambert E. Mechanisms of sympathetic activation in obesity-related hypertension. *Hypertension* 2006; 48:787-796.

18. Grassi G, Elam M. Leptin, sympathetic and baroreflex function: another step on the road to sympathetic differentiation. *J Hypertens* 2002; 20:1487-1489.

19. Earnest CP, Lavie CJ, Blair SN, Church TS. Heart rate variability characteristics in sedentary postmenopausal women following six months of exercise training: the DREW study. *PLoS ONE* 2008; 3:e2288.

20. Yang R, Barouch LA. Leptin signaling and obesity: cardiovascular consequences. *Circ Res* 2007; 101:545-559.

21. Alpert MA. Obesity cardiomyopathy: pathophysiology and evolution of the clinical syndrome. *Am J Med Sci* 2001; 321:225-236.

22. Messerli FH, Sundgaard-Riise K, Reisin ED *et al*. Dimorphic cardiac adaptation to obesity and arterial hypertension. *Ann Intern Med* 1983; 99:757-761.

23. Messerli FH, Ventura HO, Reisin E *et al*. Borderline hypertension and obesity: two prehypertensive states with elevated cardiac output. *Circulation* 1982; 66:55-60.

24. Messerli FH, Christie B, DeCarvalho JG, Aristimuno GG, Suarez DH, Frohlich ED. Obesity and essential hypertension: hemodynamics, intravascular volume, sodium excretion, and plasma renin activity. *Arch Intern Med* 1981; 141:81-85.

25. Messerli FH, Nunez BD, Ventura HO, Snyder DW. Overweight and sudden death: increased ventricular ectopy in cardiomyopathy of obesity. *Arch Intern Med* 1987; 147:1725-1728.

26. Ku CS, Lin SL, Wang DJ, Chang SK, Lee WJ. Left ventricular filling in young normotensive obese adults. *Am J Cardiol* 1994; 73:613-615.

27. Messerli FH. Cardiomyopathy of obesity: a not-so-Victorian disease. *N Engl J Med* 1986; 314:378-380.

28. Lavie CJ, Milani RV, Ventura HO, Cardenas GA, Mehra MR, Messerli FH. Disparate effects of left ventricular geometry and obesity on mortality in patients with preserved left ventricular ejection fraction. *Am J Cardiol* 2007; 100:1460-1464.

29. Steinberg JS. Atrial fibrillation: an emerging epidemic? *Heart* 2004; 90:239-240.

30. Wanahita N, Messerli FH, Bangalore S *et al*. Atrial fibrillation and obesity – results of a meta-analysis. *Am Heart J* 2008; 155:310-315.

31. Frost L, Hune LJ, Vestergaard P. Overweight and obesity as risk factors for atrial fibrillation or flutter: the Danish Diet, Cancer, and Health Study. *Am J Med* 2005; 118:489-495.

32. Lavie CJ, Amodeo C, Ventura HO, Messerli FH. Left atrial abnormalities indicating diastolic ventricular dysfunction in cardiopathy of obesity. *Chest* 1987; 92:1042-1046.

33. Chakko S, Mayor M, Allison MD, Kessler KM, Materson BJ, Myerburg RJ. Abnormal left ventricular diastolic filling in eccentric left ventricular hypertrophy of obesity. *Am J Cardiol* 1991; 68:95-98.

34. Garavaglia GE, Messerli FH, Nunez BD, Schmieder RE, Grossman E. Myocardial contractility and left ventricular function in obese patients with essential hypertension. *Am J Cardiol* 1988; 62:594-597.

35. Alpert MA, Lambert CR, Terry BE *et al*. Interrelationship of left ventricular mass, systolic function and diastolic filling in normotensive morbidly obese patients. *Int J Obes Relat Metab Disord* 1995; 19:550-557.

36. Alpert MA, Lambert CR, Terry BE *et al*. Effect of weight loss on left ventricular mass in nonhypertensive morbidly obese patients. *Am J Cardiol* 1994; 73:918-921.

37. el-Gamal A, Gallagher D, Nawras A *et al*. Effects of obesity on QT, RR, and QTc intervals. *Am J Cardiol* 1995; 75:956-959.

38. Rasmussen LH, Andersen T. The relationship between QTc changes and nutrition during weight loss after gastroplasty. *Acta Med Scand* 1985; 217:271-275.

39. Lalani AP, Kanna B, John J, Ferrick KJ, Huber MS, Shapiro LE. Abnormal signal-averaged electrocardiogram (SAECG) in obesity. *Obes Res* 2000; 8:20-28.

40. Kenchaiah S, Evans JC, Levy D *et al*. Obesity and the risk of heart failure. *N Engl J Med* 2002; 347:305-313.

41. Alpert MA, Terry BE, Mulekar M *et al*. Cardiac morphology and left ventricular function in normotensive morbidly obese patients with and without congestive heart failure, and effect of weight loss. *Am J Cardiol* 1997; 80:736-740.

42. Lavie CJ, Milani RV, Ventura HO. Obesity, heart disease, and favorable prognosis – truth or paradox? *Am J Med* 2007; 120:825-826.

43. Lavie CJ, Ventura HO, Milani RV. The 'obesity paradox' – is smoking/lung disease the explanation? *Chest* 2008; 134:896-898.

44. Sugerman HJ, Suggerman EI, Wolfe L,Kellum JM Jr, Schweitzer MA, DeMaria EJ. Risks and benefits of gastric bypass in morbidly obese patients with severe venous stasis disease. *Ann Surg* 2001; 234:41-46.

45. Mehra MR, Uber PA, Parh MH *et al*. Obesity and suppressed B-type natriuretic peptide levels in heart failure. *J Am Coll Cardiol* 2004; 43:1590-1595.

46. Horwich TB, Fonarow GC, Hamilton MA *et al*. The relationship between obesity and mortality in patients with heart failure. *J Am Coll Cardiol* 2001; 38:789-795.

47. Lavie CJ, Osman AF, Milani RV, Mehra MR. Body composition and prognosis in chronic systolic heart failure: the obesity paradox. *Am J Cardiol* 2003; 91:891-894.

48. Lavie CJ, Milani RV, Artham SM *et al*. Does body composition impact survival in patients with advanced heart failure. *Circulation* 2007; 116:ll_360.

49. Oreopoulos A, Padwal R, Kalantar-Zadeh K *et al*. Body mass index and mortality in heart failure: a meta-analysis. *Am Heart J* 2008; 156:13-22.

50. Fonarow GC, Srikanthan P, Costanzo MR *et al*. An obesity paradox in acute heart failure: analysis of body mass index and inhospital mortality for 108,927 patients in the acute decompensated heart failure national registry. *Am Heart J* 2007; 153:74-81.

51. Lavie CJ, Mehra MR, Milani RV. Obesity and heart failure prognosis: paradox or reverse epidemiology. *Eur Heart J* 2005; 26:5-7.

52. Kalantar-Zadeh K, Block G, Horwich T, Fonarow GC. Reverse epidemiology of conventional cardiovascular risk factors in patients with chronic heart failure. *J Am Coll Cardiol* 2004; 43:1439-1444.

53. Anker S, Rauchhaus M. Insights into the pathogenesis of chronic heart failure: immune activation and cachexia. *Curr Opin Cardiol* 1999; 14:211-216.

54. Anker S, Negassa A, Coats AJ *et al*. Prognostic importance of weight loss in chronic heart failure and the effect of treatment with angiotensin-converting enzyme inhibitors: an observational study. *Lancet* 2003; 361:1077-1083.

55. Mohamed-Ali V, Goodrick S, Bulmer K *et al*. Production of soluble tumor necrosis factor receptors by human subcutaneous adipose tissue in vivo. *Am J Physiol* 1999; 277:E971-E975.

56. Schrier R, Abraham WT. Hormones and hemodynamics in heart failure. *N Eng J Med* 1999; 341:577-585.

57. Weber M, Neutel JM, Smith DHG. Contrasting clinical properties and exercise responses in obese and lean hypertensive patients. *J Am Coll Cardiol* 2001; 37:169-174.

58. Mehra MR, Uber PA, Parh MH *et al*. Obesity and suppressed B-type natriuretic peptide levels in heart failure. *J Am Coll Cardiol* 2004; 43:1590-1595.

59. Rauchhaus M, Coats AJS, Anker SD. The endotoxin–lipoprotein hypothesis. *Lancet* 2000; 356:930-933.

60. Mehra MR, Lavie CJ, Milani RV. Predicting prognosis in advanced heart failure: use of exercise indices. *Chest* 1996; 110:310-312.

61. Milani RV, Lavie CJ, Mehra MR, Ventura HO. Understanding the basics of cardiopulmonary exercise testing. *Mayo Clin Proc* 2006; 81:1603:1611.

62. Mancini DM, Eisen H, Kussmaul W, Mull R, Edmunds LH Jr, Wilson JR. Value of peak exercise oxygen consumption for optimal timing of cardiac transplantation in ambulatory patients with heart failure. *Circulation* 1991; 83:773-786.

63. Artham SM, Lavie CJ, Milani RV, Ventura HO. The obesity paradox and discrepancy between peak oxygen consumption and heart failure prognosis – it's all in the fat. *Congest Heart Fail* 2007; 13:177-180.

64. Osman AF, Mehra MR, Lavie CJ, Nunez E, Milani RV. The incremental prognostic importance of body fat adjusted peak oxygen consumption in chronic heart failure. *J Am Coll Cardiol* 2000; 36:2126-2131.

65. Lavie CJ, Osman AF, Milani RV, Mehra MR. Body composition and prognosis in chronic systolic heart failure – the obesity paradox. *J Am Coll Cardiol* 2002; 39(suppl A):191A.

66. Lavie CJ, Milani RV, Mehra MR. Peak exercise oxygen pulse and prognosis in chronic heart failure. *Am J Cardiol* 2004; 93:588-593.

67. Manson JE, Colditz GA, Stampfer MJ *et al.* A prospective study of obesity and risk of coronary heart disease in women. *N Engl J Med* 1990; 322:882-889.

68. Fonarow GC, Horwich TB, Hamilton MA *et al.* Obesity, weight reduction and survival in heart failure: reply. *J Am Coll Cardiol* 2002; 39:1563-1564.

69. Allison DB, Zannolli R, Faith MS *et al.* Weight loss increases and fat loss decreases all-cause mortality rates: results from two independent cohort studies. *Int J Obes Relat Metab Disord* 1999; 23:603-611.

70. Sierra-Johnson J, Romero-Corral A, Somers VK *et al.* Prognostic importance of weight loss in patients with coronary heart disease regardless of initial body mass index. *Eur J Cardiovasc Prev Rehabil* 2008; 15:336-340.

71. Sorensen TI. Weight loss causes increased mortality: pros. *Obes Rev* 2003; 4:3-7.

72. Lavie CJ, Milani RV, Ventura HO. Obesity and cardiovascular disease – risk factor, paradox, and impact of weight loss. *J Am Coll Cardiol* 2009; 53:1925-1932.

73. Adams TD, Gress RE, Smith SC *et al.* Long-term mortality after gastric bypass surgery. *N Engl J Med* 2007; 357:753-761.

74. Sjöström L, Narbro K, Sjöström CD *et al.* Effects of bariatric surgery on mortality in Swedish obese subjects. *N Engl J Med* 2007; 357:741-752.

75. Christou NV, Sampalis JS, Liberman M *et al.* Surgery decreases long-term mortality, morbidity, and health care use in morbidly obese patients. *Ann Surg* 2004; 240:416-424.

76. Lavie CJ, Milani RV, Ventura HO, Romero-Corral A. Body composition and heart failure prevalence and prognosis: getting to the fat of the matter in the "obesity paradox". *Mayo Clin Proc* 2010; 85:605-608.

77. Artham SM, Lavie CJ, Milani RV, Ventura HO. Value of weight reduction in patients with cardiovascular disease. *Curr Treat Options Cardiovasc Med* 2010; 12:21-35.

12

The role for revascularization in asymptomatic patients with left ventricular systolic dysfunction

T. J. Mulhearn IV, J. G. Rogers

INTRODUCTION

Coronary artery disease is the most common cause of left ventricular (LV) systolic dysfunction in the developed world. Patients with ischemic LV systolic dysfunction have significantly higher mortality rates than those with ischemic heart disease associated with normal LV systolic function [1, 2]. In the United States, the attributable risk of ischemic heart disease for LV dysfunction is 67.9% in men and 55.9% in women [3]. Several large observational studies and databases, such as the Coronary Artery Surgery Study (CASS) and Duke Cardiovascular Disease Databank, have shown a significant survival advantage with revascularization in patients with LV systolic dysfunction [4, 5]. The majority of patients included in these studies had angina and symptomatic heart failure (HF), so definitive data to guide the management of patients with asymptomatic ischemic heart disease and LV systolic dysfunction are not available. It has been observed that LV dysfunction may be a reversible phenomenon when due to myocardial stunning or hibernation. This chapter will review the pathophysiology of hibernation and stunning, techniques for determination of myocardial viability, and the evidence supporting revascularization in HF patients with coronary artery disease.

OVERVIEW

Basic and clinical investigation has demonstrated that myocardial dysfunction secondary to coronary artery occlusion is not necessarily caused by infarction and that subsequent revascularization may result in significant improvements in contractile function and mortality. In other words, ischemic myocardium may respond to critical reductions in blood flow with a complex series of protective mechanisms that ultimately maintain cell viability at the expense of overall myocardial function. These observations form the conceptual basis for 'stunned' and 'hibernating' myocardium. The residual challenges for investigators and clinicians are to devise reliable tools that distinguish between viable and non-viable myocardium, to quantitate the amount of viable myocardium and determine thresholds beyond which func-

Thomas J. Mulhearn IV, MD, Fellow in Cardiovascular Medicine, Division of Cardiology, Duke University Medical Center, Durham, NC, USA.

Joseph G. Rogers, MD, Associate Professor of Medicine, Division of Cardiology, Duke University School of Medicine and the Duke Clinical Research Institute, Durham, NC, USA.

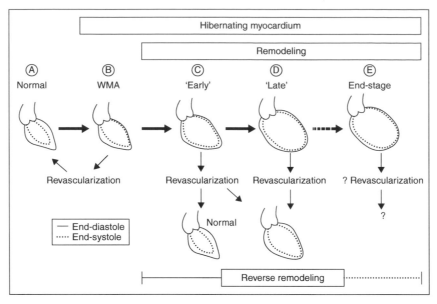

Figure 12.1 Diagrammatic representation of postulated progressive changes in a patient with hibernating myocardium and (A) no remodeling (B), mild to moderate remodeling (C and D), and end-stage (E) of the disorder. WMA=wall – motion abnormality (with permission from *J Am Coll Cardiol* 2006; 47: 978–980. ©2006, The American College of Cardiology Foundation).

tional recovery is likely following revascularization, and to design and conduct trials to determine the most appropriate treatment strategies for patients with asymptomatic ischemic cardiomyopathy. To date, the management of ischemic LV dysfunction without angina is particularly challenging as diagnostic and therapeutic choices have broadened, and there are no randomized trials to guide therapy. The majority of observational studies demonstrating benefit with revascularization have included primarily patients with angina. In patients without angina, viability testing has been proposed as a useful tool to identify those who might benefit from revascularization. However, this strategy has not been thoroughly tested in large scale clinical trials.

WHAT IS STUNNED OR HIBERNATING MYOCARDIUM?

It has been recognized for more than 30 years that LV dysfunction in the setting of significant coronary artery disease frequently improves following surgical revascularization [6, 7]. These observations form the clinical basis for the notion that ischemic LV dysfunction may result from either acute or chronic reductions in myocardial perfusion or myocardial infarction (Figure 12.1). In an attempt to explain transient myocardial dysfunction that improves with revascularization, the concepts of myocardial stunning and hibernation were developed. The unifying concept underlying myocardial stunning and hibernation is that myocardial perfusion may decrease below a level that permits normal contractile function without causing cell death. Myocardial stunning refers to acute LV dysfunction resulting from transient ischemia that may persist for weeks after restoration of adequate coronary blood flow to viable myocardium. Hibernating myocardium is characterized by myocardial dysfunction resulting from chronic reductions in coronary perfusion that similarly may improve as coronary blood flow is enhanced [8]. Hibernation is thought to be a protective

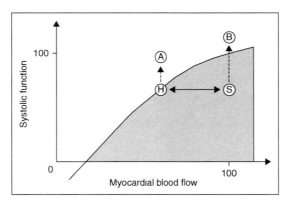

Figure 12.2 The relationship between myocardial blood flow and systolic function. The line demonstrates the relationship between myocardial blood flow and left ventricular systolic function (flow-function relationship). When myocardium is operating below this line, function is disproportionately depressed relative to flow and when it is above the line, function exceeds blood flow and ischemia is likely to result. Chronically hypoperfused myocardium, resulting from an epicardial coronary stenosis that restricts basal coronary flow, produces hibernation (H). In comparison, stunning (S), resulting from repetitive bouts of ischemia, occurs when the stenosis severely limits flow reserve but not basal coronary flow. Small variations in blood flow may result in a change in myocardial state, between H and S, without any appreciable change in systolic function. Following inotropic stimulation, myocardium operating at both H and S will increase systolic function without a substantial change in blood flow (A and B, respectively). As a result, the two situations cannot be reliably distinguished by stress echocardiography (with permission from Redwood SR, Ferrari R, Marber MS. Myocardial hibernation and stunning: from physiological principles to clinical practice. *Heart* 1998; 80: 218–222).

mechanism in which the heart reduces its need for energy substrate to maintain 'perfusion-contraction matching' [9]. Chronic reduction in coronary blood flow induces expression of myocardial cell survival proteins and morphologic changes that may also explain some of the benefit of ischemic pre-conditioning [10]. Repetitive stunning has been shown in animal studies to lead to hibernation despite restoration of normal coronary perfusion [11]. Myocardial stunning, hibernation and infarction are not distinct entities, but rather represent a continuum of LV dysfunction that are dependent on the severity and duration of reduced coronary perfusion. The relationship between coronary blood flow and myocardial systolic function is shown in Figure 12.2.

IMAGING MODALITIES AVAILABLE FOR MYOCARDIAL VIABILITY ASSESSMENT

Several techniques can be used to identify dysfunctional, yet viable myocardium. The most commonly used techniques today are dobutamine echocardiography, nuclear myocardial perfusion imaging, positron emission tomography (PET) scanning, and cardiac magnetic resonance imaging (MRI).

DOBUTAMINE ECHOCARDIOGRAPHY

Demonstration of improvements in either segmental or global myocardial function during dobutamine stress echocardiography ('contractile reserve') is useful in the assessment of viability. Low dose dobutamine (5–10 mcg/kg/min) can lead to increased contractility in dysfunctional segments. At higher doses, contractility may improve further or diminish. A biphasic response, in which contractility initially improves with low-dose dobutamine and subsequently worsens at higher dose dobutamine, is thought to represent ischemic and viable myocardium and is highly correlated with improved contractility after revascularization [12]. Improved contractile response to dobutamine appears to require > 50% myocardial viability and is associated with lesser degrees of interstitial fibrosis [13]. Dobutamine echocardiography has also been used to predict improvements in LV function following revascularization. Perrone-Filardi [14] demonstrated improved contractility after revascularization in 42 of 46 (91%) segments with contractile reserve during dobutamine infusion compared with six of 33 (18%) segments that were thought to be nonviable. The positive and negative predictive value for dobutamine echocardiography to predict improvement in LV function after revascularization was 91% and 82%, respectively. The strengths of dobutamine echocardiography include widespread availability, portability, safety, and low cost. The limitations include low spatial resolution, high inter-observer variability, and diminished diagnostic accuracy with severely depressed LV function.

NUCLEAR SPECT

Thallium-201 myocardial perfusion imaging is another commonly used technique for viability assessment. Myocardial uptake of thallium occurs via a Na/K+ ATPase-dependent process requiring cell membrane integrity and perfusion. Thallium-201 was initially introduced as a perfusion tracer, but it was subsequently demonstrated that some stress-induced perfusion defects normalize or redistribute several hours after the initial injection [15]. This normalized myocardial perfusion with delayed imaging was thought to represent ischemic, yet viable myocardium. Stress-redistribution thallium imaging subsequently became a standard protocol for assessing ischemic myocardium. However, a large proportion of 'fixed' perfusion defects seen at 4 h were found to be viable by PET scanning. This led to late redistribution reimaging 18–24 h after the initial injection of thallium. Several centers administer a second smaller dose of thallium after the redistribution images are obtained in order to increase blood levels. Thallium reinjection has been shown to increase the sensitivity for detecting viable myocardium over redistribution imaging [16]. A single injection of thallium at rest followed by redistribution images 4–24 h later can also be performed to assess viability when stress data is not necessary. Technetium-99m labeled radiotracers have also been used to assess viability, but technetium does not redistribute in the myocardium like thallium. This theoretical concern has limited the use of technetium-labeled radiotracers to assess perfusion rather than viability [17].

PET

PET is another commonly used technique for evaluating myocardial viability. PET is most commonly performed using fluorine-18 labeled deoxyglucose (FDG), which is taken up by metabolically active myocytes. FDG PET has excellent predictive accuracy in determining reversibility of wall motion abnormalities following surgical revascularization. In a study of 17 patients with ischemic cardiomyopathy, determination of viability by FDG PET with subsequent improvement in wall motion abnormalities following revascularization was correctly predicted in 35/41 segments (85 percent) whereas 24/26 segments (92 percent) were correctly identified as non-viable [18]. Furthermore, FDG PET has been used to predict improvements in LV performance and functional status after revascularization [19, 20]. The main advantage of PET over SPECT is superior spatial resolution.

The relative predictive accuracy of dobutamine echocardiography, thallium SPECT, technetium-sestamibi SPECT, and FDG PET were compared in a meta-analysis of 52 studies. For all imaging techniques, the negative predictive value was higher than the positive predictive value. Dobutamine echo had the highest positive predictive value for assessment of recovery in dysfunctional segments after revascularization. FDG PET followed by thallium

SPECT had the highest negative predictive value. Of note, most of the studies included in this meta-analysis did not compare imaging techniques in the same patient [21, 22].

MAGNETIC RESONANCE IMAGING (MRI)

Cardiac MRI has become an increasingly utilized method for assessing myocardial viability. Cine imaging with gradient echo sequencing has been used in a manner similar to dobutamine echocardiography to assess viability [23–25]. The addition of gadolinium contrast agents to detect areas of scar or non-viable myocardium has been an important advance in the use of cardiac MRI. Delayed enhancement after gadolinium administration correlates well with myocardial necrosis and thus nonviable myocardium [26, 27]. Cardiac MRI has been used to predict improvement in contractility following revascularization. An example of cine and contrast enhanced images obtained by MRI in patients with reversible and irreversible ventricular dysfunction is shown in Figure 12.3. Kim and colleagues analyzed 41 patients and 2093 myocardial segments with cardiac MRI before and after revascularization. More than 75% of dysfunctional segments without delayed enhancement demonstrated improved contractility following revascularization, and the likelihood of improvement was inversely related to the amount of transmural enhancement. Only 1/58 segments with > 75% enhancement demonstrated improved contractility. The relationship between transmural hyperhancement determined by cardiac MRI and the likelihood of contractility improvement after revascularization is shown (Figure 12.4). The total percentage of myocardium determined to be dysfunctional and viable was significantly related to the degree of improvement in ejection fraction after revascularization [28].

WHICH PATIENTS WITH LV DYSFUNCTION SHOULD BE REFERRED FOR REVASCULARIZATION?

Current clinical practice and recommendations are based on surgical studies performed nearly two decades ago. O'Connor et al. [4] reported the 25 year experience from the Duke Cardiovascular Disease Databank comparing surgical revascularization to medical therapy in 1052 patients with ischemic LV dysfunction (EF<0.40). After adjusting for covariates, survival after coronary artery bypass graft (CABG) was significantly better than medical therapy at 1 year (83% vs. 74%, $P<0.0001$), 5 years (61% vs. 37%, $P<0.0001$) and 10 years (42% vs. 13%, $P<0.0001$). The Coronary Artery Surgery Study (CASS) demonstrated a survival benefit 6 years following coronary artery bypass grafting (64%) compared to medical therapy (46%) in patients with ejection fraction<0.36 ($P=0.0007$) [29]. Bounous et al. [30] found similar results in an analysis of 710 patients with LV dysfunction (EF ≤ 0.40) and coronary artery disease. Adjusted 3 year survival for patients undergoing CABG was 86% and medical therapy survival was 68%. The majority of patients discussed in these studies had angina (Duke Database: 69%; CASS: 63%). The applicability of these data to patients without angina is less clear, but at present there are no large scale clinical trials to guide decision making in the HF patient with asymptomatic CAD.

HOW CAN VIABILITY TESTING BE USED TO SELECT PATIENTS FOR REVACULARIZATION?

The efficacy of pre-operative viability testing to guide revascularization has not been tested in large scale clinical trials, but there are several observational studies that demonstrate superior outcomes when clinical data is combined with viability testing to determine patients with ischemic and viable myocardium. A large meta-analysis of 3088 patients with LV dysfunction (EF=0.32 ± 0.08) and coronary artery disease examined the role of viability testing

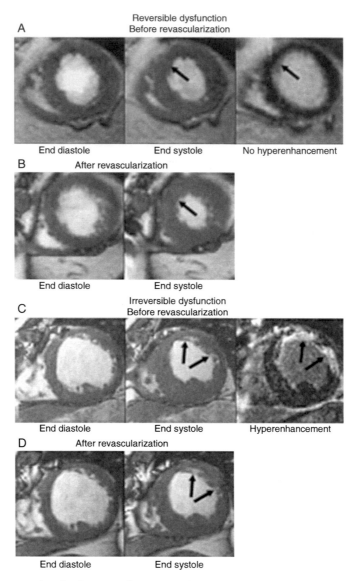

Figure 12.3 Representative cine images and contrast-enhanced images obtained by MRI in one patient with reversible ventricular dysfunction (Panels A and B) and one with irreversible ventricular dysfunction (Panels C and D). The patient with reversible dysfunction had severe hypokinesia of the anteroseptal wall (arrows), and this area was not hyperenhanced before revascularization. The contractility of the wall improved after revascularization. The patient with irreversible dysfunction had akinesia of the anterolateral wall (arrows), and this area was hyperenhanced before revascularization. The contractility of the wall did not improve after revascularization (with permission from [28]).

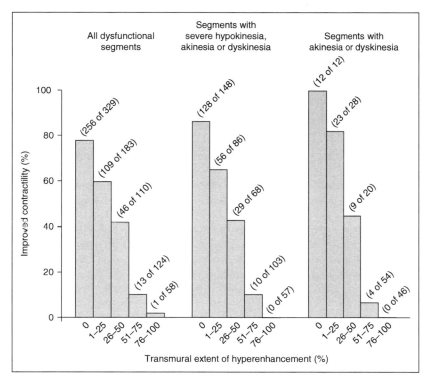

Figure 12.4 Relation between the transmural extent of hyperenhancement before revascularization and the likelihood of increased contractility after revascularization (with permission from [28]).

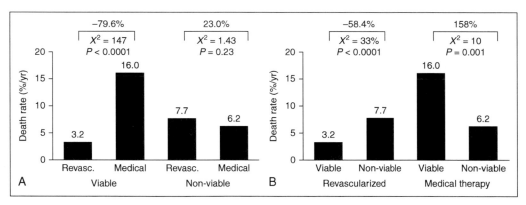

Figure 12.5 (A) Death rates for patients with and without myocardial viability treated by revascularization or medical therapy. There is 79.6% reduction in mortality for patients with viability treated by revascularization (P<0.0001). In patients without myocardial viability, there was no significant difference in mortality with revascularization versus medical therapy. (B) Same data as (A) with comparisons based on treatment strategy in patients with and without viability. Annual mortality was lower in revascularized patients when viability was present versus absent (3.2% vs. 7.7%, P<0.0001). Annual mortality was significantly higher in medically treated patients when viability was present versus absent (16% vs. 6.2%, P=0.001) (with permission from [31]). Revasc. = revascularization.

with thallium perfusion imaging, dobutamine echocardiography, or FDG PET. Patients with viable myocardium who underwent revascularization (surgical or percutaneous) experienced a 79.6 percent relative risk reduction in annual mortality (3.2% vs. 16%, $P=0.0001$) compared with those treated medically (Figure 12.5). Patients without viability that underwent revascularization had a trend toward higher mortality than those treated medically (7.7% vs. 6.2%, $P=$NS). When stratified based on treatment strategy, revascularized patients with viable myocardium had a significantly lower annual mortality than revascularized patients without viability (3.2% vs. 7.7%, $P<0.0001$). There was no difference between the three imaging modalities in predicting outcomes. A survival benefit was uniformly demonstrated for patients with viability treated with revascularization. Paradoxically, there was an incremental survival advantage following revascularization in those with the worst LV dysfunction. However, the relevance of these observations in contemporary practice is not clear. These studies were conducted between 1992 and 1999, an era that preceded the widespread use of medical therapies for patients with LV systolic dysfunction that are now considered standard-of-care including angiotensin converting enzyme inhibitors, beta adrenergic antagonists, aldosterone receptor blockers, HMG-CoA reductase inhibitors and anti-tachycardia devices [31]. In a more contemporary cohort, Camici et al. [8] analyzed the impact of viability testing and revascularization in 14 non-randomized trials conducted between 1998 and 2006. Patients were separated into four groups based on treatment (medical or revascularization) and the presence or absence of viability. Patients with viable myocardium derived a survival benefit from revascularization compared to medical therapy whereas there was no significant difference observed between revascularization and medical therapy in those without evidence of viability.

Determination of the amount of viable myocardium is another critical component of predicting improvements in LV function following revascularization. Most published studies have shown that the number of viable segments is linearly correlated with the degree of LV functional improvement [32–36]. However, comparison of the different imaging techniques is limited by a lack of standardization in nomenclature and the definition of 'viability'. The optimum criteria to predict ≥ 5% increase in left ventricular ejection fraction (LVEF) after revascularization appears to be 25% segment viability using dobutamine stress echocardiography and 38% segment viability using Thallium SPECT or PET [20, 37]. The optimal amount of viability for predicting improvement in LV function as measured by cardiac MRI is less clear. Kim et al. [28] did not find an optimal cutoff point, but rather demonstrated that 78% of all dysfunctional segments without hyperenhancement demonstrated improved contractility after revascularization. The likelihood of improved contractility was 86% and 100% in akinetic or dyskinetic segments, respectively. Thus, in contrast to other imaging techniques, cardiac MRI appears to have superior accuracy in myocardium with the most severe dysfunction [38].

THE TIMING OF REVASCULARIZATION

Prolonged waiting times between viability assessment and coronary revascularization may lead to worse outcomes and affect the postoperative recovery of LV function [39] and perioperative mortality. Beanlands et al. [40] followed 46 patients with ischemic LV dysfunction who underwent pre-operative viability testing with FDG PET and were referred for surgical revascularization. Patients were retrospectively divided into two groups based on the time between the PET scan and revascularization: an early group (< 35 days) and a late group (≥ 35 days). The preoperative mortality rate was higher in the late group versus the early group (24% vs. 0%, $P< 0.05$). LVEF increased in the early group at 3 months (24 ± 7% to 29 ± 8%, $P<0.001$), but not in the late group (27 ± 5% to 28 ± 6%, $P=$NS). Bax et al. [41] confirmed these findings in a larger study with longer follow-up. Eighty-five patients with ischemic cardiomyopathy and > 25% viability were divided into two groups based on the timing of subsequent surgical revascularization. Patients that underwent CABG in less than 1 month had improved long-term mortality versus patients that underwent CABG later than 1 month (5% vs. 20%, $P < 0.05$). Early revascularization patients experienced a significant improvement in EF ($28\pm9\%$ to $40\pm12\%$, $P < 0.05$), whereas the late revascularization group showed no improvement in ventricular function.

REVASCULARIZATION IN PATIENTS WITHOUT ANGINA

The above studies provide minimal information on the number of patients without angina undergoing revascularization. It is reasonable to assume that patients with angina would derive more benefit from revascularization, as angina may be used as a surrogate for viable myocardium. Gimelli *et al.* [42] analyzed a series of 180 patients with ischemic LV dysfunction undergoing revascularization stratified on the basis of the presence or absence of angina. Survival at 3 years was not statistically different in patients with and without angina (84% vs. 78%, P – NS). However, the intraoperative mortality was extremely high in patients with non-viable myocardium (10% in patients with angina and 20% in patients without angina), whereas intraoperative mortality was 3% in patients with mostly viable myocardium.

HOW DOES PERCUTANEOUS REVASCULARIZATION COMPARE TO SURGICAL REVASCULARIZATION?

Coronary artery bypass grafting and percutaneous coronary interventions (PCI) in patients with LV systolic dysfunction are associated with relatively high periprocedural mortality. Perioperative mortality ranges from 5 to 30% for CABG depending on the comorbidities and the degree of LV dysfunction [43]. A report from the New York State Registry compared mortality outcomes in patients with multivessel disease that underwent either CABG ($n = 37\,212$) or PCI with stent placement ($n = 22\,102$). Long-term outcomes with CABG were superior to stent placement in patients with LV dysfunction (EF < 0.40) and involvement of the proximal left anterior descending (LAD) coronary artery (mortality hazard ratio [HR] = 0.70; 95% confidence interval [CI] 0.56–0.87). In this analysis, there was no survival advantage with CABG in individuals without involvement of the proximal LAD coronary artery [44]. These findings were confirmed in another analysis examining patients undergoing CABG or PCI with a drug eluting stent between 2003 and 2004. Among patients with LV dysfunction (EF < 0.40) the rate of death or myocardial infarction was significantly lower for those treated with CABG (adjusted HR = 0.67; 95% CI 0.53–0.84; $P < 0.001$) [45]. The benefit of CABG over PCI is thought to be related to more complete revascularization, but alternative mechanisms have been proposed [46]. Some experts have hypothesized that PCI treats the current 'culprit' lesion and that CABG treats future culprit lesions by bypassing the entire diseased segment [47].

There are many limits to the observational studies discussed above in evaluating the effects of revascularization on asymptomatic patients with ischemic LV dysfunction and the role that viability testing may play in patient selection. First, observational studies are prone to selection bias in which patient characteristics may influence the choice of the therapy and ultimately impact outcomes in a manner that is difficult to quantitate. Secondly, many of these studies were performed in an earlier era and do not reflect current revascularization techniques, medical therapy, and use of implantable cardioverter defibrillators. Several ongoing randomized trials may answer some of these questions: the STICH trial (Surgical Treatment for Ischemic Heart Failure) [48], the HEART (Heart Failure Revascularization Trial) [49], and the PARR-2 study (Positron Emission Tomography and Recovery Following Revascularization-2) [50].

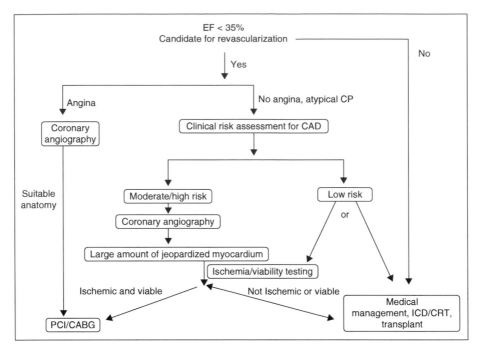

Figure 12.6 Management algorithm for patients with LV dysfunction and suspected coronary disease (with permission from [5]). CABG=coronary artery bypass graft; CAD=coronary artery disease; CP=chest pain; CRT=cardiac resynchronization therapy; ICD=implantable cardioverter/defibrillator.

CONCLUSIONS

Revascularization in asymptomatic patients with LV dysfunction remains a difficult clinical dilemma. There is extensive evidence regarding the medical management of this patient population, but there are no randomized data to guide the clinician about recommendations for revascularization. The data to support revascularization of the asymptomatic patient is inferred from a larger literature supporting this strategy in patients with symptomatic ischemic heart disease. Current observational data suggests patients who are candidates for revascularization should be referred for viability testing. The modality of viability testing should be determined by institutional availability and expertise, realizing the advantages and disadvantages of each modality. Patients with viable myocardium should be offered revascularization in addition to medical therapy. Currently coronary artery bypass grafting appears to be the preferred method over PCI in patients with multivessel disease, significant left main stenosis, left main equivalent (proximal LAD and circumflex disease) or isolated proximal LAD coronary artery involvement. An integrated approach to the diagnosis and treatment of patients with ischemic cardiomyopathy is shown (Figure 12.6). Ongoing randomized clinical trials should better define the role of revascularization and viability testing in patients with ischemic LV dysfunction.

REFERENCES

1. Emond M, Mock MB, Davis KB *et al*. Long-term survival of medically treated patients in the Coronary Artery Surgery Study (CASS) Registry. *Circulation* 1994; 90:2645-2657.

2. Muhlbaier LH, Pryor DB, Rankin JS *et al*. Observational comparison of event-free survival with medical and surgical therapy in patients with coronary artery disease. 20 years of follow-up. *Circulation* 1992; 86(5 suppl):II198-II204.
3. He J, Ogden LG, Bazzano LA, Vupputuri S, Loria C, Whelton PK. Risk factors for congestive heart failure in US men and women: NHANES I epidemiologic follow-up study. *Arch Intern Med* 2001; 161:996-1002.
4. O'Connor CM, Velazquez EJ, Gardner LH *et al*. Comparison of coronary artery bypass grafting versus medical therapy on long-term outcome in patients with ischemic cardiomyopathy (a 25-year experience from the Duke Cardiovascular Disease Databank). *Am J Cardiol* 2002; 90:101-107.
5. Phillips HR, O'Connor CM, Rogers J. Revascularization for heart failure. *Am Heart J* 2007; 153(4 suppl):65-73.
6. Dyke SH, Cohn PF, Gorlin R, Sonnenblick EH. Detection of residual myocardial function in coronary artery disease using post-extra systolic potentiation. *Circulation* 1974; 50:694-699.
7. Horn HR, Teichholz LE, Cohn PF, Herman MV, Gorlin R. Augmentation of left ventricular contraction pattern in coronary artery disease by an inotropic catecholamine. The epinephrine ventriculogram. *Circulation* 1974; 49:1063-1071.
8. Camici PG, Prasad SK, Rimoldi OE. Stunning, hibernation, and assessment of myocardial viability. *Circulation* 2008; 117:103-114.
9. Ross J Jr. Myocardial perfusion-contraction matching. Implications for coronary heart disease and hibernation. *Circulation* 1991; 83:1076-1083.
10. Heusch G, Schulz R, Rahimtoola SH. Myocardial hibernation: a delicate balance. *Am J Physiol Heart Circ Physiol* 2005; 288:H984-H999.
11. Matsuzaki M, Gallagher KP, Kemper WS, White F, Ross J Jr. Sustained regional dysfunction produced by prolonged coronary stenosis: gradual recovery after reperfusion. *Circulation* 1983; 68:170-182.
12. La Canna G, Alfieri O, Giubbini R, Gargano M, Ferrari R, Visioli O. Echocardiography during infusion of dobutamine for identification of reversibly dysfunction in patients with chronic coronary artery disease. *J Am Coll Cardiol* 1994; 23:617-626.
13. Nagueh SF, Mikati I, Weilbaecher D *et al*. Relation of the contractile reserve of hibernating myocardium to myocardial structure in humans. *Circulation* 1999; 100:490-496.
14. Perrone-Filardi P, Pace L, Prastaro M *et al*. Dobutamine echocardiography predicts improvement of hypoperfused dysfunctional myocardium after revascularization in patients with coronary artery disease. *Circulation* 1995; 91:2556-2565.
15. Pohost GM, Zir LM, Moore RH, McKusick KA, Guiney TE, Beller GA. Differentiation of transiently ischemic from infarcted myocardium by serial imaging after a single dose of thallium-201. *Circulation* 1977; 55:294-302.
16. Ohtani H, Tamaki N, Yonekura Y *et al*. Value of thallium-201 reinjection after delayed SPECT imaging for predicting reversible ischemia after coronary artery bypass grafting. *Am J Cardiol* 1990; 66:394-399.
17. Altehoefer C, vom Dahl J, Biedermann M *et al*. Significance of defect severity in technetium-99m-MIBI SPECT at rest to assess myocardial viability: comparison with fluorine-18-FDG PET. *J Nucl Med* 1994; 35:569-574.
18. Tillisch J, Brunken R, Marshall R *et al*. Reversibility of cardiac wall-motion abnormalities predicted by positron tomography. *N Engl J Med* 1986; 314:884-888.
19. Di Carli MF, Asgarzadie F, Schelbert HR *et al*. Quantitative relation between myocardial viability and improvement in heart failure symptoms after revascularization in patients with ischemic cardiomyopathy. *Circulation* 1995; 92:3436-3444.
20. Gerber BL, Ordoubadi FF, Wijns W *et al*. Positron emission tomography using (18)F-fluoro-deoxyglucose and euglycaemic hyperinsulinaemic glucose clamp: optimal criteria for the prediction of recovery of post-ischaemic left ventricular dysfunction. Results from the European Community Concerted Action Multicenter study on use of (18)F-fluoro-deoxyglucose Positron Emission Tomography for the Detection of Myocardial Viability. *Eur Heart J* 2001; 22:1691-1701.
21. Bax JJ, Poldermans D, Elhendy A, Boersma E, Rahimtoola SH. Sensitivity, specificity, and predictive accuracies of various noninvasive techniques for detecting hibernating myocardium. *Curr Probl Cardiol* 2001; 26:147-186.
22. Underwood SR, Bax JJ, vom Dahl J *et al*. Imaging techniques for the assessment of myocardial hibernation. Report of a Study Group of the European Society of Cardiology. *Eur Heart J* 2004; 25:815-836.

23. Bree D, Wollmuth JR, Cupps BP *et al*. Low-dose dobutamine tissue-tagged magnetic resonance imaging with 3-dimensional strain analysis allows assessment of myocardial viability in patients with ischemic cardiomyopathy. *Circulation* 2006; 114(1 suppl):I33-I36.

24. Kim RJ, Manning WJ. Viability assessment by delayed enhancement cardiovascular magnetic resonance: will low-dose dobutamine dull the shine? *Circulation* 2004; 109:2476-2479.

25. Wellnhofer E, Olariu A, Klein C *et al*. Magnetic resonance low-dose dobutamine test is superior to SCAR quantification for the prediction of functional recovery. *Circulation* 2004; 109:2172-2174.

26. Fieno DS, Kim RJ, Chen EL, Lomasney JW, Klocke FJ, Judd RM. Contrast-enhanced magnetic resonance imaging of myocardium at risk: distinction between reversible and irreversible injury throughout infarct healing. *J Am Coll Cardiol* 2000; 36:1985-1991.

27. Kim RJ, Fieno DS, Parrish TB *et al*. Relationship of MRI delayed contrast enhancement to irreversible injury, infarct age, and contractile function. *Circulation* 1999; 100:1992-2002.

28. Kim RJ, Wu E, Rafael A *et al*. The use of contrast-enhanced magnetic resonance imaging to identify reversible myocardial dysfunction. *N Engl J Med* 2000; 343:1445-1453.

29. Alderman EL, Fisher LD, Litwin P *et al*. Results of coronary artery surgery in patients with poor left ventricular function (CASS). *Circulation* 1983; 68:785-795.

30. Bounous EP, Mark DB, Pollock BG *et al*. Surgical survival benefits for coronary disease patients with left ventricular dysfunction. *Circulation* 1988 Sep; 78:I151-I157.

31. Allman KC, Shaw LJ, Hachamovitch R, Udelson JE. Myocardial viability testing and impact of revascularization on prognosis in patients with coronary artery disease and left ventricular dysfunction: a meta-analysis. *J Am Coll Cardiol* 2002; 39:1151-1158.

32. Baer FM, Theissen P, Crnac J *et al*. Head to head comparison of dobutamine-transoesophageal echocardiography and dobutamine-magnetic resonance imaging for the prediction of left ventricular functional recovery in patients with chronic coronary artery disease. *Eur Heart J* 2000; 21:981-991.

33. Bax JJ, Visser FC, Poldermans D *et al*. Relationship between preoperative viability and postoperative improvement in LVEF and heart failure symptoms. *J Nucl Med* 2001; 42:79-86.

34. Pace L, Perrone-Filardi P, Storto G *et al*. Prediction of improvement in global left ventricular function in patients with chronic coronary artery disease and impaired left ventricular function: rest thallium-201 SPET versus low-dose dobutamine echocardiography. *Eur J Nucl Med* 2000; 27:1740-1746.

35. Pagano D, Fath-Ordoubadi F, Beatt KJ, Townend JN, Bonser RS, Camici PG. Effects of coronary revascularisation on myocardial blood flow and coronary vasodilator reserve in hibernating myocardium. *Heart* 2001; 85:208-212.

36. Slart RH, Bax JJ, van Veldhuisen DJ *et al*. Prediction of functional recovery after revascularization in patients with chronic ischaemic left ventricular dysfunction: head-to-head comparison between 99mTc-sestamibi/18F-FDG DISA SPECT and 13N-ammonia/18F-FDG PET. *Eur J Nucl Med Mol Imaging* 2006; 33:716-723.

37. Bax JJ, Maddahi J, Poldermans D *et al*. Sequential (201)Tl imaging and dobutamine echocardiography to enhance accuracy of predicting improved left ventricular ejection fraction after revascularization. *J Nucl Med* 2002; 43:795-802.

38. Perrone-Filardi P, Pace L, Prastaro M *et al*. Assessment of myocardial viability in patients with chronic coronary artery disease. Rest-4-hour-24-hour 201Tl tomography versus dobutamine echocardiography. *Circulation* 1996; 94:2712-2719.

39. Pitt M, Dutka D, Pagano D, Camici P, Bonser R. The natural history of myocardium awaiting revascularisation in patients with impaired left ventricular function. *Eur Heart J* 2004; 25:500-507.

40. Beanlands RS, Hendry PJ, Masters RG, deKemp RA, Woodend K, Ruddy TD. Delay in revascularization is associated with increased mortality rate in patients with severe left ventricular dysfunction and viable myocardium on fluorine 18-fluorodeoxyglucose positron emission tomography imaging. *Circulation* 1998; 98(19 suppl):II51-II56.

41. Bax JJ, Schinkel AFL, Boersma E *et al*. Early versus delayed revascularization in patients with ischemic cardiomyopathy and substantial viability: impact on outcome. *Circulation* 2003; 108:II-39-II-42.

42. Gimelli A, Neto JA, Marcassa C, Ferrazzi P, Glauber M, Marzullo P. Beneficial effects of coronary revascularization in patients with ischaemic left ventricular dysfunction with and without anginal symptoms. *Interact Cardiovasc Thorac Surg* 2002; 1:9-15.

43. Baker DW, Jones R, Hodges J, Massie BM, Konstam MA, Rose EA. Management of heart failure. III. The role of revascularization in the treatment of patients with moderate or severe left ventricular systolic dysfunction. *JAMA* 1994; 272:1528-1534.

44. Hannan EL, Racz MJ, Walford G, Jones RH, Ryan TJ, Bennett E *et al*. Long-term outcomes of coronary-artery bypass grafting versus stent implantation. *N Engl J Med* 2005; 352:2174-2183.
45. Hannan EL, Wu C, Walford G *et al*. Drug-eluting stents vs. coronary-artery bypass grafting in multivessel coronary disease. *N Engl J Med* 2008; 358:331-341.
46. Chareonthaitawee P, Gersh BJ, Araoz PA, Gibbons RJ. Revascularization in severe left ventricular dysfunction: the role of viability testing. *J Am Coll Cardiol* 2005; 46:567-574.
47. Gersh BJ, Frye RL. Methods of coronary revascularization – things may not be as they seem. *N Engl J Med* 2005; 352:2235-2237.
48. Velazquez EJ, Lee KL, O'Connor CM *et al*. The rationale and design of the Surgical Treatment for Ischemic Heart Failure (STICH) trial. *J Thorac Cardiovasc Surg* 2007; 134:1540-1547.
49. Cleland JG, Freemantle N, Ball SG *et al*. The Heart Failure Revascularisation Trial (HEART): rationale, design and methodology. *Eur J Heart Fail* 2003; 5:295-303.
50. Beanlands R, Nichol G, Ruddy TD *et al*. Evaluation of outcome and cost-effectiveness using an FDG PET-guided approach to management of patients with coronary disease and severe left ventricular dysfunction (PARR-2): rationale, design, and methods. *Control Clin Trials* 2003; 24:776-794.

13

Blood based biomarkers in heart failure: where are we now?

C. deFilippi, K. B. Shah

INTRODUCTION

With the introduction of a commercially available point-of-care assay for B-type natriuretic peptide (BNP) and the publication of the Breathing Not Properly study in 2000 and 2002 respectively for the diagnosis of acute decompensated heart failure in patients with dyspnea, biomarkers for heart failure have been in the spotlight this decade. The ensuing years has seen a proliferation of interest in biomarkers in all aspects of heart failure [1]. The enthusiasm for heart failure blood based biomarkers by researchers and clinicians is not without precedent. The prior decade had seen the introduction of the cardiac troponins with the result of redefining the diagnosis of acute myocardial infarction and directing early management in patients with non-ST elevation acute coronary syndromes based on their troponin level [2, 3]. The success of the troponins generated a hope of developing a comparable marker for patients with heart failure. Chronic heart failure is the only category of cardiovascular diseases for which the prevalence, incidence, hospitalization rate, total burden of mortality, and costs have increased in the past 25 years. Furthermore, as compared to an acute coronary syndrome, the diagnosis of heart failure can be particularly challenging. As a result, and despite ongoing controversy, the use of natriuretic peptides to aid diagnosis has generally been well accepted with inclusion in the recently updated American Heart Association/ American College of Cardiology guidelines for the diagnosis of heart failure in the patient presenting with dyspnea [4]. With the relative success of the natriuretic peptides for the diagnosis of heart failure there has been a tremendous amount of research to expand the application of these tests to screening those at risk for developing a new diagnosis of heart failure, prognosticating patients with heart failure and optimizing their management. New biomarkers have also been developed to either assist or supersede the natriuretic peptides, and established cardiac biomarker assays (i.e. the cardiac troponins) have evolved to play a role in the prognostication of heart failure patients. The field of candidate markers for heart failure is quite large [5]. However, for purposes of this chapter we have focused on established and novel markers that meet at least the first and hopefully the second criteria outlined in Figure 13.1 as proposed criteria for evaluating new biomarkers for clinical application [6]. That being said it is ultimately up to the judgment of the reader as to what role cardiac biomarkers should play in the care of patients 'at-risk' or diagnosed with heart failure.

Christopher deFilippi, MD, FACC, Associate Professor of Medicine, Division of Cardiology, University of Maryland School of Medicine, Baltimore, MD, USA.

Keyur B. Shah, MD, FACC, Assistant Professor of Medicine, Division of Cardiology, Virginia Commonwealth University, Richmond, VA, USA.

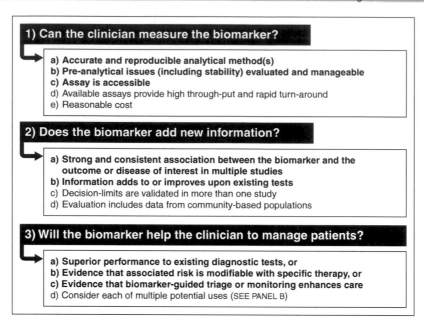

Figure 13.1 Criteria for assessment of novel cardiovascular biomarkers for clinical use (with permission from [6]).

THE NATRIURETIC PEPTIDES

MECHANISM OF ACTION

The natriuretic peptides are neurohormones that affect body fluid homeostasis by natriuresis and diuresis, as well as vascular tone by decreasing angiotensin II and norepinephrine synthesis. In large part, natriuretic peptides can be thought of as opposing regulatory hormones of the renin angiotensin aldosterone system. They also have a fundamental role in vascular function and remodeling by potentiating the effects of nitric oxide in the vascular wall, and increasing parasympathetic tone.

BNP originates from a 134-amino acid prepropeptide that is cleaved into a precursor molecule proBNP108, which is stored within secretory granules in cardiac myocytes. On release, the protease corin cleaves proBNP108 into N-terminal-proBNP (NT-proBNP), a 76-amino acid biologically inert molecule, and BNP, the biologically active counterpart (Figure 13.2). BNP is found primarily in the myocardium of the left ventricle but also in atrial tissue and right ventricular myocardial tissue. Clearance of BNP occurs via glomerular filtration, natriuretic peptide receptors, and degradation by neutral endopeptidases. The processes involved in the elimination of NT-proBNP are incompletely understood. The half-life of BNP is 18 min compared with 90–120 min for NT-proBNP. The role of renal disease on influencing natriuretic peptide clearance and therefore levels has been a source of great controversy with claims that BNP is less influenced by renal function than NT-proBNP [7]. This will be discussed in more detail below.

DIAGNOSING HEART FAILURE IN THE PATIENT WITH DYSPNEA

Many patients presenting with dyspnea to the emergency department (ED) have complicated medical histories that make diagnosis of acute decompensated heart failure challeng-

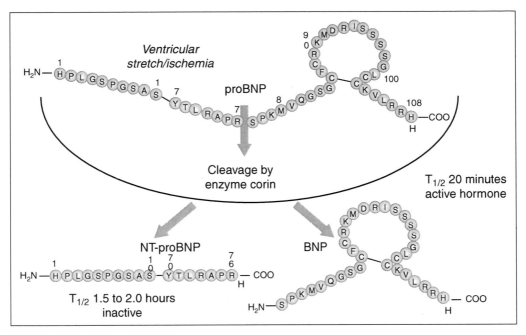

Figure 13.2 Schematic of the cleavage of intracellular proBNP to release from the myocyte of the active hormone BNP and the biologically inert N-terminal of proBNP (NT-proBNP).

ing. An example of such a case presentation is shown in Figure 13.3. Based on the Breathing Not Properly study of over 1500 dyspnea patients from seven EDs, a BNP level provides an accurate test to differentiate heart failure from those without heart failure etiologies. These investigators found the overall accuracy of BNP in this setting to be an area under the curve (AUC) of 0.90 as calculated by the receiver operator characteristic curve statistic. These investigators selected a value of 100 pg/ml to represent the optimal trade off between sensitivity and specificity (Figure 13.4) [1]. Therefore, the patient presented in Figure 13.3 would be diagnosed with heart failure in part based upon his BNP level. These investigators further sought to quantify the extent to which a BNP level aided the ED physicians' clinical judgment. The addition of the BNP level to clinical judgment increased the overall accuracy for the diagnosis of heart failure from 74% to 81% [8]. An important reference point is to consider test performance only in patients with an intermediate clinical probability of heart failure (21–79% ED clinician pre-test probability). Using a BNP cut off of 100 pg/ml, 74% of these patients were correctly classified suggesting BNP is a good, but not perfect, test in the most diagnostically complex patients. Lastly, the cost-effectiveness for measuring BNP and NT-proBNP in the ED has been established for reducing length of stay and overall costs in several studies, but this has recently been challenged [9–11].

CONTROVERSIES TO CONSIDER WHEN USING NATRIURETIC PEPTIDES TO DIAGNOSE HEART FAILURE

BNP VERSUS NT-PROBNP?

Both of these tests are clinically available from multiple vendors. Many studies have now evaluated the accuracy of NT-proBNP and BNP levels for diagnosing decompensated heart

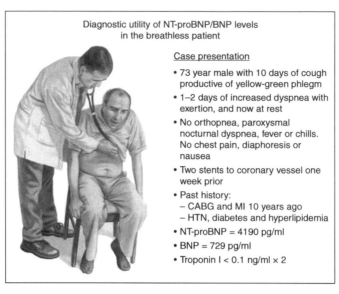

Figure 13.3 Case presentation. BNP=B-type natriuretic peptide; CABG=coronary artery bypass graft; HTN=hypertension; MI=myocardial infarction.

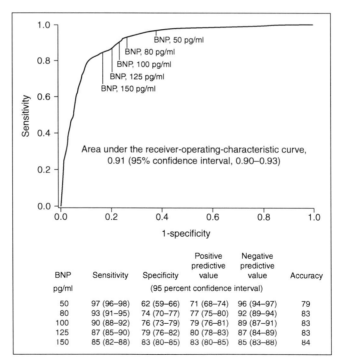

BNP	Sensitivity	Specificity	Positive predictive value	Negative predictive value	Accuracy
pg/ml		(95 percent confidence interval)			
50	97 (96–98)	62 (59–66)	71 (68–74)	96 (94–97)	79
80	93 (91–95)	74 (70–77)	77 (75–80)	92 (89–94)	83
100	90 (88–92)	76 (73–79)	79 (76–81)	89 (87–91)	83
125	87 (85–90)	79 (76–82)	80 (78–83)	87 (84–89)	83
150	85 (82–88)	83 (80–85)	83 (80–85)	85 (83–88)	84

Figure 13.4 Calculation of the diagnostic accuracy of BNP for acute decompensated heart failure in patients presenting to the emergency department with dyspnea from the Breathing Not Properly study (with permission from [1]).

Table 13.1 Optimal NT-proBNP cut-points for the diagnosis or exclusion of acute HF among dyspnoeic patients (with permission from [19])

Category	Optimal cut-point	Sensitivity (%)	Specificity (%)	PPV (%)	NPV (%)	Accuracy (%)
Confirmatory ('rule in') cut-points						
<50 years (n=184)	450 pg/ml	97	93	76	99	94
50–75 years (n=537)	900 pg/ml	90	82	83	88	85
>75 years (n=535)	1800 pg/ml	85	73	92	55	83
Rule in, overall		90	84	88	66	85
Exclusionary ('rule out') cut-point						
All patients (n=1256)	300 pg/ml	99	60	77	98	83

NPV=negative predictive value; PPV=positive predictive value.

failure in the dyspneic patient yielding a consistent conclusion [1, 12–15]. The accuracy of the two tests is comparable even after adjustment for confounding factors, such as impaired renal function [16, 17]. Although the correlation between the two tests is excellent (typically correlation coefficient, $R \geq 0.9$), and in subjects without cardiovascular disease the values for both tests can be similar, in heart failure, NT-proBNP levels are often 6–10 times greater than those for BNP [18]. The International Collaborative of NT-proBNP (ICON) Study established optimal age-based cut offs to rule in acute decompensated heart failure and a single cut off to rule out heart failure [19] (Table 13.1). At first look, NT-proBNP appears more complex to apply clinically than BNP. However, subsequent analysis of the data from the BNP study showed that a single cut off was an oversimplification and, similar to NT-proBNP, an intermediate or 'grey-zone' also exists between 'ruling out' HF (<100 pg/l) and 'ruling in' acute decompensated HF (> 500 pg/ml) [20]. The significance of the 'grey-zone' is discussed below.

INTERPRETING 'GRAY-ZONE' VALUES OF NATRIURETIC PEPTIDES

Based on the Breathing Not Properly study there appeared to be excellent sensitivity with adequate specificity using a single cut off in dyspnea patients for the diagnosis of heart failure but this hasn't endured the test of time and subsequent studies. Frankly, this shouldn't be of much surprise since prior to the publication of the Breathing Not Properly study there was the publication in the *New England Journal of Medicine* showing a BNP level was an independent prognosticator of death in the TIMI-16 study of acute coronary syndrome patients including most with an absence of signs or symptoms of heart failure [21]. A substantial body of literature has developed demonstrating that both BNP and NT-proBNP elevation in the setting of acute or chronic ischemic heart disease is a harbinger of a poor prognosis independent of left ventricular ejection fraction or symptoms of heart failure [22–24]. The NT-proBNP test has even received a Food and Drug Administration (FDA) indication for risk stratifying patients with ischemic heart disease. Cardiac ischemia is a major alternative etiology for natriuretic peptide elevation, but one of only several factors that can influence levels other than heart failure. A summary of clinical factors that can influence BNP and NT-proBNP levels is shown in Table 13.2. A natriuretic peptide level may reflect the contributions of multiple cardiac pathologies including ischemia, fibrosis and hypertrophy in addition to hemodynamic stress, such that these biomarkers reflect the

Table 13.2 Impact on NT-proBNP/BNP levels for conditions other than acute decompensated heart failure

Clinical state	Effect on (NT-pro) BNP value
Acute coronary syndrome/CAD	↑
Pulmonary embolism	↑
Right ventricular overload	↑
Obesity	↓
Age	↑
Renal failure	↑
Critical illness	↑
Chronic heart failure	↑ or ↓
CAD = coronary artery disease.	

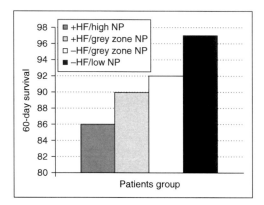

Figure 13.5 Bar graph demonstrating the 60-day survival rates of subjects included in the ICON study [105]. 'Gray-zone NP' denotes a NT-pro-BNP concentration between the rule in and rule out concentrations. 'Low NP' denotes a NT-proBNP concentration < 300 ng/l in patients without heart failure (HF) and a 'high NP' denotes a NT-proBNP result greater than the rule in cut-point for those with HF (see Table 13.1).

overall burden of clinical and subclinical cardiovascular disease [25]. However, hemodynamic stress represents the greatest perturbation to stimulate the natriuretic peptide system and can be anticipated to generate some of the highest levels. The influence of the 'grey-zone' values on prognosis was considered by the ICON investigators with NT-proBNP. They identified that irrespective of a heart failure diagnosis or not, intermediate elevations of NT-proBNP in patients with dyspnea were associated with a poorer 60-day survival than subjects with low levels of NT-proBNP (Figure 13.5). Therefore, modest elevations of natriuretic peptides should alert a clinician to a patient with underlying cardiovascular disease even if it is not acute decompensated heart failure.

THE INFLUENCE OF RENAL FUNCTION

The interpretation of NP results in either symptomatic or asymptomatic patients with chronic kidney disease (CKD) has been a source of confusion since the introduction of these assays into clinical practice. However, in the past 3–4 years numerous studies have shed

Table 13.3 Correlations between natriuretic peptide levels and eGFR (with permission from [106])

Author	Population	NT-proBNP	BNP
Mark	Amb CKD		−0.40
deFilippi	Amb CKD	−0.31	
Khan	Amb CKD	−0.45	−0.38
Vickory	Amb CKD	−0.53	−0.36
Richards	Amb ICM	−0.51	−0.51
van Kimmenade	Amb hypertension	−0.30	−0.35
Anwaruddin	ED all dyspnea	−0.55 (log)	
deFilippi	ED all dyspnea	−0.42	−0.34
Anwaruddin	ED Dx HF	−0.34 (log)	
McCullough	ED Dx HF		−0.19
Kimmenade	Dx HF	−0.34	

Amb = ambulatory; BNP = B-type natriuretic peptide; CKD = chronic kidney disease; Dx – diagnosis; ED = emergency department; eGFR = estimated glomerular filtration rate; HF = heart failure; ICM = ischemic cardiomyopathy.

considerable insight into the interpretation of these tests in the setting of impaired renal function. During the early clinical experience with NPs an assumption developed that BNP clearance was independent of renal clearance based on the findings that BNP, but not NT-proBNP was cleared by a natriuretic peptide receptor-C and degraded by neutral endepetidases [7]. Concern regarding differences in renal clearance between NT-proBNP and BNP were also identified by differences in the correlation coefficient between the NP and estimated glomerular filtration rate (eGFR). NT-proBNP level was identified as having a much stronger inverse correlation with eGFR than BNP [7]. This initial conclusion may have in part been related to a failure to account for upper limit of detection of the first generation of the BNP assay when calculating a correlation coefficient [17] as more recent studies have shown correlation coefficients between BNP and GFR vs. NT-proBNP and eGFR to be more similar than different (Table 13.3). Perhaps most definitive is a recent study evaluating 165 hypertensive patients showing the fractional extraction of BNP and NT-proBNP were essentially identical and changed minimally across a large spectrum of eGFR (Figure 13.6) [26]. The presence of elevated levels of NPs in asymptomatic patients with chronic kidney disease is more likely a function of the high prevalence of cardiovascular disease. Both NPs appear to have a similarly strong association with known 'arteriopathic' disease (peripheral and coronary vascular disease) and similar predictive accuracy for the presence of LV hypertrophy, depressed LVEF and known coronary disease [27–29]. Recently it has been recognized in ambulatory African-Americans with chronic kidney disease that an elevated NT-proBNP is associated with increased risk of several cardiovascular events including heart failure [30].

While there may be more frequent 'grey-zone' values in asymptomatic renal disease patients due to underlying cardiovascular disease, BNP and NT-proBNP can still be utilized for diagnosing heart failure. If utilizing NT-proBNP, no adjustments need to be made if utilizing the ICON proposed cut offs since in large part the age related 'rule in' cut offs account for differences in renal function. If utilizing BNP then doubling the cut off from 100 to 200 pg/ml is appropriate [17]. The caveat remains that the studies from which these numbers are derived had very few patients with an eGFR < 30 ml/min/1.73 m². Furthermore, none of these cut offs are appropriate for patients requiring dialysis, where BNP levels are commonly > 1000 pg/ml in the absence of heart failure.

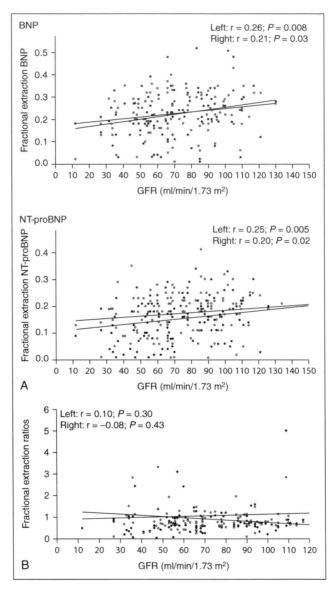

Figure 13.6 (A) The correlation between fractional extraction and GFR for BNP and NT-proBNP. Solid dots indicate left kidney, open dots indicate right kidney [26]. (B) Correlation between the ratios of FENT-proBNP/ BNP in the left and the right kidney with GFR. Solid dots indicate left kidney, open dots indicate right kidney (with permission from [26]). FE=fractional extraction.

WHAT IS BEING MEASURED IN THE LAB AND DOES IT MATTER

It is now recognized that the assays for BNP and NT-proBNP are in part measuring the same molecule. The intact or minimally modified proBNP molecule has been found at low levels in the majority of healthy subjects and at high levels in the blood of patients with asymptomatic depressed LVEF or decompensated HF [31–33]. Though biologically active, it is to a

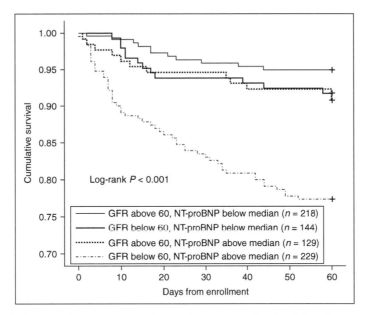

Figure 13.7 Survival curves of heart failure subjects in ICON (International Collaborative on NT-proBNP) as a function of glomerular filtration rate (GFR) and amino-terminal pro-brain natruiuretic peptide (NT-proBNP) concentration on admission (log-rank $P<0.001$) (with permission from [38]).

much lesser extent than BNP [33]. ProBNP is detected by the commercial assays for both NT-proBNP and BNP [33]. The proportion of measured NT-proBNP and BNP that is actually proBNP appears substantial and varies between patients [33, 34]. This may in part explain why patients with decompensated HF and BNP levels measured in the thousands can still respond favorably to an infusion of exogenous BNP (nesiritide). Though seemingly not as accurate as BNP or NT-proBNP for identifying patients with HF, there may be a diagnostic role for measuring intact proBNP [31]. Lastly, admission or discharge proBNP was found to be an inferior predictor of cardiovascular and all-cause death compared to NT-proBNP during a 90-day follow-up suggesting that measuring the pro hormone may add little additional information [35]. However, there is minimal correlation between the several pre commercial assays for proBNP so whether this is a biological or analytical issue has yet to be determined.

NATRIURETIC PEPTIDES AND PROGNOSIS IN PATIENT WITH HEART FAILURE

Both NT-proBNP and BNP levels can predict short and long-term mortality in patients presenting with dyspnea [19, 36, 37]. This prediction appears independent of the final diagnosis of acute decompensated HF. In the PRIDE study, an elevated NT-proBNP was an independent and the most powerful predictor of 1 year mortality irrespective of the diagnosis of acute decompensated HF [37]. As discussed above, elevated NT-proBNP levels in the absence of acute decompensated HF is not a reflection of incorrect diagnosis, but identifies other cardiac comorbidities that can have a substantial impact on survival. Such comorbidities may not be immediately identifiable clinically. In a statistical model containing clinical predictors of mortality the addition of NT-proBNP level added significantly to improve the prediction of death [37]. Furthermore, a natriuretic peptide level can provide synergistic information with respect to prognosis. The ICON investigators made an intriguing finding with respect to 60-day prognosis in patients with decompensated heart failure. The presence of renal disease and a markedly elevated NT-proBNP portended a poor prognosis, but in the absence of both, mortality was similar to patients with more normal renal function and lower NT-proBNP levels (Figure 13.7) [38].

SERIAL MEASURES

A single measure of BNP or NT-proBNP at presentation is easy to obtain and diagnostic and prognostic information is robust. Patients often improve dramatically with a variety of medical therapies over the course of hospitalization. Preliminary data suggested that BNP levels could reflect left ventricular filling pressures, as measured by the pulmonary capillary wedge pressure, in patients who responded to therapy [39]. However, as experienced by most clinicians sampling serial levels during hospitalization, there often appears to be little correlation between BNP or NT-proBNP levels, the pulmonary capillary wedge pressure, and a patient's clinical response. The poor correlation between the natriuretic peptide level, the clinical findings or pulmonary capillary wedge pressure has been confirmed in multiple subsequent studies and appears particularly relevant in medically complex patients [40–42]. Therefore, at this time there seems to be little merit to daily measurements of either natriuretic peptide test to guide acute in-hospital therapy. However, there is important prognostic information that can be gained by evaluating the change in either BNP or NT-proBNP level from admission to the time of discharge [43, 44]. Bettencourt *et al.* demonstrated despite a substantial and uniform improvement in clinical symptoms during admission an adverse 6-month outcome (predominantly driven by re-admission) could be predicted by the change in NT-proBNP levels from admission to discharge. The best prognosis was associated with a decrease in NT-proBNP level by $\geq 30\%$ and the poorest prognosis associated with an increase from admission to discharge of $\geq 30\%$ [44]. However, not all studies have replicated this finding that a change from admission to discharge in BNP or NT-proBNP level is prognostic [35].

Lastly, the prognostic value of natriuretic peptides for HF extends beyond patients with acute dyspnea presentations. Both NT-proBNP and BNP are independent prognosticators of mortality in ambulatory patients with compensated HF (New York Heart Association [NYHA] classes II–IV) and patients with known ischemic cardiomyopathies [18, 45–48]. In ambulatory patients with stable HF symptoms or asymptomatic severely depressed LVEF, NT-proBNP and BNP, when compared head-to-head, are generally equivalent prognosticators [18, 46]. In addition to just a single value, the Valsartan Heart Failure Trial (Val-HEFT) investigators showed that change in natriuretic peptide level over time (4 months) also additionally stratifies those at risk, similar to the in patient changes seen in other studies [43–45, 49].

CAN NATRIURETIC PEPTIDES GUIDE CHRONIC HEART FAILURE THERAPY?

Individualizing heart failure medications based on continuous feedback from a biomarker sensitive to myocardial function may optimize therapy and ultimately improve symptoms and survival. While ample data support the prognostic and diagnostic potential of natriuretic peptides for heart failure patients, only recently have data surfaced suggesting serial measurements of BNP or NT-proBNP could guide more effective medical therapy.

In an early study pre-dating widespread acceptance of beta blockers and spironolactone for heart failure, Troughton *et al.* compared a treatment strategy for medication titration guided by NT-proBNP (goal < 200 pg/ml) versus one guided by symptoms and clinical exam. After randomizing patients ($n = 69$) with LV dysfunction (LVEF < 40%), they found

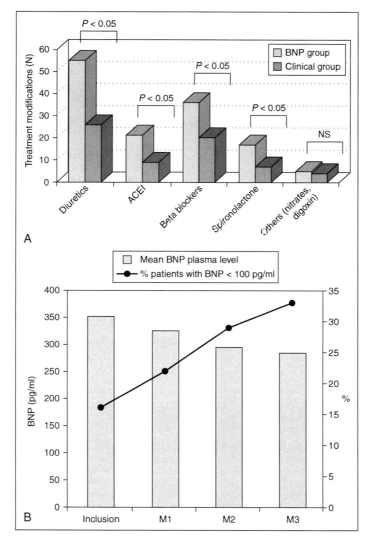

Figure 13.8 (A) Changes in medical therapy during the titration phase in BNP group and clinical group in a strategy to guide therapy with BNP levels versus usual care. (B) Plasma BNP level in BNP group during titration phase and percent of patients reaching target BNP value (with permission from [51]). ACEI = angiotensin-converting-enzyme inhibitor; BNP = B-type natriuretic peptide; M = month; NS = not significant.

after a median follow-up of 9.5 months that therapy guided by serial measurements of NT-proBNP led to more aggressive therapy with angiotensin-converting-enzyme (ACE) inhibitors and subsequently improved cardiovascular outcome (cardiovascular death *or* cardiovascular hospital admission *or* out-patient episode of heart failure) [50]. While the difference in outcome was primarily due to decreased congestion that was managed in the out patient setting, the study highlighted that signs and symptoms alone may not adequately guide optimal therapy.

In the Systolic Heart Failure Treatment Supported by BNP (STARS-BNP) trial, heart failure specialists cared for patients ($n = 220$) with systolic dysfunction (LVEF < 45%) randomized to routine care or BNP guided therapy (BNP < 100 pg/ml). Patients received more beta block-

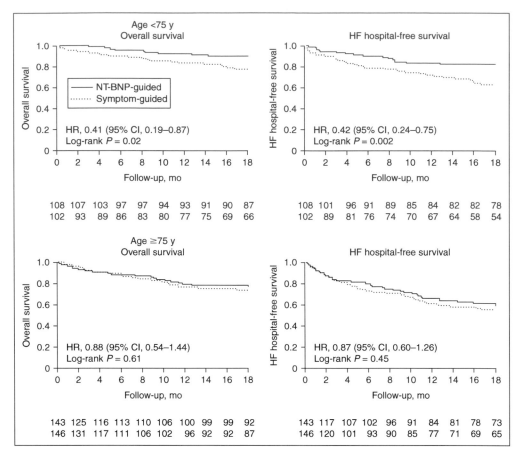

Figure 13.9 Evaluating the outcomes of heart failure patients guided by following NT-proBNP levels versus usual care. Treatment effects on main outcomes in younger (age 60–74 years) compared with older patients (age ≥75 years). The differences between treatment groups were observed only in younger but not older patients (with permission from [52]). CI = confidence interval; HF = heart failure; HR = hazard ratio; NT-BNP = N-terminal brain natriuretic peptide.

ers, spironolactone, loop diuretics and ACE-inhibitors or angiotensin receptor blockers (ARBs) when treatment was guided by BNP. Despite heart failure experts caring for both the BNP guided and standard therapy group, the BNP guided group suffered less hospitalization for heart failure (median follow-up 15 months) [51]. Interestingly, despite substantially more changes in beta blockers, ACE inhibitors/angiotensin receptor blockers and spironolactone in the BNP guided cohort the decrease in BNP levels was modest and few obtained the prespecified goal of < 100 pg/ml (Figure 13.8). This suggests that simply the addition of an objective measure such as a BNP level is potentially motivating to physicians to obtain guideline levels of medication and improve patient compliance despite no obvious change in symptoms or physical findings.

Heart failure is in large part a disease of the elderly and the largest trial to address natriuretic peptide guided therapy, the Trial of Intensified Versus Standard Medical Therapy in Elderly Patients with Congestive Heart Failure (TIME-CHF) randomized trial, specifically addressed this difficult to treat population [52]. NT-proBNP guided therapy was examined in an elderly population with a heart failure admission in the last year (499 patients, $\geq$ 60 years old). Patients enrolled had symptomatic heart failure (NYHA $\geq$ class III in 74%, 80% with an LVEF < 45%) and an elevated NT-proBNP concentration (2 x upper limit of age based normal). While comparisons of the entire study population only showed less heart failure related hospitalization for NT-proBNP guided therapy, prespecified subgroup analysis of those less than 75 years of age revealed significant benefits for survival. In contrast, those $\geq$ 75 years of age had no benefit with respect to heart failure admissions or death despite more frequently achieving guideline levels of beta blockers and ACE inhibitors/ARBs compared to those managed by signs and symptoms (Figure 13.9). In fact, investigators judged more serious adverse events to be related to N-terminal BNP-guided therapy vs. symptom-guided therapy in patients aged 75 years or older (10.5% vs. 5.5%, respectively; $P = 0.12$) Interestingly, the age dependent benefits were corroborated with preliminary data from the BNP Assisted Treatment to Lessen Serial Cardiac Readmission or Death (BATTLESCARRED) Trial [53]. One hypothesis may be that aggressive medical therapy is less tolerated by the elderly precluding clinical benefit or the benefits from medical therapy diminish as heart failure progresses. Regardless of the explanation, these trials suggest natriuretic peptide guided therapy is of no additional clinical benefit in the elderly ($\geq$75 years of age).

Further re-enforcing a limited application for serial natriuretic peptide testing to guide heart failure therapy in recently discharged patients are the results from the Can Pro-Brain-Natriuretic Peptide Guided Therapy of Chronic Heart Failure Improve Heart Failure Morbidity and Mortality? (PRIMA) study ($n = 345$; median follow-up 702 days) [54]. Again, there was no difference in mortality between those targeted to their own nadir NT-proBNP level versus clinically guided therapy. However, like TIME-CHF there is an intriguing subgroup suggesting that specific circumstances may warrant following serial levels to guide therapy. In the PRIMA study, individuals who stayed near their target level $\geq$75% of the time had a mortality of only 10.9% vs. 33.3% of the clinically guided group. Whether this reflects an intrinsic characteristic of these patients, the pathology of their heart failure or the ability by medical management to keep them at target has yet to be determined.

While guided therapy leads to more aggressive medication titration and decreased hospitalizations in select populations, the data supporting routine use of natriuretic peptides for the chronic management of heart failure are inconclusive. The concept of utilizing a biomarker to adjudicate and guide clinical decisions is appealing; however, as with any other diagnostic tools, the clinician must be wary of its limitations. Natriuretic peptide levels are affected by age, gender, renal function, body composition and acute non-cardiovascular illness [55–59]. Until additional data become available, clinicians should not mandate titration of medications based on ambulatory natriuretic peptide levels without consideration of additional clinical information.

CARDIAC TROPONINS: ACUTE CORONARY SYNDROMES TO HEART FAILURE

The cardiac troponin assays are the backbone of the diagnosis of acute coronary syndromes [60]. However, it is also well recognized that there are multiple non-acute coronary syndrome etiologies for troponin elevation including both chronic and acute decompensated heart failure [60, 61]. In both settings elevated troponin levels portend a poor prognosis in proportion to their levels [62–64]. Furthermore, troponin levels are not static and following serial levels over time in out patients either by identifying newly detectable levels or increases in levels in those with already elevated levels confers a poor prognosis [64, 65]. In addition, troponin testing can be used synergistically with natriuretic peptide levels as part of multi-marker strategy to enhance prognostication based on biomarker levels [62, 65, 66]. Troponin assays are rapidly evolving, for lack of a better term, to high sensitivity assays that can detect levels an order of magnitude lower than the current generation's most sensitive test [67]. Little has yet to be published with respect to these new assays particularly in the

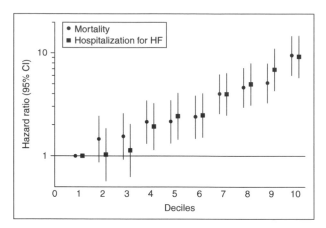

Figure 13.10 Unadjusted HRs and 95% CIs for mortality and for hospitalization for heart failure (HF) by deciles of hsTnT at baseline. The concentration range for hsTnT, rate of events (death [circles], hospitalization for HF [squares]), and number of patients with detectable cTnT are reported for each decile of hsTnT (with permission from [66]). The hazard ratios for mortality was significantly higher for decile 4 (0.00717 to 0.00978 ng/ml) than for the reference category (decile 1). CI = confidence intervals; HF = heart failure.

area of heart failure. Several specific recent studies will be reviewed below that give hints as to the potential directions for troponin testing in heart failure.

PROGNOSTIC SIGNIFICANCE OF MINOR TROPONIN ELEVATIONS

Data from the ADHERE registry in nearly 85000 patients presenting with acute heart failure found 6.2% had a 'positive' troponin result using a variety of troponin assays and cut off values specific to the many hospitals in the registry. Despite this heterogeneity in testing, a positive result was associated with markedly higher in-hospital mortality (8.0% vs. 2.7%) [63]. Consistent with this finding, the Val-HeFT investigators found that the 10% of their chronic stable heart failure patients with a detectable troponin T using the lower limit of detection of this clinically available third generation assay had a poorer prognosis than those without a detectable level. However, when they tested the same patients with a next generation high sensitivity troponin T assay that had a ten-fold lower limit of detection (0.001 ng/ml vs. 0.01 ng/ml for the current assay), 92% of the patients now had detectable levels with a gradient of risk for adverse outcomes throughout the spectrum of these low levels that were previously undetectable, starting as low as 0.007 ng/ml (Figure 13.10) [66]. It should therefore be anticipated that as these newer assays are introduced into clinical care most heart failure patients, irrespective of the setting, will have detectable troponin levels and that these levels will provide a gradient of risk for prognosticating death and heart failure hospitalizations. What remains uncertain is whether this information will provide incremental information for patient management [68].

SCREENING FOR 'AT-RISK' INDIVIDUALS FOR NEW ONSET HEART FAILURE WITH CARDIAC TROPONIN

Due to assay low-end detection limitations considering screening the general population with troponin testing has not been practical. Despite this finding, there is recognition that an elevated level is associated with cardiac comorbities [69]. Using a newer more sensitive (but not yet 'high sensitive') cTnI assay in a cohort of 1089 elderly Swedish men a cTnI ≥ 0.03 ng/ ml (8.2% of subjects) was associated with an incidence rate of heart failure of 25.5 per 1000 patient-years compared to an incidence rate of 4.6 for those with a cTnI < 0.01 ng/ml [70]. Such findings will need to be still put in the context of other biomarkers and most importantly if such findings can trigger preventive measures to prevent progression to symptomatic heart failure.

ST2 RECEPTOR

The ST2 receptor is a member of the interleukin-1 receptor family which is expressed by cardiomyocytes and has both soluble (sST2) and transmembrane (ST2L) isoforms [71, 72]. IL-33, the recently discovered functional ligand of the ST2 receptor, activates the NF-κB and mitogen-activated protein kinase (MAPK) signaling pathways [73]. In a mouse model, binding of IL-33 to ST2L was protective and prevented hypertrophy in the presence of angiotensin II or phenylephrine. In other words, activation of the membrane bound ST2 receptor exerts cardioprotective effect against adverse neurhormonal stimulation from the renin-angiotensin axis and sympathetic system. However, high circulating concentrations of the *soluble* receptor sST2 muted the protective effects of IL-33, possibly by binding available IL-33 and competitively preventing activation of ST2L [74]. These and other data suggest that the interactions of IL-33 and the ST2 receptors play an important role in directing myocardial remodeling and function. Gene expression of ST2, much like BNP, increases in response to mechanical stretch, which has stimulated interest for its role as a clinical biomarker for patients with heart failure [75].

Investigations of ST2 in humans have focused on patients with acute coronary syndrome or acute heart failure. After myocardial infarction, serum concentrations of sST2 increase early (peak value at 12 h) and predict development of congestive heart failure and death [75, 76]. Januzzi *et al.* measured sST2 in acute dyspnea patients enrolled in the Pro-Brain Natriuretic Peptide Investigation of Dyspnea in the Emergency Department (PRIDE) study. They found that sST2 concentrations ≥ 0.20 ng/ml predicted mortality in patients with heart failure at 1 year of follow-up (hazard ratio [HR] = 9.3; 95% CI; 1.3–17.8; $P = 0.03$). ST2 levels correlate with the severity of heart failure symptoms and inversely with LVEF. However, it remains equally predictive of 1 year mortality in those with depressed or preserved systolic function. Furthermore, the prognostic value of the test is synergistic with natriuretic peptides such that those with high levels of NT-proBNP and ST2 have the highest 1 year mortality (42%) and in those with low ST2 and NT-proBNP levels mortality was only 10% [77]. Despite a comparable or superior prognostic accuracy compared to natriuretic peptides, ST2 is not as an accurate test for diagnosing heart failure in a dyspnea cohort and can't be considered a substitute for this diagnostic application [78].

The data for ST2 in ambulatory heart failure patients is limited. Weinberg *et al.* [79] evaluated non-ischemic patients with severe symptomatic chronic heart failure (NYHA class III/ VI) and found that increases in ST2 concentrations over a 2 week interval identified those at greater risk of death or heart transplantation.

ST2 is also expressed in fibroblasts and modulates T-cell response. ST2 plays a role in inflammation and elevated levels have been observed in non-cardiac inflammatory disease states, including sepsis, trauma, asthma, and malignancy. While increased concentrations are not exclusive to heart failure, measurement of ST2 in selected heart failure patients may identify individuals that benefit from increased clinical surveillance or transplantation. Ultimately how this marker may be used in heart failure requires further investigation.

MARKERS OF INFLAMMATION

Myocardial injury and remodeling is a pro-inflammatory process. The prevailing theory suggests the myocardium releases cytokines which activate monocytes and increase sympathetic tone, further perpetuating systemic cytokine release and further myocardial dysfunction [80]. Tumor necrosis factor α (TNF-α), interleukin (IL) 1, and IL-6 are key cytokines implicated in the progression of chronic heart failure. *In vitro*, they increase myocyte hypertrophy, induce myocyte apoptosis, promote left ventricular dilation, and depress myocardial contractility [81]. Elevated levels have been observed in patients with depressed systolic function or congestive heart and higher levels are associated with cachexia and poor prognosis [82–84].

As the pathophysiology of heart failure seems to closely involve inflammatory mediators, considerable effort has been put forth to incorporate markers of inflammation into the prognostic evaluation of heart failure patients. C-reactive protein (CRP) is a non-specific acute phase reactant synthesized and secreted from the liver in response to IL-6 [85]. Early observations associated CRP increased with heart failure severity [86]. Measuring CRP or, more specifically, the contemporary high sensitive CRP (hsCRP), is akin to measuring erythrocyte sedimentation rate (ESR). Both laboratory studies have been shown to predict future development heart failure in aysmptomatic patients and mortality in patients with heart failure [87–91].

In a post hoc analysis of the Val-HeFT study, Anand and colleagues found that increased hsCRP in stable heart failure patient (> 3.23 mg/l) predicted mortality (HR of 1.23 [1.05–1.44]; $P = 0.009$) [89]. In a prospective study, Lamblin *et al.* evaluated hsCRP in 546 ambulatory heart failure patients with depressed LV systolic function. They found after a multivariate analysis that included natriuretic peptides, age, *and* peak oxygen consumption (VO_2), hsCRP ≥ 3 mg/dl predicted increased death or transplantation (HR of 1.55 [1.02–2.38]; $P = 0.04$) at a median follow-up of 2.7 years [92]. Furthermore, CRP levels have been shown to predict new onset heart failure in the community dwelling elderly [90, 91]. In the cardiovascular health study a serum CRP level ≥ 5 mg/dl was associated with a 2.8-fold increased risk of congestive heart failure (CHF) ($P = 0.02$) [91].

Incorporating measurements of systemic inflammation, be it TNF-α, ESR or hsCRP, is not routine practice, although it seems to be a reasonable method of surveying disease progression. The ability of the inflammatory biomarkers to alter clinician behavior and more importantly improve symptoms and outcomes is yet to be proven for patients with heart failure.

MYELOPEROXIDASE

Myeloperoxidase (MPO) is released from activated neutrophils and monocytes during inflammation and increases the oxidative potential of hydrogen peroxide by conversion to hydrochlorous acid [93]. In coronary artery disease, MPO has been implicated in initiating and propagating atherosclerosis, and has prognostic utility for patients with chest pain or acute coronary syndromes [94–99]. After a myocardial infarction, increased MPO levels predict higher mortality independent of LVEF and NT-proBNP level [100].

The role of MPO in heart failure is less well defined. Inflammatory mediators increase oxidative stress which worsens myocardial function by causing protein dysfunction, fibrosis, nitric-oxide depletion, and myocyte apoptosis [101]. We studied serum MPO concentrations in patients presenting to the ED with acute dyspnea. We found MPO did not provide diagnostic or prognostic information alone, or provide additive information to BNP or NT-proBNP concentrations [102]. However, in patients with compensated severe systolic heart failure, serum MPO concentrations predict mortality and heart transplantation [103, 104]. Higher levels of MPO are also associated with an increased prevalence of severe diastolic dysfunction and right ventricular systolic dysfunction [104]. Thus MPO concentrations, while nonspecific in the general dyspnea population may help identify those with characteristics of late stage heart failure who warrant closer consideration for heart transplantation.

CONCLUSIONS

With the introduction of natriuretic peptide tests into clinical practice in 2000–2002, blood based biomarkers have become an established part of care of patients with heart failure [4]. Though well accepted by ED physicians for their diagnostic role in identifying dyspnea patients with heart failure, the additional value of natruretic peptide testing for risk stratification and guiding therapy remains a source of controversy particularly among physicians with expertise in heart failure. The role of other cardiac markers is evolving and new markers such as ST2 and older markers with newer generation sensitive assays such as the cardiac troponins may find a place to complement or supersede the natriuretic peptide tests. Ultimately, the role for heart failure biomarkers may be to add more quantification to a field in which there is as much art as science applied to the management of these complex patients.

REFERENCES

1. Maisel AS, Krishnaswamy P, Nowak RM *et al*. Rapid measurement of B-type natriuretic peptide in the emergency diagnosis of heart failure. *N Engl J Med* 2002; 347:161-167.
2. Alpert JS, Thygesen K, Antman E, Bassand JP. Myocardial infarction redefined – a consensus document of The Joint European Society of Cardiology/American College of Cardiology Committee for the redefinition of myocardial infarction. *J Am Coll Cardiol* 2000; 36:959-969.
3. Anderson JL, Adams CD, Antman EM *et al*. ACC/AHA 2007 guidelines for the management of patients with unstable angina/non ST-elevation myocardial infarction: a report of the American College of Cardiology/American Heart Association Task Force on Practice Guidelines (Writing Committee to Revise the 2002 Guidelines for the Management of Patients With Unstable Angina/Non ST-Elevation Myocardial Infarction): developed in collaboration with the American College of Emergency Physicians, the Society for Cardiovascular Angiography and Interventions, and the Society of Thoracic Surgeons: endorsed by the American Association of Cardiovascular and Pulmonary Rehabilitation and the Society for Academic Emergency Medicine. *Circulation* 2007; 116:e148-e304.
4. Hunt SA, Abraham WT, Chin MH *et al*. 2009 Focused update incorporated into the ACC/AHA 2005 Guidelines for the Diagnosis and Management of Heart Failure in Adults: A Report of the American College of Cardiology Foundation/American Heart Association Task Force on Practice Guidelines Developed in Collaboration With the International Society for Heart and Lung Transplantation. *J Am Coll Cardiol* 2009; 53:e1-e90.
5. Braunwald E. Biomarkers in heart failure. *N Engl J Med* 2008; 358:2148-2159.
6. Morrow DA, de Lemos JA. Benchmarks for the assessment of novel cardiovascular biomarkers. *Circulation* 2007; 115:949-952.
7. McCullough PA, Sandberg KR. Sorting out the evidence on natriuretic peptides. *Rev Cardiovasc Med* 2003; 4(suppl 4):S13-S19.
8. McCullough PA, Nowak RM, McCord J *et al*. B-type natriuretic peptide and clinical judgment in emergency diagnosis of heart failure: analysis from Breathing Not Properly (BNP) Multinational Study. *Circulation* 2002; 106:416-422.
9. Moe GW, Howlett J, Januzzi JL, Zowall H. N-terminal pro-B-type natriuretic peptide testing improves the management of patients with suspected acute heart failure: primary results of the Canadian prospective randomized multicenter IMPROVE-CHF study. *Circulation* 2007; 115:3103-3110.
10. Mueller C, Scholer A, Laule-Kilian K *et al*. Use of B-type natriuretic peptide in the evaluation and management of acute dyspnea. *N Engl J Med* 2004; 350:647-654.
11. Schneider H-G, Lam L, Lokuge A *et al*. B-type natriuretic peptide testing, clinical outcomes, and health services use in emergency department patients with dyspnea. *Ann Intern Med* 2009; 150:365-371.
12. Januzzi JL Jr, Camargo CA, Anwaruddin S *et al*. The N-terminal Pro-BNP Investigation of Dyspnea in the Emergency Department (PRIDE) study. *Am J Cardiol* 2005; 95:948-954.

13. Lainchbury JG, Campbell E, Frampton CM, Yandle TG, Nicholls MG, Richards AM. Brain natriuretic peptide and n-terminal brain natriuretic peptide in the diagnosis of heart failure in patients with acute shortness of breath. *J Am Coll Cardiol* 2003; 42:728-735.

14. Mueller T, Gegenhuber A, Poelz W, Haltmayer M. Diagnostic accuracy of B type natriuretic peptide and amino terminal proBNP in the emergency diagnosis of heart failure. *Heart (British Cardiac Society)* 2005; 91:606-612.

15. Zaphiriou A, Robb S, Murray-Thomas T *et al*. The diagnostic accuracy of plasma BNP and NTproBNP in patients referred from primary care with suspected heart failure: results of the UK natriuretic peptide study. *Eur J Heart Fail* 2005; 7:537-541.

16. Anwaruddin S, Lloyd-Jones DM, Baggish A *et al*. Renal function, congestive heart failure, and amino-terminal pro-brain natriuretic peptide measurement: results from the ProBNP Investigation of Dyspnea in the Emergency Department (PRIDE) Study. *J Am Coll Cardiol* 2006; 47:91-97.

17. McCullough PA, Duc P, Omland T *et al*. B-type natriuretic peptide and renal function in the diagnosis of heart failure: an analysis from the Breathing Not Properly Multinational Study. *Am J Kidney Dis* 2003; 41:571-579.

18. Richards M, Nicholls MG, Espiner EA *et al*. Comparison of B-type natriuretic peptides for assessment of cardiac function and prognosis in stable ischemic heart disease. *J Am Coll Cardiol* 2006; 47:52-60.

19. Januzzi JL, van Kimmenade R, Lainchbury J *et al*. NT-proBNP testing for diagnosis and short-term prognosis in acute destabilized heart failure: an international pooled analysis of 1256 patients: the International Collaborative of NT-proBNP Study. *Eur Heart J* 2006; 27:330-337.

20. Knudsen CW, Clopton P, Westheim A *et al*. Predictors of elevated B-type natriuretic peptide concentrations in dyspneic patients without heart failure: an analysis from the breathing not properly multinational study. *Ann Emerg Med* 2005; 45:573-580.

21. de Lemos JA, Morrow DA, Bentley JH *et al*. The prognostic value of B-type natriuretic peptide in patients with acute coronary syndromes. *N Engl J Med* 2001; 345:1014-1021.

22. James SK, Lindahl B, Siegbahn A *et al*. N-terminal pro-brain natriuretic peptide and other risk markers for the separate prediction of mortality and subsequent myocardial infarction in patients with unstable coronary artery disease: a Global Utilization of Strategies To Open occluded arteries (GUSTO)-IV substudy. *Circulation* 2003; 108:275-281.

23. Morrow DA, de Lemos JA, Blazing MA *et al*. Prognostic value of serial B-type natriuretic peptide testing during follow-up of patients with unstable coronary artery disease. *JAMA* 2005; 294:2866-2871.

24. Morrow DA, de Lemos JA, Sabatine MS *et al*. Evaluation of B-type natriuretic peptide for risk assessment in unstable angina/non-ST-elevation myocardial infarction: B-type natriuretic peptide and prognosis in TACTICS-TIMI 18. *J Am Coll Cardiol* 2003; 41:1264-1272.

25. Konstam MA. Natriuretic peptides and cardiovascular events: more than a stretch. *JAMA* 2007; 297:212-214.

26. van Kimmenade RR, Januzzi JL Jr, Bakker JA *et al*. Renal clearance of B-type natriuretic peptide and amino terminal pro-B-type natriuretic peptide a mechanistic study in hypertensive subjects. *J Am Coll Cardiol* 2009; 53:884-890.

27. Khan IA, Fink J, Nass C, Chen H, Christenson R, deFilippi CR. N-terminal pro-B-type natriuretic peptide and B-type natriuretic peptide for identifying coronary artery disease and left ventricular hypertrophy in ambulatory chronic kidney disease patients. *Am J Cardiol* 2006; 97:1530-1534.

28. Luchner A, Hengstenberg C, Lowel H, Riegger GA, Schunkert H, Holmer S. Effect of compensated renal dysfunction on approved heart failure markers: direct comparison of brain natriuretic peptide (BNP) and N-terminal pro-BNP. *Hypertension* 2005; 46:118-123.

29. Vickery S, Price CP, John RI *et al*. B-type natriuretic peptide (BNP) and amino-terminal proBNP in patients with CKD: relationship to renal function and left ventricular hypertrophy. *Am J Kidney Dis* 2005; 46:610-620.

30. Astor BC, Yi S, Hiremath L *et al*. N-terminal prohormone brain natriuretic peptide as a predictor of cardiovascular disease and mortality in blacks with hypertensive kidney disease: the African American Study of Kidney Disease and Hypertension (AASK). *Circulation* 2008; 117:1685-1692.

31. Lam CS, Burnett JC Jr, Costello-Boerrigter L, Rodeheffer RJ, Redfield MM. Alternate circulating pro-B-type natriuretic peptide and B-type natriuretic peptide forms in the general population. *J Am Coll Cardiol* 2007; 49:1193-1202.

32. Giuliani I, Rieunier F, Larue C *et al*. Assay for measurement of intact B-type natriuretic peptide prohormone in blood. *Clin Chem* 2006; 52:1054-1061.

33. Liang F, O'Rear J, Schellenberger U *et al*. Evidence for functional heterogeneity of circulating B-type natriuretic peptide. *J Am Coll Cardiol* 2007; 49:1071-1078.

34. Seferian KR, Tamm NN, Semenov AG *et al*. The brain natriuretic peptide (BNP) precursor is the major immunoreactive form of BNP in patients with heart failure. *Clin Chem* 2007; 53:866-873.

35. Waldo SW, Beede J, Isakson S *et al*. Pro-B-type natriuretic peptide levels in acute decompensated heart failure. *J Am Coll Cardiol* 2008; 51:1874-1882.

36. Harrison A, Morrison LK, Krishnaswamy P *et al*. B-type natriuretic peptide predicts future cardiac events in patients presenting to the emergency department with dyspnea. *Ann Emerg Med* 2002; 39:131-138.

37. Januzzi JL Jr, Sakhuja R, O'Donoghue M *et al*. Utility of amino-terminal pro-brain natriuretic peptide testing for prediction of 1-year mortality in patients with dyspnea treated in the emergency department. *Arch Intern Med* 2006; 166:315-320.

38. van Kimmenade RR, Januzzi JL Jr, Baggish AL *et al*. Amino-terminal pro-brain natriuretic peptide, renal function, and outcomes in acute heart failure: redefining the cardiorenal interaction? *J Am Coll Cardiol* 2006; 48:1621-1627.

39. Kazanegra R, Cheng V, Garcia A *et al*. A rapid test for B-type natriuretic peptide correlates with falling wedge pressures in patients treated for decompensated heart failure: a pilot study. *J Card Fail* 2001; 7:21-29.

40. Forfia PR, Watkins SP, Rame JE, Stewart KJ, Shapiro EP. Relationship between B-type natriuretic peptides and pulmonary capillary wedge pressure in the intensive care unit. *J Am Coll Cardiol* 2005; 45:1667-1671.

41. Dokainish H, Zoghbi WA, Lakkis NM *et al*. Optimal noninvasive assessment of left ventricular filling pressures: a comparison of tissue Doppler echocardiography and B-type natriuretic peptide in patients with pulmonary artery catheters. *Circulation* 2004; 109:2432-2439.

42. Jefic D, Lee JW, Jefic D, Savoy-Moore RT, Rosman HS. Utility of B-type natriuretic peptide and N-terminal pro B-type natriuretic peptide in evaluation of respiratory failure in critically ill patients. *Chest* 2005; 128:288-295.

43. Logeart D, Thabut G, Jourdain P *et al*. Predischarge B-type natriuretic peptide assay for identifying patients at high risk of re-admission after decompensated heart failure. *J Am Coll Cardiol* 2004; 43:635-641.

44. Bettencourt P, Azevedo A, Pimenta J, Frioes F, Ferreira S, Ferreira A. N-terminal-pro-brain natriuretic peptide predicts outcome after hospital discharge in heart failure patients. *Circulation* 2004; 110:2168-2174.

45. Anand IS, Fisher LD, Chiang YT *et al*. Changes in brain natriuretic peptide and norepinephrine over time and mortality and morbidity in the Valsartan Heart Failure Trial (Val-HeFT). *Circulation* 2003; 107:1278-1283.

46. Masson S, Latini R, Anand IS *et al*. Direct comparison of B-type natriuretic peptide (BNP) and amino-terminal proBNP in a large population of patients with chronic and symptomatic heart failure: the Valsartan Heart Failure (Val-HeFT) data. *Clin Chem* 2006; 52:1528-1538.

47. Hartmann F, Packer M, Coats AJ *et al*. Prognostic impact of plasma N-terminal pro-brain natriuretic peptide in severe chronic congestive heart failure: a substudy of the Carvedilol Prospective Randomized Cumulative Survival (COPERNICUS) trial. *Circulation* 2004; 110:1780-1786.

48. Richards AM, Doughty R, Nicholls MG *et al*. Plasma N-terminal pro-brain natriuretic peptide and adrenomedullin: prognostic utility and prediction of benefit from carvedilol in chronic ischemic left ventricular dysfunction. Australia-New Zealand Heart Failure Group. *J Am Coll Cardiol* 2001; 37:1781-1787.

49. Masson S, Latini R, Anand IS *et al*. Prognostic value of changes in N-terminal pro-brain natriuretic peptide in Val-HeFT (Valsartan Heart Failure Trial). *J Am Coll Cardiol* 2008; 52:997-1003.

50. Troughton RW, Frampton CM, Yandle TG, Espiner EA, Nicholls MG, Richards AM. Treatment of heart failure guided by plasma aminoterminal brain natriuretic peptide (N-BNP) concentrations. *Lancet* 2000; 355:1126-1130.

51. Jourdain P, Jondeau G, Funck F *et al*. Plasma brain natriuretic peptide-guided therapy to improve outcome in heart failure: the STARS-BNP Multicenter Study. *J Am Coll Cardiol* 2007; 49:1733-1739.

52. Pfisterer M, Buser P, Rickli H *et al*. BNP-guided vs symptom-guided heart failure therapy: the Trial of Intensified vs Standard Medical Therapy in Elderly Patients With Congestive Heart Failure (TIME-CHF) randomized trial. *JAMA* 2009; 301:383-392.

53. Richards AM, Lainchbury JG, Troughton RW *et al*. Abstract 5946: Ntprobnp guided treatment for chronic heart failure: results from the BATTLESCARRED Trial. *Circulation* 2008; 118:S_1035-c-6.
54. Eurlings L. Can Pro-Brain-Natriuretic Peptide Guided Therapy of Chronic Heart Failure Improve Heart Failure Morbidity and Mortality? www.theheart.org/article/952927.do (Accessed May 14 2009).
55. Berdague P, Caffin PY, Barazer I *et al*. Use of N-terminal prohormone brain natriuretic peptide assay for etiologic diagnosis of acute dyspnea in elderly patients. *Am Heart J* 2006; 151:690-698.
56. Maisel AS, Clopton P, Krishnaswamy P *et al*. Impact of age, race, and sex on the ability of B-type natriuretic peptide to aid in the emergency diagnosis of heart failure: results from the Breathing Not Properly (BNP) multinational study. *Am Heart J* 2004; 147:1078-1084.
57. Mehra MR, Uber PA, Park MH *et al*. Obesity and suppressed B-type natriuretic peptide levels in heart failure. *J Am Coll Cardiol* 2004; 43:1590-1595.
58. Shah KB, Nolan MM, Rao K *et al*. The characteristics and prognostic importance of NT-ProBNP concentrations in critically ill patients. *Am J Med* 2007; 120:1071-1077.
59. Taylor JA, Christenson RH, Rao K, Jorge M, Gottlieb SS. B-type natriuretic peptide and N-terminal pro B-type natriuretic peptide are depressed in obesity despite higher left ventricular end diastolic pressures. *Am Heart J* 2006; 152:1071-1076.
60. Thygesen K, Alpert JS, White HD *et al*. Universal definition of myocardial infarction. *Circulation* 2007; 116:2634-2653.
61. Jeremias A, Gibson CM. Narrative review: alternative causes for elevated cardiac troponin levels when acute coronary syndromes are excluded. *Ann Intern Med* 2005; 142:786-791.
62. Horwich TB, Patel J, MacLellan WR, Fonarow GC. Cardiac troponin I is associated with impaired hemodynamics, progressive left ventricular dysfunction, and increased mortality rates in advanced heart failure. *Circulation* 2003; 108:833-838.
63. Peacock WFIV, De Marco T, Fonarow GC *et al*. Cardiac troponin and outcome in acute heart failure. *N Engl J Med* 2008; 358:2117-2126.
64. Perna ER, Macin SM, Canella JPC *et al*. Ongoing myocardial injury in stable severe heart failure: value of cardiac troponin T monitoring for high-risk patient identification. *Circulation* 2004; 110:2376-2382.
65. Miller WL, Hartman KA, Burritt MF *et al*. Serial biomarker measurements in ambulatory patients with chronic heart failure: the importance of change over time. *Circulation* 2007; 116:249-257.
66. Latini R, Masson S, Anand IS *et al*. Prognostic value of very low plasma concentrations of troponin T in patients with stable chronic heart failure. *Circulation* 2007; 116:1242-1249.
67. Morrow DA, Antman EM. Evaluation of high-sensitivity assays for cardiac troponin. *Clin Chem* 2009; 55:5-8.
68. Wang TJ. Significance of circulating troponins in heart failure: if these walls could talk. *Circulation* 2007; 116:1217-1220.
69. Wallace TW, Abdullah SM, Drazner MH *et al*. Prevalence and determinants of troponin T elevation in the general population. *Circulation* 2006; 113:1958-1965.
70. Sundstrom J, Ingelsson E, Berglund L *et al*. Cardiac troponin-I and risk of heart failure: a community-based cohort study. *Eur Heart J* 2009; 30:773-781.
71. Bergers G, Reikerstorfer A, Braselmann S, Graninger P, Busslinger M. Alternative promoter usage of the Fos-responsive gene Fit-1 generates mRNA isoforms coding for either secreted or membrane-bound proteins related to the IL-1 receptor. *EMBO J* 1994; 13:1176-1188.
72. Iwahana H, Yanagisawa K, Ito-Kosaka A *et al*. Different promoter usage and multiple transcription initiation sites of the interleukin-1 receptor-related human ST2 gene in UT-7 and TM12 cells. *Eur J Biochem/FEBS* 1999; 264:397-406.
73. Schmitz J, Owyang A, Oldham E *et al*. IL-33, an interleukin-1-like cytokine that signals via the IL-1 receptor-related protein ST2 and induces T helper type 2-associated cytokines. *Immunity* 2005; 23:479-490.
74. Sanada S, Hakuno D, Higgins LJ, Schreiter ER, McKenzie AN, Lee RT. IL-33 and ST2 comprise a critical biomechanically induced and cardioprotective signaling system. *J Clin Invest* 2007; 117:1538-1549.
75. Weinberg EO, Shimpo M, De Keulenaer GW *et al*. Expression and regulation of ST2, an interleukin-1 receptor family member, in cardiomyocytes and myocardial infarction. *Circulation* 2002; 106:2961-2966.
76. Shimpo M, Morrow DA, Weinberg EO *et al*. Serum levels of the interleukin-1 receptor family member ST2 predict mortality and clinical outcome in acute myocardial infarction. *Circulation* 2004; 109:2186-2190.

77. Rehman SU, Mueller T, Januzzi JL Jr. Characteristics of the novel interleukin family biomarker ST2 in patients with acute heart failure. *J Am Coll Cardiol* 2008; 52:1458-1465.

78. Januzzi JL Jr, Peacock WF, Maisel AS *et al*. Measurement of the interleukin family member ST2 in patients with acute dyspnea: results from the PRIDE (Pro-Brain Natriuretic Peptide Investigation of Dyspnea in the Emergency Department) study. *J Am Coll Cardiol* 2007; 50:607-613.

79. Weinberg EO, Shimpo M, Hurwitz S, Tominaga S, Rouleau JL, Lee RT. Identification of serum soluble ST2 receptor as a novel heart failure biomarker. *Circulation* 2003; 107:721-726.

80. Anker SD, von Haehling S. Inflammatory mediators in chronic heart failure: an overview. *Heart* 2004; 90:464-470.

81. Mann DL. Inflammatory mediators and the failing heart: past, present, and the foreseeable future. *Circ Res* 2002; 91:988-998.

82. Levine B, Kalman J, Mayer L, Fillit HM, Packer M. Elevated circulating levels of tumor necrosis factor in severe chronic heart failure. *N Engl J Med* 1990; 323:236-241.

83. Tsutamoto T, Hisanaga T, Wada A *et al*. Interleukin-6 spillover in the peripheral circulation increases with the severity of heart failure, and the high plasma level of interleukin-6 is an important prognostic predictor in patients with congestive heart failure. *J Am Coll Cardiol* 1998; 31:391-398.

84. Raymond RJ, Dehmer GJ, Theoharides TC, Deliargyris EN. Elevated interleukin-6 levels in patients with asymptomatic left ventricular systolic dysfunction. *Am Heart J* 2001; 141:435-438.

85. Castell JV, Gomez-Lechon MJ, David M, Fabra R, Trullenque R, Heinrich PC. Acute-phase response of human hepatocytes: regulation of acute-phase protein synthesis by interleukin-6. *Hepatology* 1990; 12:1179-1186.

86. Elster SK, Braunwald E, Wood HF. A study of C-reactive protein in the serum of patients with congestive heart failure. *Am Heart J* 1956; 51:533-541.

87. Ingelsson E, Arnlov J, Sundstrom J, Lind L. Inflammation, as measured by the erythrocyte sedimentation rate, is an independent predictor for the development of heart failure. *J Am Coll Cardiol* 2005; 45:1802-1806.

88. Sharma R, Rauchhaus M, Ponikowski PP *et al*. The relationship of the erythrocyte sedimentation rate to inflammatory cytokines and survival in patients with chronic heart failure treated with angiotensin-converting enzyme inhibitors. *J Am Coll Cardiol* 2000; 36:523-528.

89. Anand IS, Latini R, Florea VG *et al*. C-reactive protein in heart failure: prognostic value and the effect of valsartan. *Circulation* 2005; 112:1428-1434.

90. Vasan RS, Sullivan LM, Roubenoff R *et al*. Inflammatory markers and risk of heart failure in elderly subjects without prior myocardial infarction: the Framingham Heart Study. *Circulation* 2003; 107:1486-1491.

91. Gottdiener JS, Arnold AM, Aurigemma GP *et al*. Predictors of congestive heart failure in the elderly: the Cardiovascular Health Study. *J Am Coll Cardiol* 2000; 35:1628-1637.

92. Lamblin N, Mouquet F, Hennache B *et al*. High-sensitivity C-reactive protein: potential adjunct for risk stratification in patients with stable congestive heart failure. *Eur Heart J* 2005; 26:2245-2250.

93. Nicholls SJ, Hazen SL. Myeloperoxidase and cardiovascular disease. *Arterioscler Thromb Vasc Biol* 2005; 25:1102-1111.

94. Hazen SL, Heinecke JW. 3-Chlorotyrosine, a specific marker of myeloperoxidase-catalyzed oxidation, is markedly elevated in low density lipoprotein isolated from human atherosclerotic intima. *J Clin Invest* 1997; 99:2075-2081.

94. Thukkani AK, McHowat J, Hsu FF, Brennan ML, Hazen SL, Ford DA. Identification of alpha-chloro fatty aldehydes and unsaturated lysophosphatidylcholine molecular species in human atherosclerotic lesions. *Circulation* 2003; 108:3128-3133.

96. Fu X, Kassim SY, Parks WC, Heinecke JW. Hypochlorous acid generated by myeloperoxidase modifies adjacent tryptophan and glycine residues in the catalytic domain of matrix metalloproteinase-7 (matrilysin): an oxidative mechanism for restraining proteolytic activity during inflammation. *J Biol Chem* 2003; 278:28403-28409.

97. Sugiyama S, Okada Y, Sukhova GK, Virmani R, Heinecke JW, Libby P. Macrophage myeloperoxidase regulation by granulocyte macrophage colony-stimulating factor in human atherosclerosis and implications in acute coronary syndromes. *Am J Pathol* 2001; 158:879-891.

98. Baldus S, Heeschen C, Meinertz T *et al*. Myeloperoxidase serum levels predict risk in patients with acute coronary syndromes. *Circulation* 2003; 108:1440-1445.

99. Brennan ML, Penn MS, Van Lente F *et al*. Prognostic value of myeloperoxidase in patients with chest pain. *N Engl J Med* 2003; 349:1595-1604.

100. Mocatta TJ, Pilbrow AP, Cameron VA *et al*. Plasma concentrations of myeloperoxidase predict mortality after myocardial infarction. *J Am Coll Cardiol* 2007; 49:1993-2000.
101. Ferrari R, Guardigli G, Mele D, Percoco GF, Ceconi C, Curello S. Oxidative stress during myocardial ischaemia and heart failure. *Curr Pharm Des* 2004; 10:1699-1711.
102. Shah KB, Kop WJ, Christenson RH *et al*. Lack of diagnostic and prognostic utility of circulating plasma myeloperoxidase concentrations in patients presenting with dyspnea. *Clin Chem* 2009; 55:59-67.
103. Tang WH, Brennan ML, Philip K *et al*. Plasma myeloperoxidase levels in patients with chronic heart failure. *Am J Cardiol* 2006; 98:796-799.
104. Tang WH, Tong W, Troughton RW *et al*. Prognostic value and echocardiographic determinants of plasma myeloperoxidase levels in chronic heart failure. *J Am Coll Cardiol* 2007; 49:2364-2370.
105. van Kimmenade RR, Pinto YM, Bayes-Genis A, Lainchbury JG, Richards AM, Januzzi JL Jr. Usefulness of intermediate amino-terminal pro-brain natriuretic peptide concentrations for diagnosis and prognosis of acute heart failure. *Am J Cardiol* 2006; 98:386-390.
106. DeFilippi C, van Kimmenade RR, Pinto YM. Amino-terminal pro-B-type natriuretic peptide testing in renal disease. *Am J Cardiol* 2008; 101:82-88.

14

Atrial fibrillation in patients with heart failure: the cart or the horse?

K. B. Shah, T. M. Dickfeld

INTRODUCTION

The association between congestive heart failure (CHF) and atrial fibrillation (AF) has been repeatedly observed. Several studies reported an increasing prevalence of AF with worsening New York Heart Association (NYHA) functional class [1–5]. Conversely, an analysis of the Framingham Heart Study revealed that nearly 40% of patients with pre-existing AF eventually developed CHF. Regardless of which occurs first, the development of both, AF and CHF, portends a poor prognosis [6, 7].

During AF, the hemodynamic consequences related to persistent tachycardia, irregular filling intervals and loss of atrial contribution in late diastole have been well characterized. The loss of atrial contraction and AV-synchrony have been shown to decrease the cardiac index and to increase the pulmonary capillary wedge pressure regardless of ventricular function [8]. Furthermore, an irregular ventricular rhythm itself may lead to a diminished cardiac output [9]. The correlation between insufficient rate-control in AF and occurrence of tachycardia-induced cardiomyopathy has been well described [10, 11]. In patients with AF and depressed LV systolic function, ventricular rate control with medical therapy or AV nodal ablation increased LV ejection fraction [10, 12–14].

In this chapter, we will examine the coexistence of both diseases and the rationale for treating AF in patients with CHF.

WHY DOES HEART FAILURE (HF) GIVE RISE TO AF?

Current evidence suggests that AF could arise from single re-entrant, multiple re-entrant or ectopic foci [15]. In models of rapid atrial pacing or increased sympathetic stimulation, AF appears to be initiated and maintained by re-entry promoting changes in cycle length or atrial tissue refractoriness [16]. In CHF, however, alternative mechanisms such as structural remodeling and intracellular calcium regulation may play more significant roles.

In CHF, atrial remodeling provides a substrate for the increased incidence of arrhythmias. In a study comparing AF induced by rapid atrial pacing versus a HF based model, Li *et al.* [17] showed that the conduction and histological properties of the atria differed in both models. In the pacing model, the atria tissue exhibited decrease in wavelength and short-

Keyur B. Shah, MD, FACC, Assistant Professor of Medicine, Division of Cardiology, Virginia Commonwealth University, Richmond, VA, USA.

Timm M. Dickfeld, MD, PhD, FACC, Associate Professor of Medicine, Division of Cardiology, University of Maryland School of Medicine, Baltimore, MD, USA.

ened effective refractory period, both promoting re-entry and AF. In the CHF model, the investigators identified conduction defects caused by fibrosis thoughout the atrial tissue. The notion that diffuse fibrosis and the resulting conduction heterogeneity rather than atrial electrical properties play a key role in the HF associated AF has been observed in subsequent studies [18, 19].

In addition to structural changes, unique ion channel modifications are observed with CHF compared to traditional pacing models. In atrial tachycardia and acute atrial stretch, atrial ionic remodeling decreases transient outward and L-type Ca^{2+} currents in turn reducing the tissue's refractory period [20, 21]. Heterogeneous changes in the tissue refractory period creates substrate for re-entry and allows the tachyarrhythmia to continue. With CHF, however, the refractory period of the tissue is often unchanged due to decreased inward current and increased outward current generated by enhanced activity of the sodium-calcium exchanger [22].

Molecular changes associated specifically with HF may also play a role in arrhythmogenesis. Dysregulation of calcium handling is a well described feature of ventricular myocyte dysfunction in CHF [23]. In addition to blunting contractile efficiency, abnormal calcium handling and release from sarcoplasmic reticulum predisposes the myocyte to be delayed after depolarizations and triggered arrhythmias [24]. It has been observed that atrial myocytes in dilated HF models also exhibit signs of calcium overload and mishandling, thus offering an additional mechanism to initiate and propagate AF [25].

Activation of the renin-angiotensin-aldosterone axis, which is instrumental in the pathophysiology of CHF, may promote AF. In animal models, angiotensin II promotes arrhythmia sustaining atrial fibrosis via a transforming growth factor (TGF)-β1 pathway [26, 27]. Additionally, increased angiotensin II induces arterial vasoconstriction and LV hypertrophy, increasing intracavitary pressures. Through mechano-electrical interactions, atrial wall stretch shortens the atrial refractory period and predisposes HF patients to AF [20]. Angiotensin II has been observed to alter ion channel activity *in vitro*, however, the clinical relevance of this finding in humans is not clear [28].

In fact, medications designed to inhibit the renin-angiotensin-aldosterone pathway to treat CHF have been effective for reducing AF [29]. In a dog model of HF, treatment with an angiotensin-converting-enzyme (ACE) inhibitor decreased atrial fibrosis and occurrence of AF [30]. In a meta-analysis, Healey *et al.* reported that ACE inhibitors or angiotensin receptor blockers (ARBs) reduced the incidence of AF. Interestingly, the benefit was only realized in patients who had depressed LV systolic function or significant LV hypertrophy [31].

Inflammation and oxidative stress have been associated with AF. Patients with AF are likely to have higher C-reactive protein (CRP) concentrations [32]. Conversely, patients with high CRP levels are more likely to develop AF *de novo* or suffer recurrence after cardioversion [33, 34]. Interventions with anti-inflammatory medications including nitric oxide donors, statins, and glucocorticoids may reduce the occurrence of AF [35–38]. Omega-3 polyunsaturated fatty acid (PUFA), which have recently been proven to improve outcomes in HF, may reduced AF by attenuating atrial fibrosis in a canine model for CHF [38, 39]. Given that myocardial remodeling in chronic CHF is a dynamic, pro-inflammatory condition, inflammation resulting from the natural progression of HF may give rise to AF [40].

In CHF, atrial fibrosis, inflammation and abnormal calcium regulation promote and maintain arrhythmias. Additionally, molecular pathways are beginning to emerge. Future studies will have to determine if this may allow more specific therapeutic strategies in regard to prevention and treatment of AF in HF.

RATE OR RHYTHM CONTROL FOR PATIENTS WITH HF?

In asymptomatic patients, Atrial Fibrillation Follow-up Investigation of Rhythm Management (AFFIRM) and the Rate Control versus Electrical Cardioversion (RACE) showed comparable outcomes with a rate-control strategy in patients unselected for HF [41, 42]. Observations of improved survival in HF patients converting to sinus rhythm with amiodarone prompted subsequent prospective trials to examine antiarrhythmic medications for AF in selected patients with HF [3]. However, clinical trials have repeatedly shown disappointing results for antiarrhythmic medications in CHF patients [43–45]. In patients with CHF, further delay of repolarization of the diseased ventricular myocardium predisposes the patient to *torsades de pointes*. In fact, only class III agents have been shown to not increase mortality in patients with LV dysfunction [46–48]. Among those, dofetilide and sotalol significantly increases the risk of *torsades de pointes* to approximately 3%. Therefore, in-patient monitoring for 3 days is mandated when starting dofetilide and sotalol with assessment of the QT interval [48]. Amiodarone, which has been proven in unselected patients with AF to be more effective than sotolal for maintaining sinus rhythm, is generally the first-line antiarrhythmic in patients with HF [49].

Prospective evaluation of a rhythm control strategy in patients with LV dysfunction was performed in the Atrial Fibrillation and Congestive Heart Failure (AF-CHF) study. In this randomized controlled trial, 1376 HF patients with severe LV dysfunction (LV ejection fraction ≤ 35%), receiving contemporary therapy, were randomized to either rhythm control with amiodarone or rate control. Rate control therapy consisted of beta blockers, digitalis, and, if required, AV node ablation with biventricular pacing. The results showed no effect of rhythm control on progression of HF or incidence of stroke or mortality with a mean follow-up period of 37 months [50]. It is important to note that the study population excluded overt, unstable HF and nearly 70% of patients were < NYHA class III at enrollment.

Based on available data, a rhythm control strategy should mostly be targeted at HF patients with a likely component of tachycardia-mediated cardiomyopathy or if the patient is obviously symptomatic from the arrhythmia. Initial management with a class III agent is appropriate, assuming the clinician will perform vigilant surveillance for potential side-effects.

HOW ABOUT ABLATION, SURGERY OR PACEMAKER IMPLANTATION?

AV NODE ABLATION WITH PACEMAKER IMPLANTATION

Ablation of the AV node with insertion of a pacemaker has been shown to improve NYHA functional class and quality of life scores in patients with otherwise uncontrollable symptomatic AF [51]. However, studies have shown that chronic right ventricular pacing can lead to ventricular dyssynchrony in up to 50% of patients, which can deteriorate LV systolic function and eventually worsen HF [52, 53]. Those that develop LV dyssynchrony have lower LV ejection fractions ($48 \pm 7\%$ to $43 \pm 7\%$), increased ventricular volumes (116 ± 39 ml to 130 ± 52 ml) and worsening NYHA classification (1.8 ± 0.6 to 2.2 ± 0.7) [53]. In the Post AV Nodal Ablation Evaluation (the PAVE study), biventricular pacing, compared to right ventricular pacing, after AV node ablation for AF had greater improvements in LV ejection fraction ($46 \pm 13\%$ vs. $41 \pm 13\%$) and 6 min walk distance (82.9 ± 94.7 m vs. 61.2 ± 90.0 m) [54]. Upgrade of a pre-exisiting RV pacemaker or *de novo* implantation of a biventricular pacemaker following AV node ablation is an option for HF patients with drug refractory AF [55–57].

Curiously, while CRT improves HF status, ejection fraction, chamber size and mitral regurgitation, the Cardiac Resynchronization in Heart Failure (CARE-HF) trial did not show a difference in the incidence (16% vs. 14%, $P = 0.79$) or time to onset of AF with CRT [58, 59]. In a patient receiving CRT without AV node ablation or developing AF with CRT, adequate rate control is essential to deliver effective therapy and maximize the therapeutic benefit of CRT. If rate control is not achieved there will be insufficient biventricular pacing, necessitating eventual AV node ablation [55].

ABLATION

Haissaguerre *et al.* demonstrated the initiating triggers of AF could be found within or near the pulmonary veins (PV) in over 90% of the patients [60, 61]. Early techniques that targeted ablation of the PV foci were abandonded when high rates of pulmonary stenosis were observed [62, 63].

Currently, several different approaches to AF ablation exist including segmental or antral pulmonary vein isolation, circumferential pulmonary vein ablation, ablation of fractionated atrial electrograms as well as denervation/targeting of ganglionated plexus [64–67]. Success rates have varied from 11 to 99% with most investigators reporting results in the range of 70–90% [68, 69]. However, the need for repeat ablations and the incidence of post-procedural atrial flutter or atrial tachycardia remain significant [70, 71].

Initial retrospective data suggested that ablation strategies in patients with impaired LV function were less successful, possibly related to the extensive fibrosis associated with HF [72]. Strategies have since been studied prospectively in patients with CHF with depressed left ventricular systolic function. Hsu *et al.* evaluated segmental ostial PV isolation in patients with predominantly NYHA class II/III HF. In a non-randomized study, 58 patients with an LV ejection fraction of 35±7% were matched with patients with normal ejection fraction. After 12±7 months of follow-up, 78% of the low ejection fraction group and 84% of the controls remained in sinus rhythm (69% and 71% independent of antiarrhythmic drugs, 50% re-ablation rate). In subjects with CHF, they reported an improvement in LV ejection fraction symptom score, NYHA functional class and exercise capacity [73].

The only prospective *randomized* study compared the efficacy of PV antral isolation to AV node ablation + biventricular pacemaker implantation in patients with drug refractory AF, LV ejection fraction < 40% and NYHA class II/III symptoms. The investigators reported an over-all success rate of 88% (71% without antiarrhythmic medications) for maintaining sinus rhythm at 6-month follow-up. After 6 months patients randomized to an ablation strategy had greater LV ejection fractions (35±9% vs. 28±6%), increased 6 min walk distance (340±49 m vs. 297±36) and lower Minnesota Living with Hearth Failure Score (60±8 vs. 82±14) [74].

While ablation may offer improved quality of life and exercise capacity compared to AV-nodal ablation, data for long-term follow-up are lacking. Considering the progressive nature of chronic HF, one can expect continued atrial fibrosis and remodeling. Thus, the intervention's durability and long-term success is a valid concern. Additionally, AF ablation is a technically difficult procedure and the published data reflects complication rates at only experienced centers and adverse events are expected to be higher in the 'real world' experience.

SURGERY

A successful surgical treatment for AF was first developed by Cox *et al.* [75] who described the electrical 'compartmentalization' of the atria with multiple suture lines (Maze procedure). The reported rate of sinus rhythms after 8.5 years is > 90% in patients without significant LV dysfunction [76]. Retrospective data characterizing selected patients with depressed LV function undergoing an isolated Maze procedure suggests sustained long-term success is feasible. In one surgical study 37 patients with abnormal ejection fractions (65% with symptomatic HF) underwent a surgical Maze procedure without adjuvant therapy. After a follow-up of 63 months only one patient experienced symptomatic atrial fibrillation and all had improvement in their LV ejection fractions [77]. Previous studies evaluating the role of surgical AF therapies in HF were confounded by concomitant cardiac surgeries [78, 79].

Compartmentalization techniques have expanded to include ablation with radiofrequency and microwave energy and cryothermy. Less invasive surgical approaches implementing robotics and epicardial ablation are currently being investigated. While isolated surgical PV ablation is currently performed in several centers, it is mostly considered in patients also requiring concomitant coronary artery bypass or valve surgery. Trials evaluating a 'primary' Maze procedure are currently ongoing.

IS AF SIMPLY A MARKER OF DISEASE SEVERITY IN PATIENTS WITH CHF?

Atrial fibrillation in the presence of CHF is associated with unique structural and electrical atrial remodeling. The diffuse atrial fibrosis that promotes multiple foci of re-entry is irreversible, while the ion channel remodeling may revert to normal once that tachycardia stimulus or CHF is resolved [19, 80]. A patient with CHF is at an increasing risk of developing AF once sufficient remodeling has taken place. Furthermore, it seems that therapy aimed to slow the progression of HF prevents atrial fibrosis and the eventual occurrence of AF. In this regard, AF can be considered as a marker of HF progression and severity, and therapies limiting progression of HF may prevent AF.

REFERENCES

1. Effects of enalapril on mortality in severe congestive heart failure. Results of the Cooperative North Scandinavian Enalapril Survival Study (CONSENSUS). The CONSENSUS Trial Study Group. *N Engl J Med* 1987; 316:1429-1435.
2. Carson PE, Johnson GR, Dunkman WB, Fletcher RD, Farrell L, Cohn JN. The influence of atrial fibrillation on prognosis in mild to moderate heart failure. The V-HeFT Studies. The V-HeFT VA Cooperative Studies Group. *Circulation* 1993; 87:VI102-VI110.
3. Deedwania PC, Singh BN, Ellenbogen K, Fisher S, Fletcher R, Singh SN. Spontaneous conversion and maintenance of sinus rhythm by amiodarone in patients with heart failure and atrial fibrillation: observations from the Veterans Affairs Congestive Heart Failure Survival Trial of Antiarrhythmic Therapy (CHF-STAT). The Department of Veterans Affairs CHF-STAT Investigators. *Circulation* 1998; 98:2574-2579.
4. Maisel WH, Stevenson LW. Atrial fibrillation in heart failure: epidemiology, pathophysiology, and rationale for therapy. *Am J Cardiol* 2003; 91:2D-8D.
5. Middlekauff HR, Stevenson WG, Stevenson LW. Prognostic significance of atrial fibrillation in advanced heart failure. A study of 390 patients. *Circulation* 1991; 84:40-48.
6. Wang TJ, Larson MG, Levy D et al. Temporal relations of atrial fibrillation and congestive heart failure and their joint influence on mortality: the Framingham Heart Study. *Circulation* 2003; 107:2920-2925.
7. Olsson LG, Swedberg K, Ducharme A et al. Atrial fibrillation and risk of clinical events in chronic heart failure with and without left ventricular systolic dysfunction: results from the Candesartan in Heart failure-Assessment of Reduction in Mortality and morbidity (CHARM) program. *J Am Coll Cardiol* 2006; 47:1997-2004.
8. Mukharji J, Rehr RB, Hastillo A et al. Comparison of atrial contribution to cardiac hemodynamics in patients with normal and severely compromised cardiac function. *Clin Cardiol* 1990; 13:639-643.
9. Daoud EG, Weiss R, Bahu M et al. Effect of an irregular ventricular rhythm on cardiac output. *Am J Cardiol* 1996; 78:1433-1436.
10. Grogan M, Smith HC, Gersh BJ, Wood DL. Left ventricular dysfunction due to atrial fibrillation in patients initially believed to have idiopathic dilated cardiomyopathy. *Am J Cardiol* 1992; 69:1570-1573.
11. Shinbane JS, Wood MA, Jensen DN, Ellenbogen KA, Fitzpatrick AP, Scheinman MM. Tachycardia-induced cardiomyopathy: a review of animal models and clinical studies. *J Am Coll Cardiol* 1997; 29:709-715.
12. Morady F, Hasse C, Strickberger SA et al. Long-term follow-up after radiofrequency modification of the atrioventricular node in patients with atrial fibrillation. *J Am Coll Cardiol* 1997; 29:113-121.
13. Redfield MM, Kay GN, Jenkins LS, Mianulli M, Jensen DN, Ellenbogen KA. Tachycardia-related cardiomyopathy: a common cause of ventricular dysfunction in patients with atrial fibrillation referred for atrioventricular ablation. *Mayo Clin Proc* 2000; 75:790-795.

14. Twidale N, Manda V, Nave K, Seal A. Predictors of outcome after radiofrequency catheter ablation of the atrioventricular node for atrial fibrillation and congestive heart failure. *Am Heart J* 1998; 136:647-657.

15. Nattel S. New ideas about atrial fibrillation 50 years on. *Nature* 2002; 415:219-226.

16. Gaspo R, Bosch RF, Talajic M, Nattel S. Functional mechanisms underlying tachycardia-induced sustained atrial fibrillation in a chronic dog model. *Circulation* 1997; 96:4027-4035.

17. Li D, Fareh S, Leung TK, Nattel S. Promotion of atrial fibrillation by heart failure in dogs: atrial remodeling of a different sort. *Circulation* 1999; 100:87-95.

18. Cha TJ, Ehrlich JR, Zhang L, Nattel S. Atrial ionic remodeling induced by atrial tachycardia in the presence of congestive heart failure. *Circulation* 2004; 110:1520-1526.

19. Cha TJ, Ehrlich JR, Zhang L *et al*. Dissociation between ionic remodeling and ability to sustain atrial fibrillation during recovery from experimental congestive heart failure. *Circulation* 2004; 109:412-418.

20. Ravelli F, Allessie M. Effects of atrial dilatation on refractory period and vulnerability to atrial fibrillation in the isolated Langendorff-perfused rabbit heart. *Circulation* 1997; 96:1686-1695.

21. Yue L, Feng J, Gaspo R, Li GR, Wang Z, Nattel S. Ionic remodeling underlying action potential changes in a canine model of atrial fibrillation. *Circ Res* 1997; 81:512-525.

22. Cha TJ, Ehrlich JR, Zhang L, Nattel S. Atrial ionic remodeling induced by atrial tachycardia in the presence of congestive heart failure. *Circulation* 2004; 110:1520-1526.

23. Armoundas AA, Rose J, Aggarwal R *et al*. Cellular and molecular determinants of altered Ca2+ handling in the failing rabbit heart: primary defects in SR Ca2+ uptake and release mechanisms. *Am J Physiol Heart Circ Physiol* 2007; 292:H1607-H1618.

24. Pogwizd SM, Qi M, Yuan W, Samarel AM, Bers DM. Upregulation of Na(+)/Ca(2+) exchanger expression and function in an arrhythmogenic rabbit model of heart failure. *Circ Res* 1999; 85:1009-1019.

25. Yeh YH, Wakili R, Qi XY *et al*. Calcium-handling abnormalities underlying atrial arrhythmogenesis and contractile dysfunction in dogs with congestive heart failure. *Circ Arrhythmia Electrophysiol* 2008; 1:93-102.

26. Verheule S, Sato T, Everett T IV *et al*. Increased vulnerability to atrial fibrillation in transgenic mice with selective atrial fibrosis caused by overexpression of TGF-{beta}1. *Circ Res* 2004; 94:1458-1465.

27. Nakajima H, Nakajima HO, Salcher O *et al*. Atrial but not ventricular fibrosis in mice expressing a mutant transforming growth factor-{beta}1 transgene in the heart. *Circ Res* 2000; 86:571-579.

28. Ehrlich JR, Hohnloser SH, Nattel S. Role of angiotensin system and effects of its inhibition in atrial fibrillation: clinical and experimental evidence. *Eur Heart J* 2006; 27:512-518.

29. Belluzzi F, Sernesi L, Preti P, Salinaro F, Fonte ML, Perlini S. Prevention of recurrent lone atrial fibrillation by the angiotensin-II converting enzyme inhibitor ramipril in normotensive patients. *J Am Coll Cardiol* 2009; 53:24-29.

30. Li D, Shinagawa K, Pang L *et al*. Effects of angiotensin-converting enzyme inhibition on the development of the atrial fibrillation substrate in dogs with ventricular tachypacing-induced congestive heart failure. *Circulation* 2001; 104:2608-2614.

31. Healey JS, Baranchuk A, Crystal E *et al*. Prevention of atrial fibrillation with angiotensin-converting enzyme inhibitors and angiotensin receptor blockers: a meta-analysis. *J Am Coll Cardiol* 2005; 45:1832-1839.

32. Chung MK, Martin DO, Sprecher D *et al*. C-reactive protein elevation in patients with atrial arrhythmias: inflammatory mechanisms and persistence of atrial fibrillation. *Circulation* 2001; 104:2886-2891.

33. Aviles RJ, Martin DO, Apperson-Hansen C *et al*. Inflammation as a risk factor for atrial fibrillation. *Circulation* 2003; 108:3006-3010.

34. Liu T, Li G, Li L, Korantzopoulos P. Association Between C-reactive protein and recurrence of atrial fibrillation after successful electrical cardioversion: a meta-analysis. *J Am Coll Cardiol* 2007; 49:1642-1648.

35. Cavolli R, Kaya K, Aslan A *et al*. Does sodium nitroprusside decrease the incidence of atrial fibrillation after myocardial revascularization?: a pilot study. *Circulation* 2008; 118:476-481.

36. Dernellis J, Panaretou M. Effect of C-reactive protein reduction on paroxysmal atrial fibrillation. *Am Heart J* 2005; 150:1064.

37. Halonen J, Halonen P, Jarvinen O *et al*. Corticosteroids for the prevention of atrial fibrillation after cardiac surgery: a randomized controlled trial. *JAMA* 2007; 297:1562-1567.

38. Sakabe M, Shiroshita-Takeshita A, Maguy A *et al*. Omega-3 polyunsaturated fatty acids prevent atrial fibrillation associated with heart failure but not atrial tachycardia remodeling. *Circulation* 2007; 116:2101-2109.
39. GISSI-HF Investigators, Tavazzi L, Maggioni AP, Marchioli R *et al*. I. Effect of n-3 polyunsaturated fatty acids in patients with chronic heart failure (the GISSI-HF trial): a randomised, double-blind, placebo-controlled trial. *Lancet* 2008; 372:1223-1230.
40. Radauceanu A, Ducki C, Virion JM *et al*. Extracellular matrix turnover and inflammatory markers independently predict functional status and outcome in chronic heart failure. *J Card Fail* 2008; 14:467-474.
41. Van Gelder IC, Hagens VE, Bosker HA *et al*. A comparison of rate control and rhythm control in patients with recurrent persistent atrial fibrillation. *N Engl J Med* 2002; 347:1834-1840.
42. Wyse DG, Waldo AL, DiMarco JP *et al*. A comparison of rate control and rhythm control in patients with atrial fibrillation. *N Engl J Med* 2002; 347:1825-1833.
43. Echt DS, Liebson PR, Mitchell LB *et al*. Mortality and morbidity in patients receiving encainide, flecainide, or placebo. The Cardiac Arrhythmia Suppression Trial. *N Engl J Med* 1991; 324:781-788.
44. Kober L, Torp-Pedersen C, McMurray JJV *et al*. Increased mortality after dronedarone therapy for severe heart failure. *N Engl J Med* 2008; 358:2678-2687
45. Waldo AL, Camm AJ, deRuyter H *et al*. Effect of d-sotalol on mortality in patients with left ventricular dysfunction after recent and remote myocardial infarction. The SWORD Investigators. Survival With Oral d-Sotalol. *Lancet* 1996; 348:7-12.
46. Julian DG, Camm AJ, Frangin G *et al*. Randomised trial of effect of amiodarone on mortality in patients with left-ventricular dysfunction after recent myocardial infarction: EMIAT. European Myocardial Infarct Amiodarone Trial Investigators. *Lancet* 1997; 349:667-674.
47. Singh SN, Fletcher RD, Fisher SG *et al*. Amiodarone in patients with congestive heart failure and asymptomatic ventricular arrhythmia. *N Engl J Med* 1995; 333:77-82.
48. Torp-Pedersen C, Moller M, Bloch-Thomsen PE *et al*. Dofetilide in patients with congestive heart failure and left ventricular dysfunction. *N Engl J Med* 1999; 341:857-865.
49. Singh BN, Singh SN, Reda DJ *et al*. Amiodarone versus sotalol for atrial fibrillation. *N Engl J Med* 2005; 352:1861-1872.
50. Roy D, Talajic M, Nattel S *et al*. Rhythm control versus rate control for atrial fibrillation and heart failure. *N Engl J Med* 2008; 358:2667-2677.
51. Kay GN, Ellenbogen KA, Giudici M *et al*. The Ablate and Pace Trial: a prospective study of catheter ablation of the AV conduction system and permanent pacemaker implantation for treatment of atrial fibrillation. APT Investigators. *J Interv Card Electrophysiol* 1998; 2:121-135.
52. Brignole M, Menozzi C, Gianfranchi L *et al*. Assessment of Atrioventricular Junction Ablation and VVIR Pacemaker Versus Pharmacological Treatment in Patients With Heart Failure and Chronic Atrial Fibrillation : A Randomized, Controlled Study. *Circulation* 1998; 98:953-960.
53. Tops LF, Schalij MJ, Holman ER, van Erven L, van der Wall EE, Bax JJ. Right ventricular pacing can induce ventricular dyssynchrony in patients with atrial fibrillation after atrioventricular node ablation. *J Am Coll Cardiol* 2006; 48:1642-1648.
54. Doshi RN, Daoud EG, Fellows C *et al*. Left ventricular-based cardiac stimulation Post AV Nodal Ablation Evaluation (the PAVE study). *J Cardiovasc Electrophysiol* 2005; 16:1160-1165.
55. Gasparini M, Auricchio A, Regoli F *et al*. Four-year efficacy of cardiac resynchronization therapy on exercise tolerance and disease progression: the importance of performing atrioventricular junction ablation in patients with atrial fibrillation. *J Am Coll Cardiol* 2006; 48:734-743.
56. Leon AR, Greenberg JM, Kanuru N *et al*. Cardiac resynchronization in patients with congestive heart failure and chronic atrial fibrillation: effect of upgrading to biventricular pacing after chronic right ventricular pacing. *J Am Coll Cardiol* 2002; 39:1258-1263.
57. Upadhyay GA, Choudhry NK, Auricchio A, Ruskin J, Singh JP. Cardiac resynchronization in patients with atrial fibrillation: a meta-analysis of prospective cohort studies. *J Am Coll Cardiol* 2008; 52:1239-1246.
58. Cleland JG, Daubert JC, Erdmann E *et al*. The effect of cardiac resynchronization on morbidity and mortality in heart failure. *N Engl J Med* 2005; 352:1539-1549.
59. Hoppe UC, Casares JM, Eiskjaer H *et al*. Effect of cardiac resynchronization on the incidence of atrial fibrillation in patients with severe heart failure. *Circulation* 2006; 114:18-25.
60. Haissaguerre M, Jais P, Shah DC *et al*. Spontaneous initiation of atrial fibrillation by ectopic beats originating in the pulmonary veins. *N Engl J Med* 1998; 339:659-666.

61. Jais P, Haissaguerre M, Shah DC *et al*. A focal source of atrial fibrillation treated by discrete radiofrequency ablation. *Circulation* 1997; 95:572-576.
62. Haissaguerre M, Jais P, Shah DC *et al*. Electrophysiological end point for catheter ablation of atrial fibrillation initiated from multiple pulmonary venous foci. *Circulation* 2000; 101:1409-1417.
63. Chen SA, Hsieh MH, Tai CT *et al*. Initiation of atrial fibrillation by ectopic beats originating from the pulmonary veins: electrophysiological characteristics, pharmacological responses, and effects of radiofrequency ablation. *Circulation* 1999; 100:1879-1886.
64. Haissaguerre M, Shah DC, Jais P *et al*. Electrophysiological breakthroughs from the left atrium to the pulmonary veins. *Circulation* 2000; 102:2463-2465.
65. Marrouche NF, Martin DO, Wazni O *et al*. Phased-array intracardiac echocardiography monitoring during pulmonary vein isolation in patients with atrial fibrillation: impact on outcome and complications. *Circulation* 2003; 107:2710-2716.
66. Nademanee K, McKenzie J, Kosar E *et al*. A new approach for catheter ablation of atrial fibrillation: mapping of the electrophysiologic substrate. *J Am Coll Cardiol* 2004; 43:2044-2053.
67. Pappone C, Rosanio S, Oreto G *et al*. Circumferential radiofrequency ablation of pulmonary vein ostia: a new anatomic approach for curing atrial fibrillation. *Circulation* 2000; 102:2619-2628.
68. Elayi CS, Verma A, Di BL *et al*. Ablation for longstanding permanent atrial fibrillation: results from a randomized study comparing three different strategies. *Heart Rhythm* 2008; 5:1658-1664.
69. Pappone C, Santinelli V, Manguso F *et al*. Pulmonary vein denervation enhances long-term benefit after circumferential ablation for paroxysmal atrial fibrillation. *Circulation* 2004; 109:327-334.
70. Oral H, Pappone C, Chugh A *et al*. Circumferential pulmonary-vein ablation for chronic atrial fibrillation. *N Engl J Med* 2006; 354:934-941.
71. Pappone C, Manguso F, Vicedomini G *et al*. Prevention of iatrogenic atrial tachycardia after ablation of atrial fibrillation: a prospective randomized study comparing circumferential pulmonary vein ablation with a modified approach. *Circulation* 2004; 110:3036-3042.
72. Chen MS, Marrouche NF, Khaykin Y *et al*. Pulmonary vein isolation for the treatment of atrial fibrillation in patients with impaired systolic function. *J Am Coll Cardiol* 2004; 43:1004-1009.
73. Hsu LF, Jais P, Sanders P *et al*. Catheter ablation for atrial fibrillation in congestive heart failure. *N Engl J Med* 2004; 351:2373-2383.
74. Khan MN, Jais P, Cummings J *et al*. Pulmonary-vein isolation for atrial fibrillation in patients with heart failure. *N Engl J Med* 2008; 359:1778-1785.
75. Cox JL, Schuessler RB, D'Agostino HJ Jr. *et al*. The surgical treatment of atrial fibrillation. III. Development of a definitive surgical procedure. *J Thorac Cardiovasc Surg* 1991; 101:569-583.
76. Cox JL, Schuessler RB, Lappas DG, Boineau JP. An 8 1/2-year clinical experience with surgery for atrial fibrillation. *Ann Surg* 1996; 224:267-273.
77. Stulak JM, Dearani JA, Daly RC, Zehr KJ, Sundt TM III, Schaff HV. Left ventricular dysfunction in atrial fibrillation: restoration of sinus rhythm by the Cox-maze procedure significantly improves systolic function and functional status. *Ann Thorac Surg* 2006; 82:494-500.
78. Romano MA, Bach DS, Pagani FD, Prager RL, Deeb GM, Bolling SF. Atrial reduction plasty Cox maze procedure: extended indications for atrial fibrillation surgery. *Ann Thorac Surg* 2004; 77:1282-1287.
79. Tanaka H, Narisawa T, Mori T, Masuda M, Suzuki T, Takaba T. Pulmonary vein isolation for chronic atrial fibrillation associated with mitral valve disease: the midterm results. *Ann Thorac Cardiovasc Surg* 2002; 8:88-91.
80. Shinagawa K, Shi YF, Tardif JC, Leung TK, Nattel S. Dynamic nature of atrial fibrillation substrate during development and reversal of heart failure in dogs. *Circulation* 2002; 105:2672-2678.

15

Nutraceuticals in heart failure: the good (fish oil), the bad (licorice) and ugly (ginseng)?

G. V. Ramani, P. A. Uber, M. R. Mehra

INTRODUCTION

An over the counter (OTC) drug is designated and regulated by authorities as a general sale medication and does not require pharmacy handling. Nutraceuticals are herbal or nutritional supplements, which are neither classifiable as foods nor drugs and are not subjected to traditional regulation. Herbs can be any form of a plant or plant product, including leaves, stems, flowers, roots, and seeds. The use of herbal medicine dates back more than 5000 years. In 1890, 59% of the agents in the US Pharmacopeia were from herbal products [1]. The attraction for herbal products stems from the fact that approximately a third to half of currently used drugs originated from plants. Today, one in five US adults report using an herbal product with this number escalating to 40% worldwide. A 2002 National Health Interview Survey was analyzed for non-vitamin dietary supplements and prescription medication use in the prior 12 months and 21% of adult prescription medication users reported using these products and more importantly, 69% did not disclose such a use to their medical practitioner [1, 2]. Thus, the problem of nutraceuticals is vast and in heart failure (HF) where polypharmacy is a norm, the potential for pharmacokinetic and pharmacodynamic interactions is amplified.

EXTENT OF NUTRACEUTICAL USE

A recent survey of patients who participated in the Hawthorn Extract Randomized Blinded Chronic Heart Failure Trial and from patients in an outpatient HF specialty clinic suggested broad use of nutraceuticals within 6 months of questioning. Of 252 surveys received, a third of respondents used nutraceuticals with several possessing the potential to interact negatively with traditional HF medications. The most common reasons cited for their use included perceptions of their benefits in heart problems, anxiety, weight loss, and arthritis related disorders [3].

A formal gap in training of healthcare providers exists with lack of a structured education that stems largely from a poor evidence base of studies supporting nutraceutical use. As a result of this, interactions and adverse reactions are under-reported and not always known.

Gautam V. Ramani, MD, Assistant Professor of Medicine, Division of Cardiology, University of Maryland School of Medicine, Baltimore, MD, USA.

Patricia A. Uber, BS, PharmD, Assistant Professor of Medicine, Division of Cardiology, University of Maryland School of Medicine, Baltimore, MD, USA.

Mandeep R. Mehra, MBBS, FACC, FACP, Dr Herbert Berger Professor of Medicine and Head of Cardiology, Assistant Dean for Clinical Services, Division of Cardiology, University of Maryland School of Medicine, Baltimore, MD, USA.

On the contrary, patients are exposed to unregulated marketing and have inherent beliefs in the safety of herbal medications. In fact 31% of patients believe that the use of nutraceuticals are extremely important to the maintenance of their health while 80% firmly endorse the importance of the addition of such herbal agents to traditional pharmacotherapy in the misguided belief of augmented benefit of their therapeutic regimen. Perhaps most important is the fact that patients feel in control of their own health when self-prescribing nutraceuticals [4, 5].

UNREGULATED LANDSCAPE

The Dietary Supplement Health and Education Act (DSHEA) of 1994 classified herbs as dietary supplements and although regulatory standards included restricting any claims for disease prevention, treatment, or cure manufacturers can make certain 'structure or function' claims – often vaguely worded health benefit claims. Thus, these agents can be produced, sold, and marketed without first demonstrating safety and efficacy. The US Food and Drug Administration (FDA) bears the regulatory burden of proving that a dietary supplement is unsafe before it can be removed from the market. Thus, this regulatory structure has created problems with the consistency and safety of herbal products [1].

As an example, ginseng products found a 15–200 fold variation in the concentration of two important ingredients. Similarly, inconsistencies in the labeling of such products create safety concerns. A study of 74 different St. John's wort products were evaluated for labeling that included drug interactions, contraindications, therapeutic duplication and general warnings regarding product use. No product label provided information for all of these evaluation criteria. Three products (4.1%) provided information on all but one of the evaluation criteria while four products provided no safety information at all [6].

Would regulation of labeling matter? Certainly, the inclusion of drug interaction information on product labels may help lower the incidence of inappropriate advice given by pharmacists and health store clerks and force more patients to read the label and seek advice.

The Center for Food Safety and Applied Nutrition's Adverse Event Reporting System (CAERS) reported data from 1999–2003 involving adverse effects reported on six common nutraceuticals: echinacea, ginseng, garlic, ginkgo biloba, St. John's wort, and peppermint [7]. Ginseng had the most adverse effect reports whereas reports involving St. John's wort were the least. Most reports involved multiple-ingredient nutraceuticals, and 3–13% of the reports involved multiple nutraceuticals. In this regard, gastrointestinal and neurologic problems were the most common clinical adverse effects among single-ingredient nutraceuticals. Despite the availability of such adverse event reporting mechanisms, this is a passive surveillance method, the number of reports is relatively small, validation is incomplete, and inconsistencies within reports are common.

The Poison Control Center's toxic exposure surveillance system received 356 exposures involving St. John's wort in 1 year with 13% of exposures reported as 'suspected suicidal' [8].

POTENTIAL ADVERSE EFFECTS OF NUTRACEUTICALS

There are four potential adverse outcomes of nutraceutical use in HF. These include a) drug – nutraceutical – pharmacokinetic interaction; b) nutraceutical – laboratory interaction; c) pharmacological interaction; d) nutraceutical adverse reaction. As an example of such outcomes, St. John's wort (*Hypericum perforatum*) possesses the ability to interfere at all four such levels of clinical effect. (Table 15.1)

Nutraceuticals such as ginseng interfere with pharmacological intention and can cause diuretic resistance while many such agents increase the risk of bleeding with warfarin or

Table 15.1 St John's wort (*Hypericum perforatum*) and interactions (drug, interaction and clinical effects)

Serotonin reuptake inhibitors	Synergy-additive serotonin like effects	Risk of serotonin syndrome; avoid concurrent use
Warfarin	Decrease in INR	Requires frequent monitoring; risk of thrombosis
Digoxin	Reduces blood level Lowers drug effect	Interaction worsens with prolonged use; induction of P-glycoprotein
Oral contraceptives	Possibly reduces drug level and lowers drug effect	Intermenstrual bleeding and unplanned pregnancies
Cyclosporine	Reduces blood level Lowers drug effect	Transplant rejection has been reported
Simvastatin Atorvastatin	Reduces blood levels	Increase in lipids

INR = international normalized ratio.

Table 15.2 Selected nutraceuticals and toxicity

Agents	Toxicity
Ginseng	Diuretic resistance Interference with digoxin immunoassay Increased warfarin toxicity
Kava extracts	Hepatotoxicity
Black Cohosh	Hepatotoxicity
Licorice	Hypokalemia, hypertension and ventricular tachycardia
Bitter orange (*Citrus Aurantium*)	Acute MI, angina equivalent, ischemic colitis

MI = myocardial infarction.

antiplatelet drugs (coenzyme Q10, ginger, gingko, garlic, ginseng) [9]. Similarly, others interfere with laboratory data. Thus, Asian and Siberian ginseng interfere with digoxin measurements by immunoassays [10]. *Crataegus oxycantha* (Hawthorn berry) possesses anti-inflammatory and antioxidant properties, and has been the subject of extensive research. A meta-analysis of 13 randomized studies suggested improved exercise tolerance tolerability [11]. However, more recent clinical trials suggest the addition of Hawthorn berry to standard HF therapy was either associated with clinical worsening [12], or no significant benefit in 6 minute walk distance, functional capacity and QoL measures, but a modest improvement in LVEF [13]. Therefore at this time routine use of Hawthorn berry in HF is discouraged.

Many nutraceuticals possess internal toxicity and those widely recognized include kava extracts, black cohosh, licorice and bitter orange (Table 15.2).

POTENTIAL BENEFICIAL NUTRACEUTICALS IN HF

1. **Coenzyme Q10:** A prospective double-blind trial in 32 patients with end-stage HF awaiting heart transplantation randomized patients to either 60 mg/day CoQ10 or placebo for 3 months. Improvement in the 6 min walk test and a decrease in dyspnea,

functional class severity and fatigue were noted. However, no significant changes were seen in structural remodeling parameters or cytokine levels reflecting inflammation [14]. Other studies have not supported these findings and decreased enthusiasm for such an agent [15].

2. **L-Carnitine:** Primary carnitine deficiency is an autosomal recessive disorder of fatty acid oxidation due to lack of functional OCTN2 carnitine transporter. Most of the reported cases first present between 1 to 7 years of age with progressive HF and generalized muscle weakness [16]. Although the outcome is usually very good with carnitine therapy, the cardiac failure can rapidly progress to death without this specific treatment. Some have taken this to mean that all patients with cardiomyopathy may benefit from such an agent but this remains unsupported except for small studies depicting improvements in surrogate endpoints [17].

3. **Omega-3 fatty acids:** Perhaps the best studied nutraceutical now approved as a pharmacological agent for treatment of lipid disorders (hypertriglyceridemia) has a well supported safety profile and modest benefit in HF. Perhaps the most widespread nutraceutical encountered in clinical practice, it deserves a more detailed analysis as a distinct agent and will be discussed in more depth herein.

A PRIMER ON FISH OILS AND HF

Ever since the initial observations from the 1970s that native Eskimos who consumed large quantities fish had a reduced incidence of heart disease compared to the general population, fish oils have become an area of intensive research in the cardiovascular community [18]. Several large, observational, cohort studies confirmed that increased dietary fish consumption was correlated with a dose related reduction in cardiovascular disease, regardless of gender, or ethnicity [19–22]. These findings subsequently were confirmed in randomized controlled clinical trials [23, 24] leading the American Heart Association to endorse the use of fish oils for the secondary prevention of cardiovascular disease [25]. The potential role for fish oils in congestive HF (CHF) remains less well established. We shall now explore potential beneficial mechanisms of fish oils in HF, and review the available literature regarding optimal dosing and efficacy. A recently published large European randomized controlled trial found no benefits of fish oil supplementation in the secondary prevention of coronary artery disease [26]. The dose of fish oils studied was lower than in other clinical trials, and therefore caution must be exercised when interpreting the results of this study.

MECHANISM OF ACTION

Fish oils or n-3 (omega-3) fatty acids are polyunsaturated fatty acids (PUFA's) that are produced by marine plant life, and subsequently found in fish that feed on these plants. The fish oils that have been most widely studied in clinical practice are docosahexaenoic acid (DHA) and eicosapentaenoic acid (EPA). Dietary omega-3 fatty acids are ultimately incorporated into the cellular membrane phospholipid core, with maximal incorporation typically occurring 2 weeks following initial consumption [27]. Multiple mechanisms have been identified that contribute to the observed clinical beneficial effects of fish oils. Fish oil consumption is associated with improved arterial endothelial function, improved nitric oxide (NO) production, and reduced platelet aggregation [28, 29]. Fish oil supplementation is also associated with reductions in blood pressure, and restoration of vagal tone in HF patients [30, 31]. Fish oils modulate cytokine levels, and supplementation is correlated with reductions in levels of TNF-α and proinflammatory interleukins [32]. Rodent models, utilizing a model of left ventricular pressure overload, suggest fish oil supplementation mitigates left ventricular hypertrophy, and improves serum cytokine profile, with reductions in TNF-α and urinary thromboxane B2 levels, and increases in serum adiponectin levels [33]. Finally, randomized controlled primate studies have demonstrated that fish oils are associated with an increased threshold for potentially lethal ventricular arrhythmias, and improved left ventricular diastolic filling [34, 35].

FISH OILS AND VENTRICULAR ARRHYTHMIA RISK IN HF

Sudden cardiac death (SCD) represents a major cause of mortality in CHF. Dietary consumption of fish oils, as well as blood levels of n-3 fatty acids, has been correlated with a reduced risk of SCD in humans. This observation is supported by extensive research in animal and cellular models, demonstrating the membrane stabilizing effects of fish oils [36]. Several recently completed randomized clinical trials have attempted to shed further light on this observation. A small study randomized 26 patients with ICD placement and LV dysfunction (median LVEF approximately 40%) to 3 g/day encapsulated fish oil (540 g/day EPA and 360 mg/day DHA). The authors found a significant reduction in inducible ventricular tachycardia [37]. However, larger and adequately powered randomized clinical trials have failed to demonstrate benefits in ventricular arrhythmia reduction with fish oil supplementation. One large clinical trial which randomized 200 patients who either had a pre-existing ICD and received a therapy for VT/VF, or who had an ICD implanted for documented VT/VF to receive either 1.8 g/day fish oil (756 mg EPA and 540 mg DHA) or placebo. The mean LVEF was 36%, and fish oil supplementation did not reduce the incidence of VT/VF. Surprisingly, there was a trend towards increased ventricular arrhythmias in the treatment group [38]. Similar results were reported in the SOFA trial, which randomized 546 patients with prior documented VT/VT and an ICD with mean LVEF 36% to therapy with 2 g/day fish oil (464 mg EPA and 335 mg DHA) or placebo, and found no increased protection from ventricular arrhythmias [39]. Taken together, these large clinical trials suggest that a daily dose of approximately 800 mg EPA/DHA at is not associated with any clinically relevant reduction in life threatening ventricular arrhythmias in patients with systolic HF.

GISSI-HF TRIAL

The largest and most extensive randomized investigation of fish oils in HF is the recently published GISSI-HF study [40]. This European study randomized 7046 patients, with mean LVEF 33%, to treatment with 1 g n-3 PUFA (400 mg DHA, 488 mg EPA) or placebo, and followed patients for a median of 3.9 years. Medical therapy was adequate in the GISSI-HF study, with 93% of patients on ACE/ARB therapy, and 65% on beta blocker therapy. Importantly, only 7% of patients had an ICD. There was a small but statistically significant reduction in all-cause mortality (absolute risk reduction 1.8%, number needed to treat [NNT] 56), and a combined reduction in the co-primary endpoints of death or hospital admission by 9%. However, half the absolute risk reduction of first admission to hospital for cardiovascular reasons was due to a reduction in ventricular arrhythmias, and the reduction in total mortality was presumed to be driven by a reduction in arrhythmic deaths. It remains unclear if this small cardiovascular benefit would be erased had a larger percentage of patients received ICDs.

FISH OIL PREPARATIONS

DHA and EPA are present in high concentrations in most oily fish, including tuna, salmon, and trout, and to a much lesser extent in catfish and shrimp, and typically contain higher levels of DHA than EPA [41]. In the native myocardium, DHA levels are much more abundant. Both fatty acids are equally incorporated into cell membranes and are postulated to have stabilizing effects on cellular membrane potentials. DHA may be converted to EPA *in vivo*, but humans lack the necessary enzymes to convert EPA to DHA. The n-3 fatty acid alpha linoleic acid (ALA), which is derived from plant sources, and found in flaxseed oil and walnuts, has not been shown to produce similar cardioprotective, possibly because humans cannot effectively convert ALA to either EPA or DHA.

Tremendous uncertainty remains regarding the optimal dose and ratios of EPA/DHA for dietary supplementation. Data suggest that doses required for benefit are lower for anti-inflammatory and antithrombotic effects, but higher for anti arrhythmic effects, which are far and away more relevant in the HF population [32]. What are we left to conclude regarding the treatment of fish oils in systolic HF? A plethora of basic science and animal data suggest a biochemical and physiologic benefit, and multiple observational human studies demonstrate various anti-inflammatory and anti arrhythmic benefits. However, only one large, randomized clinical trial has been published to date, and this study demonstrated a small mortality reduction. This small reduction is significant because most recently studied pharmacological agents, in the current era of extensive background pharmacotherapy, have proved to be disappointing. Clinical applicability is further compounded by remaining uncertainty regarding optimal dose and ratios of various fish oils in the HF patient. The dietary supplement industry generates several billion dollars of revenue, and therefore recommendations of such therapeutic agents have broad personal and public health implications. Current guideline based pharmacologic therapy for HF remains complex, and addition of additional agents requires careful scrutiny and analysis of the potential risks and benefits.

REFERENCES

1. Bent S, Ko R. Commonly used herbal medicines in the United States: a review. *Am J Med* 2004; 116:478-485.
2. Gardiner P, Graham RE, Legedza AT, Eisenberg DM, Phillips RS. Factors associated with dietary supplement use among prescription medication users. *Arch Intern Med* 2006; 166:1968-1974.
3. Zick SM, Blume A, Aaronson KD. The prevalence and pattern of complementary and alternative supplement use in individuals with chronic heart failure. *J Card Failure* 2005; 11:586-589.
4. Yeh GY, Davis RB, Phillips RS. Use of complementary therapies in patients with cardiovascular disease. *Am J Cardiol* 2006; 98:673-680.
5. Hermann DD. Naturoceutical agents in the management of cardiovascular disease. *Am J Cardiovasc Drugs* 2002; 2:173-196.
6. Clauson KA, Santamarina ML, Rutledge JC. Clinically relevant safety issues associated with St. John's wort product labels. *BMC Complement Altern Med* 2008; 8:42.
7. Wallace RB, Gryzlak BM, Zimmerman MB, Nisly NL. Application of FDA adverse event report data to the surveillance of dietary botanical supplements. *Ann Pharmacother* 2008; 42:653-660.
8. Gryzlak BM, Wallace RB, Zimmerman MB, Nisly NL. National surveillance of herbal dietary supplement exposures: the poison control center experience. *Pharmacoepidemiol Drug Saf* 2007; 16:947-957.
9. Pal D, Mitra AK. MDR- and CYP3A4-mediated drug-herbal interactions. *Life Sci* 2006; 78:2131-2145.
10. Hu Z, Yang X, Ho PC *et al*. Herb–drug interactions: a literature review. *Drugs* 2005; 65:1239-1282.
11. Pittler MH, Schmidt K, Ernst E. Hawthorn extract for treating chronic heart failure: meta-analysis of randomized trials. *Am J Med* 2003; 114:665-675.
12. Zick SM, Gillespie B, Aaronson KD. The effect of Crataegus oxycantha Special Extract WSS 1442 on clinical progression in patients with mild to moderate symptoms of heart failure. *Eur J Heart Failure* 2008; 10:587-593.
13. Zick SM, Vautaw BM, Gillespie B, Aaronson KD. Hawthorn Extract Randomized Blinded Chronic Heart Failure (HERB CHF) trial. *Eur J Heart Failure* 2009; 11:990-999.
14. Berman M, Erman A, Ben-Gal T *et al*. Coenzyme Q10 in patients with end-stage heart failure awaiting cardiac transplantation: a randomized, placebo-controlled study. *Clin Cardiol* 2004; 27:295-299.
15. Khatta M, Alexander BS, Krichten CM *et al*. The effect of coenzyme Q10 in patients with congestive heart failure. *Ann Intern Med* 2000; 132:636-640.
16. Cano A, Ovaert C, Vianey-Saban C, Chabrol B. Carnitine membrane transporter deficiency: a rare treatable cause of cardiomyopathy and anemia. *Pediatr Cardiol* 2008; 29:163-165.
17. Kumar A, Singh RB, Saxena M *et al*. Effect of carni Q-gel (ubiquinol and carnitine) on cytokines in patients with heart failure in the Tishcon study. *Acta Cardiol* 2007; 62:349-354.

18. Bang HO, Dyerberg J, Hjoorne N. The composition of food consumed by Greenland Eskimos. *Acta Med Scand* 1976; 200:69-73.

19. Kromhout D, Bosschieter EB, de Lezenne Coulander C. The inverse relation between fish consumption and 20-year mortality from coronary heart disease. *N Engl J Med* 1985; 312:1205-1209.

20. Yuan JM, Ross RK, Gao YT, Yu MC. Fish and shellfish consumption in relation to death from myocardial infarction among men in Shanghai, China. *Am J Epidemiol* 2001; 154:809-816.

21. Hu FB, Bronner L, Willett WC *et al*. Fish and omega-3 fatty acid intake and risk of coronary heart disease in women. *JAMA* 2002; 287:1815-1821.

22. He K, Song Y, Daviglus ML *et al*. Accumulated evidence on fish consumption and coronary heart disease mortality: a meta-analysis of cohort studies. *Circulation* 2004; 109:2705-2711.

23. Burr ML, Fehily AM, Gilbert JF *et al*. Effects of changes in fat, fish, and fibre intakes on death and myocardial reinfarction: Diet and Reinfarction Trial (DART). *Lancet* 1989; 2:757-761.

24. GISSI-Prevenzione. Dietary supplementation with n-3 polyunsaturated fatty acids and vitamin E after myocardial infarction: results of the GISSI-Prevenzione trial. Gruppo Italiano per lo Studio della Sopravvi-venza nell'Infarto miocardico. *Lancet* 1999; 354:447-455.

25. Kris-Etherton PM, Harris WS, Appel LH. American Heart Association Nutrition Committee. Fish consumption, fish oil, omega-3 fatty acids, and cardiovascular disease. *Circulation* 2002; 106:2747-2757.

26. Kromhout D, Gitlay EJ, Geleijnse JM *et al*. n-3 fatty acids and Cardiovascular events after myocardial infarction. *N Engl J Med* 2010; *published online*.

27. Masson S, Latini R, Tacconi M, Bernasconi R. Incorporation and washout of n-3 polyunsaturated fatty acids after diet supplementation in clinical studies. *J Cardiovasc Med (Hagerstown)* 2007; 8(suppl 1):S4-S10.

28. Morgan DR, Dixon LJ, Hanratt CG *et al*. Effects of dietary omega-3 fatty acid supplementation on endothelium-dependent vasodilation in patients with chronic heart failure. *Am J Cardiol* 2006; 97:547-551.

29. Hornstra G. Influence of dietary fat type on arterial thrombosis tendency. *J Nutr health Aging* 2001; 5:160-166.

30. Geleijnse JM, Giltay EJ, Grobbee DE, Donders AR, Kok FJ. Blood pressure response to fish oil supplementation: metaregression analysis of randomized trials. *J Hypertens* 2002; 20:1493-1499.

31. O'Keefe JH, Abuissa H, Sastre A, Steinhaus DM, Harris WS. Effects of omega-3 fatty acids on restng heart rate, heart rate recovery after exercise, and heart rate variability in men with healed myocardial infarction and depressed ejection fractions. *Am J Cardiol* 2006; 97:1127-1130.

32. Mehra MR, Lavie CJ, Ventura HO, Milani RV. Fish oils produce antiinflammatory effects and improve body weight in severe heart failure. *J Heart Lung Transplant* 2006; 25:834-838.

33. Duda MK, O-Shea KM, Lei B *et al*. Dietary supplementation with omega-3 PUFA increases adiponectin and attenuates ventricular remodeling and dysfunction with pressure overload. *Cardiovasc Res* 2007; 72:303-310.

34. Charnock JS, McLennan PL, Abeywardena MY. Dietary modulation of lipid metabolism and mechanical performance of the heart. *Mol Cell Biochem* 1992; 116:19-25.

35. McLellan PL, Barnden LR, Bridle TM, Abeywardena MY, Charnock JS. Dietary fat modulation of left ventricular ejection fraction due to enhanced filling. *Cardiovasc Res* 1992; 26:871-877.

36. Matthan NR, Jordan H, Chung M, Lichtenstein AH, Lathrop DA, Lau J. A systematic review and meta-analysis of the impact of omega-3-fatty acids on selected arrhythmia outcomes in animal models. *Metabolism* 2005; 54:1557-1565.

37. Metcalf RG, Sanders P, James MJ, Cleland LG, Young GD. Effect of dietary n-3 polyunsaturated fatty acids on the inducibility of ventricular tachycardia in patients with ischemic cardiomyopathy. *Am J Cardiol* 2008; 101:758-761.

38. Raitt MH, Connor WE, Morris D *et al*. Fish oil supplementation and risk of ventricular tachycardia and ventricular fibrillation in patients with implantable defibrillators: a randomized clinical trial. *JAMA* 2005; 293:2884-2891.

39. Brouwer IA, Zock PL, Camm JA *et al*. Effect of fish oil on ventricular tacharrhythmia and death in patients with implantable cardioverter defibrillatiors. *JAMA* 2006; 295:2613-2619.

40. Gissi-HF Investigators, Tavazzi L, Maggioni AP, Marchioli R *et al*. Effect of n-3 polyunsaturated fatty acids in patients with chronic heart failure (the GISSI-HF trial): a randomised, double-blind, placebo-controlled trial. *Lancet* 2008; 372:1223-1230.

41. Mozaffarian D, Rimm EB. Fish intake, contaminants, and human health: evaluating the risks and benefits. *JAMA* 2006; 296:1885-1899.

16

Statins and chronic heart failure: a failed hypothesis?

P. A. Uber, M. R. Mehra

INTRODUCTION

There has been much controversy developed around the notion of hyperlipidemia in chronic heart failure (HF). On one hand, hyperlipidemia is a sentinel risk marker for the development of coronary artery disease, a key arbiter of left ventricular dysfunction [1]. On the other hand, a reverse epidemiology has been described that denotes lower cholesterol and its lipid fractions as biomarkers of an adverse prognosis [2]. While the lowering of blood lipids in preventing HF by reducing ischemic events appears conclusive, once the clinical syndrome of HF is established, doubts are raised on the value of lipid lowering, particularly with statins. This chapter will tackle four key issues: Is there a biological rationale for statins in HF? Have we evaluated the rationale appropriately? Did CORONA and GISSI-HF 'put the nail in the coffin'? How should we use this information clinically?

IS THERE A BIOLOGICAL RATIONALE FOR STATINS IN HF?

Statins exhibit pleiotropic effects that may influence the syndrome of left ventricular failure favorably [3]. These effects include benefits on myocardial cellular function, down regulation of tissue renin-angiotensin-aldosterone system (RAAS) activation, restoration of autonomic function, neoangiogenesis and inhibition of pro-inflammatory cytokines. All of these non-lipid effects are expected to have a favorable influence on the natural history of clinical HF. Using a transgenic rat model that over expresses renin and angiotensin II, Dechend and colleagues [4] demonstrated amelioration of the deleterious effects of these neurohormones by using cerivastatin and showed that Ang II-induced hypertension, cardiac hypertrophy, fibrosis, and remodeling were favorably affected independent of lipid effects. Nickenig and colleagues [5] demonstrated that treatment with statins reversed angiotensin II infusion related elevated blood pressure responses and also downregulated AT1 receptor density. Hayashidani *et al.* [6] studied a rat coronary ligation model of HF and demonstrated amelioration of left ventricular structural remodeling in tandem with attenuation of increased extracellular matrix activity. Statins possess powerful anti-inflammatory properties and these are exhibited by a reduction of the activation of the transcription factor nuclear factor kappa-B, a player in regulating genes encoding proinflammatory cytokines and adhesion

Patricia A. Uber, BS, PharmD, Assistant Professor of Medicine, Division of Cardiology, University of Maryland School of Medicine, Baltimore, MD, USA.

Mandeep R. Mehra, MBBS, FACC, FACP, Herbert Berger Professor of Medicine and Head of Cardiology, University of Maryland School of Medicine, Baltimore, MD, USA.

molecules [7]. Similarly, statins decrease vascular cell adhesion molecule-1 levels in HF [8]. Expanding these effects into the heart transplantation realm, statins have been shown to inhibit the expression of major histocompatibility complex class II molecules on endothelial cells and monocytes, resulting in inhibition of T-cell activation [9]. Additionally, circulating cholesterol and triglyceride-rich lipoproteins have the capacity to detoxify bacterial lipopoly-saccharides (endotoxin), which stimulate the release of inflammatory cytokines in patients with HF [10]. This factor has caused us to rethink cholesterol lowering since it may reduce the capacity to bind gut translocation derived endotoxins. Taken in aggregate, the rationale for using statins in HF is on solid footing although mechanistically, some concerns exist for those patients that have transitioned to advanced stages of HF.

HAS THE STATIN HYOTHESIS BEEN EVALUATED APPROPRIATELY?

While a reverse epidemiology has been encountered in HF, with demonstration that individuals with the lowest levels of cholesterol with HF exhibit the worst clinical outcomes, other observational studies have pointed towards a disease modifying effect of statins in either ischemic or non-ischemic cardiomyopathy. Horwich and colleagues [11] described a potential disease modifying effect of statins in HF and systolic dysfunction in endpoints pertaining to sudden death or progression of HF. Ramasubbu *et al.* [12] compiled data from 13 observational trials to ascertain the effects of statins on clinical HF and, in a meta-analysis, demonstrated that these drugs provided a disease ameliorating effect that was independent of etiology of HF. Such lines of observational evidence have led to the development of the hypothesis that statins ought to be examined in the robust context of a randomized and placebo-controlled study design. This led to the performance of the CORONA and GISSI-HF trials, two unique studies of the drug rosuvastatin in syndromes of HF and reduced ejection fraction.

CORONA AND GISSI-HF – WHAT DO THEY TELL US?

The CORONA trial [13] specifically evaluated rosuvastatin in elderly patients with chronic HF. A total of 5011 patients at least 60 years of age with ischemic HF in New York Heart Association (NYHA) class II (EF < 0.36, 40% of the cohort); III-IV (EF <0.41, 60% of the cohort), were assigned to receive 10 mg of rosuvastatin or placebo per day. The primary composite outcome measure of death from cardiovascular causes, non-fatal myocardial infarction, or non-fatal stroke was no different between the placebo and rosuvastatin groups, despite significant lipid lowering and anti-inflammatory effects demonstrated by a reduction of high-sensitivity C-reactive protein. However, a prespecified secondary analysis suggested fewer hospitalizations for cardiovascular causes in the rosuvastatin group than placebo.

The GISSI-HF trial [14] was a randomized, double-blind, placebo-controlled trial in patients aged 18 years or older with chronic HF of New York Heart Association class II–IV, irrespective of cause and left ventricular ejection fraction, assigned to rosuvastatin 10 mg daily (*n*=2285) or placebo (*n*=2289). At a median follow-up of 3.9 years, the primary endpoint of time to death, and time to death or admission to hospital for cardiovascular reasons was no different in placebo and rosuvastatin groups.

There are unique aspects to these trials that must be kept in mind as clinicians interpret these findings and translate them into patient care. CORONA enrolled an elderly patient cohort who had a large proportion of 'vascular events' pre-randomization. These patients were in predominantly NYHA III HF and the clinical trial was 'event driven'. In this regard, the results of CORONA were uniquely driven by total mortality rather than other sub-components of the endpoint such as non-fatal MI and stroke. Furthermore, the trial enrolled patients with an unusually low rate of use of antiarrhythmic device therapy. Most likely, competing outcomes 'closed' the trial too early before vascular events were 'collected' since the study was an event driven trial. There is probably a real effect on vascular biology which also translates into the hospitalization reduction observed. With regard to GISSI-HF, there are similar nuances that deserve discussion. In our opinion, the trial enrolled a population exposed to too short a follow-up with very low rates of clinical 'vascular events'. Furthermore, patients already on statins were excluded from enrollment.

HOW SHOULD WE USE THIS INFORMATION CLINICALLY?

The observational trials and recent randomized trials that examine statins in HF support the rationale for their use. However, there does not appear to be a biological effect of statins on HF specific outcomes, thus challenging a 'disease modifying effect'. Importantly, the randomized trials reveal safety in HF with a low rate of adverse events. Based on the GISSI-HF trial, there is no rationale for using statins in non-ischemic HF. It is our opinion that statins should not be avoided in HF patients with prior vascular events, especially if they have 'early' HF. In addition, statins should continue to be prescribed for HF with preserved LV function, as long as a 'vascular or lipid' indication exists. Advanced systolic HF patients are unlikely to benefit from statins and it would not be unethical to discontinue them in this population, especially as cholesterol lowers significantly.

REFERENCES

1. Ducharme A, Rouleau JL. Do statins prevent heart failure in patients after myocardial infarction? *Curr Heart Fail Rep* 2004; 1:156-160.
2. Kalantar-Zadeh K, Block G, Horwich T *et al*. Reverse epidemiology of conventional cardiovascular risk factors in patients with chronic heart failure. *J Am Coll Cardiol* 2004; 43:1439-1444.
3. Paraskevas KI, Stathopoulos V, Mikhailidis DP. Pleiotropic effects of statins: implications for a wide range of diseases. *Curr Vasc Pharmacol* 2008; 6:237-239.
4. Dechend R, Fiebeler A, Park JK *et al*. Amelioration of angiotensin II-induced cardiac injury by a 3-hydroxy-3-methylglutaryl coenzyme a reductase inhibitor. *Circulation* 2001; 104:576-581.
5. Nickenig G, Bäumer AT, Temur Y, Kebben D, Jockenhövel F, Böhm M. Statin-sensitive dysregulated AT1 receptor function and density in hypercholesterolemic men. *Circulation* 1999; 100:2131-2134.
6. Hayashidani S, Tsutsui H, Shiomi T *et al*. Fluvastatin, a 3-hydroxy-3-methylglutaryl coenzyme a reductase inhibitor, attenuates left ventricular remodeling and failure after experimental myocardial infarction. *Circulation* 2002; 105:868-873.
7. Kim YS, Ahn Y, Hong MH *et al*. Rosuvastatin suppresses the inflammatory responses through inhibition of c-Jun N-terminal kinase and nuclear factor-kappaB in endothelial cells. *J Cardiovasc Pharmacol* 2007; 49:376-383.
8. Nachtigal P, Jamborova G, Pospisilova N *et al*. Atorvastatin has distinct effects on endothelial markers in different mouse models of atherosclerosis. *J Pharm Pharm Sci* 2006; 9:222-230.
9. Mehra MR, Uber PA, Vivekananthan K *et al*. Comparative beneficial effects of simvastatin and pravastatin on cardiac allograft rejection and survival. *J Am Coll Cardiol* 2002; 40:1609-1614.
10. Rauchhaus M, Coats AJ, Anker SD. The endotoxin-lipoprotein hypothesis. *Lancet* 2000; 356:930-933.
11. Horwich TB, MacLellan WR, Fonarow GC. Statin therapy is associated with improved survival in ischemic and non-ischemic heart failure. *J Am Coll Cardiol* 2004; 43:642-648.
12. Ramasubbu K, Estep J, White DL, Deswal A, Mann DL. Experimental and clinical basis for the use of statins in patients with ischemic and nonischemic cardiomyopathy. *J Am Coll Cardiol* 2008; 51:415-426.
13. Kjekshus J, Apetrei E, Barrios V *et al*. CORONA Group. Rosuvastatin in older patients with systolic heart failure. *N Engl J Med* 2007; 357:2248-2261.
14. Gissi-HF Investigators, Tavazzi L, Maggioni AP, Marchioli R *et al*. Effect of rosuvastatin in patients with chronic heart failure (the GISSI-HF trial): a randomised, double-blind, placebo-controlled trial. *Lancet* 2008; 372:1231-1239.

Abbreviations

6MWD	6 min walk distance
ACC	American College of Cardiology
ACE	angiotensin-converting-enzyme
ACE-I	Angiotensin-converting-enzyme inhibitors
ACS	acute coronary syndrome
ADHERE	Acute Decompensated Heart Failure National Registry
AF	atrial fibrillation
AF-CHF	Atrial Fibrillation and Congestive Heart Failure trial
AFFIRM	Atrial Fibrillation Follow-up Investigation of Rhythm Management
Afib	atrial fibrillation
Aflu	atrial flutter
AHA	American Heart Association
A-HeFT	African-American Heart Failure Trial
AHF	acute heart failure
AHFS	acute heart failure syndrome
AIRE	Acute Infarction Ramipril Efficacy trial
ALA	alpha linoleic acid
ALLHAT	Antihypertensive and Lipid-Lowering Treatment to Prevent Heart Attack Trial
AMI	acute myocardial infarction
ANA	antinuclear antibody
ANP	atrial natriuretic peptide
APAH	associated pulmonary arterial hypertension
ARB	angiotensin receptor blocker
ARVD	arrhythmogenic right ventricular dysplasia
ASA	acetyl salicylic acid
ASCEND-HF	Acute Study of Clinical Effectiveness of Nesiritide in Subjects in Decompensated Heart Failure
ATP	Adult Treatment Panel
AUC	area under the curve
AV	atrioventricular
AVP	arginine vasopressin
BATTLESCARRED	B-type Natriuretic Peptide Assisted Treatment to Lessen Serial Cardiac Readmission or Death Trial
BEST	Beta Blocker Evaluation of Survival Trial
BID	twice a day
BM	bone marrow
BMI	body mass index
BMMNC	bone marrow-derived mononuclear cell
BMPR2	bone morphogenetic protein receptor II
BNP	B-type natriuretic peptide

BNP-CARDS	B-Type Natriuretic Peptide in Cardiorenal Decompensation Syndrome trial
BOOST	BOne marrOw transfer to enhance ST-elevation infarct regeneration trial
BP	blood pressure
BUN	blood urea nitrogen
CABG	coronary artery bypass graft
CAD	coronary artery disease
CAERS	Center for Food Safety and Applied Nutrition's Adverse Event Reporting System
cAMP	cyclic adenosine monophosphate
CARE-HF	Cardiac Resynchronization in Heart Failure
CASS	Coronary Artery Surgery Study
CCB	calcium channel blocker
cGMP	cyclic guanosine monophosphate
CHD	coronary heart disease
CHF	congestive heart failure
CI	cardiac index
CI	confidence interval
CIBIS	Cardiac Insufficiency Bisoprolol Study
CKD	chronic kidney disease
CM	cardiomyopathy
CNP	c-type natriuretic peptide
CNS	central nervous system
CO	cardiac output
COMPASS-HF	Chronicle® Offers Management to Patients with Advanced Signs and Symptoms of Heart Failure trial
CONSENSUS	Cooperative North Scandinavian Enalapril Survival Study
COPD	chronic obstructive pulmonary disease
CP	chest pain
CPX	cardiopulmonary stress testing
CREST	calcinosis, Raynaud's phenomenon, espophageal dysmotility, sclerodactyly, telangiectasis
CRP	C-reactive protein
CSC	cardiac stem cells
CT	computerized tomography
CTD	connective tissue disease
CTEPH	chronic thrombo-embolic pulmonary hypertension
CV	cardiovascular
CVA	cerebrovascular accident
CVP	central venous pressure
CXR	chest X-ray
DCM	dilated cardiomyopathy
DHA	docosahexaenoic acid
D/I	deletion/insertion
DIG	Digitalis Investigation Group study
DM	diabetes mellitus
DNP	*Dendroaspis* natriuretic peptide
DSHEA	Dietary Supplement Health and Education Act
DSMB	Data Safety and Monitoring Board
DVT	deep vein thrombosis
Dx	diagnosis

ED	emergency department
EF	ejection fraction
eGFR	estimated glomerular filtration rate
EGIR	European Group for study of Insulin Resistance
EKG	electrocardiogram
EPA	eicosapentaenoic acid
EPC	endothelial progenitor stem cell
ERA	endothelin receptor antagonist
ESC	embryonic stem cells
ESC	European Society of Cardiology
ESR	erythrocyte sedimentation rate
ETRA	endothelin receptor antagonist
ET-1	endothelin-1
EVEREST	Efficacy of Vasopressin Antagonism in Heart Failure Outcome Study with Tolvaptan trial
FC	functional class
FDA	US Food and Drug Administration
FDC I/H	fixed-dose combination of isosorbide dinitrate/hydralazine
FDG	fluorine-18 labeled deoxyglucose
FE	fractional extraction
FPA	plasma fibrinopeptide A
G-CSF	granulocyte-colony stimulating factor
GFR	glomerular filtration rate
GI	gastrointestinal
GRACE	Genetic Risk Assessment of Cardiac Events
GRAHF	Genetic Risk in African Americans with Heart Failure
GTP	guanosine triphosphate
GWAS	Genome-Wide Association Studies
HEART	Heart Failure Revascularization Trial
HELAS	Heart failure Long-term Antithrombotic Study
HF	heart failure
HF-ACTION	Heart Failure and A Controlled Trial Investigating Outcomes of Exercise TraiNing trial
HIV	human immunodeficiency virus
HLA	human leukocyte antigen
HMG-CoA	3-hydroxy-3-methylglutaryl-coenzyme A
HPAH	heritable pulmonary arterial hypertension
HR	hazard ratio
HR	heart rate
HRR	heart rate reserve
HRT	hormone replacement therapy
HSC	hematopoietic stem cell
hsCRP	high sensitive c-reactive protein
HT	heart transplantation
HTN	hypertension
ICD	implantable cardioverter defibrillator
ICM	ischemic cardiomyopathy
ICON	International Collaborative of NT-proBNP Study.
ICOPER	International Cooperative Pulmonary Embolism Registry
ICSS	International Carotid Stenting Study
IDF	International Diabetes Federation
IL	interleukin

INR	international normalized ratio
IPAH	idiopathic pulmonary arterial hypertension
IPH	idiopathic pulmonary hypertension
iPS	induced Pluripotent Stem cell
IS	insulin sensitivity
ISD-HYD	isosorbide dinitrate and hydralazine
IV	intravenous
JNC 7	The Seventh Report of the Joint National Committee on Prevention, Detection, Evaluation, and Treatment of High Blood Pressure
KDR	kinase insert domain-containing receptor
LA	left atrium/atrial
LAD	left anterior descending
LDL	low-density lipoprotein
LFT	liver function test
LV	left ventricle/ventricular
LVAD	left ventricular assist device
LVD	left ventricular systolic dysfunction
LVEDP	left ventricular end diastolic pressure
LVEF	left ventricular ejection fraction
LVH	left ventricular hypertrophy
MAGIC	Myoblast Autologous Grafting in Ischemic Cardiomyopathy trial
MAPC	multipotent adult progenitor stem cell
MAPK	mitogen-activated protein kinase
MDCT	multidetector computed tomography
MDR-1	Multidrug Resistance protein-1
MEDENOX	Medical Patients With Enoxaparin Trial
MERIT-HF	Metoprolol CR/XL Randomized Intervention Trial in Congestive Heart Failure
MESA	Multi-Ethnic Study of Atherosclerosis
MHC	major histocompatibility complex
MI	myocardial infarction
MIAMI	multi-lineage inducible stem cell
MIDHeFT	Medtronic Impedance Diagnostics in Heart Failure Patients Trial
mPAP	mean pulmonary arterial pressure
MPO	myeloperoxidase
MRI	magnetic resonance imaging
mRNA	message ribonucleic acid
MSC	mesenchymal stem cell
NCEP	National Cholesterol Education Program
NHDS	National Hospital Discharge Survey
NIH	National Institutes of Health
NNT	number needed to treat
NO	nitric oxide
NOS3	nitric oxide synthase
NP	natriuretic peptide
NPV	negative predictive value
NR	not reported
NS	not significant
NSAID	non-steroidal anti-inflammatory drug
NT	N-terminal
NTG	nitroglycerin
NT pro-BNP	N-terminal prohormone brain natriuretic peptide

NYHA	New York Heart Association
NYHA FC	New York Heart Association Functional Class
O_2	oxygen
OPTIMAAL	Optimal Trial in Myocardial Infarction with the Angiotensin II Antagonist Losartan
OPTIME-CHF	Outcomes of a Prospective Trial of Intravenous Milrinone for Exacerbations of Chronic Heart Failure
OPTIMIZE-HF	Organized Program to Initiate Lifesaving Treatment in Hospitalized Patients With Heart Failure
OTC	over the counter
PA	pulmonary artery
PAH	pulmonary arterial hypertension
PAI-1	plasminogen activator inhibitor-1
PAP	pulmonary artery pressure
PARR-2	Positron Emission Tomography and Recovery Following Revascularization-2
PASP	pulmonary artery systolic pressure
PAVE	Post AV Nodal Ablation Evaluation study
PBMC	peripheral blood mononuclear cell
PCH	pulmonary capillary hemangiomatosis
PCI	percutaneous coronary intervention
PCR	polymerase chain reaction
PCWP	pulmonary capillary wedge pressure
PDE	phosphodiesterase
PE	pulmonary emboli
PECAM-1	platelet/endothelial cell adhesion molecule-1
PET	positron emission tomography
PFT	pulmonary function test
PH	pulmonary hypertension
PM	pacemaker
PPH	primary pulmonary hypertension
PPV	positive predictive value
PRIDE	Pro-Brain Natriuretic Peptide Investigation of Dyspnea in the Emergency Department study
PRIMA	Can Pro-Brain- Natriuretic Peptide Guided Therapy of Chronic Heart Failure Improve Heart Failure Morbidity and Mortality?
PROMISE	Prospective Randomized Milrinone Survival Evaluation trial
PROTECT	Placebo-controlled Randomized study of rolofylline for patients hOspitalised with acute HF and volume Overload to assess Treatment Effect on Congestion and renal funcTion
PROVED	Prospective Randomized study Of Ventricular failure and Efficacy of Digoxin study
PUFA	polyunsaturated fatty acid
PV	pulmonary vein
PVH	pulmonary venous hypertension
PVOD	pulmonary veno-occlusive disease
PVR	pulmonary vascular resistance
QD	once a day
QoL	quality of life
RA	right atrium
RAAS	renin-angiotensin-aldosterone systems
RACE	Rate Control versus Electrical Cardioversion trial

RADIANCE	Randomized Assessment of Digoxin on Inhibitors of Angiotensin-Converting Enzyme study
RAE	right atrial enlargement
RAP	right atrial pressure
RAS	renin-angiotensin system
REACH-UP	Placebo-controlled Randomized Study of rolofylline for Patients Hospitalized with Worsening Renal Heart Failure Requiring Intravenous Therapy
REPAIR-AMI	Reinfusion of Enriched Progenitor Cells and Infarct Remodeling in Acute Myocardial Infarction trial
RHC	right heart catheterization
RIETE	Registro Informatizado de la Enfermedad TromboEmbólica
RITZ	Randomized Intervention of TeZosentan
RPE	Rate of Perceived Exertion
RR	relative risk
RV	right ventricle
RVD	right ventricular dysfunction
RVSP	right ventricular systolic pressure
SAVE	Survival and Ventricular Enlargement trial
SC	subcutaneous
Sca-1	Stem cell antigen-1
SCD	sudden cardiac death
SCD-HeFT	Sudden Cardiac Death in Heart Failure Trial
SCF	Stem Cell Factor
SCr	serum creatinine
SD	sudden death
SNP	single nucleotide polymorphism *or* sodium nitroprusside (*check context*)
SNS	sympathetic nervous system
SOFA	Study on Omega-3 Fatty acids and ventricular Arrhythmia
SOLVD	Studies of Left Ventricular Dysfunction
SP	side population
SPAF	Stroke Prevention and Atrial Fibrillation III
SPECT	single photon emission computed tomography
STARS-BNP	Systolic Heart Failure Treatment Supported by B-type Natriuretic Peptide
STICH	Surgical Treatment for Ischemic Heart Failure
SUPER	Sildenafil Use in Pulmonary Arterial Hypertension study group
SVR	systemic vascular resistance
T-Ag	T antigen
TAT	thrombin–antithrombin complex
TE	thromboembolism
TEE	transesophageal echocardiography
TGF-ß	transforming growth factor beta
TGF	tubuloglomerular feedback
TID	three times a day
TIME-CHF	Trial of Intensified Versus Standard Medical Therapy in Elderly Patients with Congestive Heart Failure randomized trial
TNF	tumor necrosis factor
TNFα	tumor necrosis factor alpha
TR	tricuspid regurgitation
TSH	thyroid stimulating hormone

TTCW	time to clinical worsening
ULSAM	Uppsala Longitudinal Study of Adult Men
UNLOAD	Ultrafiltration Versus IV Diuretics for Patients Hospitalized for Acute Decompensated Heart Failure trial
Val-HeFT	Valsartan Heart Failure Trial
VAS	visual analogue scale
VEGF-R2	Vascular Endothelial Growth Factor receptor 2
VERITAS	Value of Endothelin Receptor Inhibition with Tezosentan in Acute Heart Failure Studies
V-HeFT	Veterans Affairs Vasodilator Heart Failure Trials
VMA	vanillylmandelic acid
VMAC	Vasodilatation in the Management of Acute Congestive Heart Failure study
VO_2	oxygen consumption
VQ	ventilation perfusion
VSEL	Very Small Embryonic Like stem cell
VT/VF	ventricular fibrillation/ventricular tachycardia
vWF	von Willebrand factor
WARCEF	Warfarin vs Aspirin in Reduced Cardiac Ejection Fraction study
WASCOPS	West of Scotland Coronary Prevention Study
WASH	Warfarin/Aspirin Study in Heart Failure study
WATCH	Warfarin and Antiplatelet Therapy in Chronic Heart Failure trial
WHS	Women's Health Study
WHO	World Health Organization
WMA	wall motion abnormality

Index